RN

Expert
Guides

Cardiovascular
Care

Wolters Kluwer | Lippincott Williams & Wilkins
Health

Philadelphia · Baltimore · New York · London
Buenos Aires · Hong Kong · Sydney · Tokyo

STAFF

EXECUTIVE PUBLISHER
Judith A. Schilling McCann, RN, MSN

EDITORIAL DIRECTOR
H. Nancy Holmes

CLINICAL DIRECTOR
Joan M. Robinson, RN, MSN

ART DIRECTOR
Elaine Kasmer

EDITORIAL PROJECT MANAGER
Christiane L. Brownell, ELS

CLINICAL PROJECT MANAGER
Jennifer Meyering, RN, BSN, MS, CCRN

EDITOR
Louise Quinn

COPY EDITORS
Kimberly Bilotta (supervisor),
Scotti Cohn, Jeannine Fielding,
Dona Perkins, Dorothy P. Terry

DESIGNERS
Linda Jovinelly Franklin

DIGITAL COMPOSITION SERVICES
Diane Paluba (manager),
Joyce Rossi Biletz, Donald G. Knauss

MANUFACTURING
Beth J. Welsh

EDITORIAL ASSISTANTS
Karen J. Kirk, Jeri O'Shea, Linda K.
Ruhf

INDEXER
Dianne Prewitt

RNEGC010707

**Library of Congress
Cataloging-in-Publication Data**

RN expert guides. Cardiovascular care.
   p. ; cm.
   Includes bibliographical references and index.
   1. Cardiovascular system—Diseases—Nursing—Handbooks, manuals, etc.   I. Lippincott Williams & Wilkins. II. Title: Cardiovascular care.
   [DNLM: 1. Cardiovascular Diseases—nursing. 2. Nursing Care—methods. WY 152.5 R627 2008]
   RC674.R63 2008
   616.1'0231—dc22
ISBN-13: 978-1-58255-704-5 (alk. paper)
ISBN-10: 1-58255-704-7 (alk. paper)
                               2007012523

Contents

Contributors and consultants

Lisa A. Brennan, RN, MS, CCRN
Clinical Nurse Specialist, Cardiology Services
Miami Valley Hospital
Dayton, Ohio

Taletha Carter, RN, MS, CCRN
Clinical Project Leader
Cleveland Clinic

Todd Isbell, RN, BSN, CCRN-CSC
Director, Critical Care
MountainView Hospital
Las Vegas

Peggy Thweatt, RN, MSN, DrPHc
Nursing Instructor
Medical Careers Institute
Newport News, Va.

Leigh Ann Trujillo, RN, BSN
Nurse Educator
St. James Hospital and Health Centers
Olympia Fields, Ill.

Demetra C. Zalman, RN, BSN, CCRN
Staff Nurse, Level III, SICU CT/GS
Hospital of the University of Pennsylvania
Philadelphia

Anatomy and physiology

The cardiovascular system's job is to deliver oxygenated blood to tissues and remove waste products. The heart pumps blood to all organs and tissues of the body, and the autonomic nervous system (ANS) controls how the heart pumps.

CARDIOVASCULAR ANATOMY

Consisting of the arteries and veins, the vascular network:
- carries blood throughout the body
- keeps the heart filled with blood
- maintains blood pressure.

Structures of the heart

The heart is a hollow, muscular organ about the size of a closed fist. It's about 5" (12.5 cm) long, 3½" (9 cm) in diameter at its widest point and weighs 1 to 1¼ lb (453.5 to 567 g). The heart is located between the lungs in the mediastinum, behind and to the left of the sternum.

The heart spans the area from the second to the fifth intercostal space. The heart's right border lines up with the right border of the sternum. The heart's left border lines up with the left midclavicular line. The heart's base, its posterior surface, is the widest part of the heart. It's formed mainly by the left atrium, which is located at the top of the heart. The apex, formed mainly by the left ventricle, is located at the fifth left intercostal space at the bottom of the heart. The apex is the point of maximum impulse, where heart sounds are the loudest. (See *Locating the heart,* page 2.)

Leading into and out of the heart are the great vessels:
- inferior vena cava
- superior vena cava

1

LOCATING THE HEART

The heart lies beneath the sternum within the mediastinum. In most people, two-thirds of the heart extends to the left of the body's midline, close to the left midclavicular line. The heart rests obliquely so that its broad part, the base, is at its upper right and the pointed end, the apex, is at its lower left.

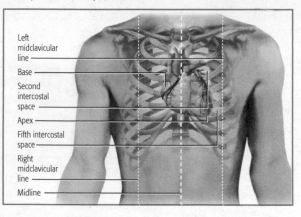

Left midclavicular line

Base

Second intercostal space

Apex

Fifth intercostal space

Right midclavicular line

Midline

- aorta
- pulmonary artery
- four pulmonary veins.

HEART WALL

The heart wall consists of three layers:
- endocardium, a thin layer of endothelial tissue
- myocardium, composed of interlacing bundles of thick cardiac muscle fibers, which forms most of the heart wall
- epicardium, which makes up the outside layer and is made of connective tissue covered by the epithelium.

The pericardium is a fibroserous sac that surrounds the heart and the roots of the great vessels. It consists of the serous pericardium and the fibrous pericardium. The serous pericardium contains two layers:
- parietal layer, which lines the inside of the fibrous pericardium
- visceral layer, which adheres to the surface of the heart.

The fibrous pericardium is a thicker layer that protects the heart. The space between the two layers, called the pericardial space, con-

A LOOK AT THE LAYERS OF THE HEART WALL

This cross section of the heart wall shows its various layers.

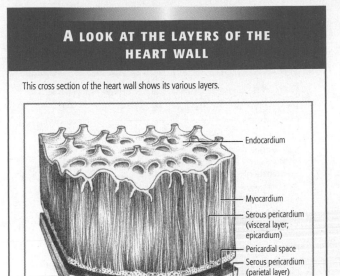

- Endocardium
- Myocardium
- Serous pericardium (visceral layer; epicardium)
- Pericardial space
- Serous pericardium (parietal layer)
- Fibrous pericardium

tains 10 to 30 ml of serous fluid, which prevents friction between the layers as the heart pumps. (See *A look at the layers of the heart wall*.)

HEART CHAMBERS

The heart contains four hollow chambers: two atria and two ventricles. The right atrium lies in front of and to the right of the smaller but thicker-walled left atrium. An interatrial septum separates the two chambers and helps them contract. The right and left atria serve as volume reservoirs for blood being sent into the ventricles. The right atrium receives deoxygenated blood returning from the body through the inferior and superior vena cavae and from the heart through the coronary sinus. The left atrium receives oxygenated blood from the lungs through the four pulmonary veins. Contraction of the atria forces blood into the ventricles. (See *A look at the internal structures of the heart*, page 4.)

The right and left ventricles make up the two lower chambers. The right ventricle:

- lies behind the sternum

A LOOK AT THE INTERNAL STRUCTURES OF THE HEART

The heart's internal structure consists of the four chambers and four valve walls.

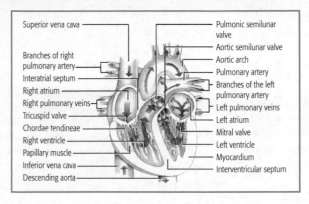

- forms the largest part of the sternocostal surface and inferior border of the heart
- receives deoxygenated blood from the right atrium
- pumps the deoxygenated blood through the pulmonary arteries to the lungs where it's reoxygenated.

The left ventricle:
- forms the apex and most of the left border of the heart and its posterior and diaphragmatic surfaces
- receives oxygenated blood from the left atrium
- pumps oxygenated blood through the aorta into the systemic circulation.

The interventricular septum separates the ventricles and helps them pump.

The thickness of a chamber's walls is determined by the amount of pressure needed to eject its blood. Because the atria act as reservoirs for the ventricles and pump the blood a shorter distance, their walls are considerably thinner than the walls of the ventricles. Likewise, the left ventricle has a much thicker wall than the right ventricle because the left ventricle pumps blood against the higher pressures in the aorta. The right ventricle pumps blood against the lower pressures in the pulmonary circulation.

BLOOD FLOW THROUGH THE HEART

Deoxygenated venous blood returns to the right atrium through three vessels:

- superior vena cava, which carries blood from the upper body
- inferior vena cava, which carries blood from the lower body
- coronary sinus, which carries blood from the heart muscle.

The increasing volume of blood in the right atrium raises the pressure in that chamber above the pressure in the right ventricle. Then the tricuspid valve opens, allowing blood to flow into the right ventricle.

The right ventricle pumps blood through the pulmonic valve into the pulmonary arteries and lungs, where oxygen is picked up and excess carbon dioxide is released. From the lungs, the oxygenated blood flows through the pulmonary veins and into the left atrium. This completes a circuit called *pulmonary circulation.*

As the volume of blood in the left atrium increases, the pressure in the left atrium exceeds the pressure in the left ventricle. The mitral valve opens, allowing blood to flow into the left ventricle. The ventricle contracts and ejects the blood through the aortic valve into the aorta. The blood is distributed throughout the body, releasing oxygen to the cells and picking up carbon dioxide. Blood then returns to the right atrium through the veins, completing a circuit called *systemic circulation.*

Coronary circulation

Like the brain and other organs, the heart needs an adequate supply of oxygenated blood to survive. The main coronary arteries lie on the surface of the heart, with smaller arterial branches penetrating the surface into the cardiac muscle mass. The heart receives its blood supply almost entirely through these arteries. Only a small percentage of the heart's endocardial surface can obtain sufficient amounts of nutrition directly from the blood in the cardiac chambers. (See *A look at coronary circulation,* page 6.)

Understanding coronary blood flow can help you provide better care to a patient with coronary artery disease because you'll be able to predict which areas of the heart will be affected by a narrowing or occlusion of a particular coronary artery.

The left main and right coronary arteries arise from the coronary ostia, small orifices located just above the aortic valve cusps. The right coronary artery fills the groove between the atria and ventricles, giving

A LOOK AT CORONARY CIRCULATION

The coronary circulation involves the arterial system of blood vessels that supply oxygenated blood to the heart and the venous system that removes oxygen-depleted blood from it.

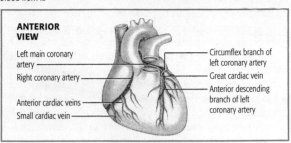

ANTERIOR VIEW

Left main coronary artery
Right coronary artery
Anterior cardiac veins
Small cardiac vein

Circumflex branch of left coronary artery
Great cardiac vein
Anterior descending branch of left coronary artery

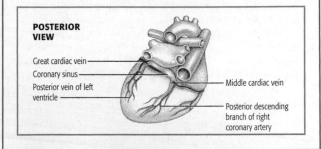

POSTERIOR VIEW

Great cardiac vein
Coronary sinus
Posterior vein of left ventricle

Middle cardiac vein
Posterior descending branch of right coronary artery

rise to the acute marginal artery and ending as the posterior descending artery. The right coronary artery supplies blood to:

- right atrium
- right ventricle
- inferior wall of the left ventricle
- sinoatrial (SA) node in about 50% of the population
- atrioventricular (AV) node in about 90% of the population.

The posterior descending artery supplies the posterior wall of the left ventricle in most people.

The left main coronary artery varies in length from a few millimeters to a few centimeters. It splits into two major branches, the left anterior descending (also known as the *interventricular*) and the left circumflex arteries. The left anterior descending artery runs down the anterior surface of the heart toward the apex. This artery and its branches—the diagonal arteries and the septal perforators—supply blood to:

- anterior wall of the left ventricle
- anterior interventricular septum
- bundle of His
- right bundle branch
- anterior fasciculus of the left bundle branch.

The circumflex artery circles the left ventricle, ending on its posterior surface. The obtuse marginal artery arises from the circumflex artery. The circumflex artery provides oxygenated blood to:

- lateral wall of the left ventricle
- left atrium
- posterior wall of the left ventricle in 10% of people
- posterior fasciculus of the left bundle branch
- SA node in about 50% of people
- AV node in about 10% of people.

In most people, the right coronary artery is the dominant vessel, meaning the right coronary artery supplies the posterior wall via the posterior descending artery. This is called *right coronary dominance* or a *dominant right coronary artery*. Likewise, when the left coronary artery supplies the posterior wall via the posterior descending artery, the terms *left coronary dominance* or *dominant left coronary artery* are used.

When two or more arteries supply the same region, they usually connect through anastomoses, junctions that provide alternative routes of blood flow. This network of smaller arteries, called *collateral circulation,* provides blood to capillaries that directly feed the heart muscle. Collateral circulation often becomes so strong that even if major coronary arteries become narrowed with plaque, collateral circulation can continue to supply blood to the heart.

In contrast to the other vascular beds in the body, the heart receives its blood supply primarily during ventricular relaxation or diastole, when the left ventricle is filling with blood. This is because the coronary ostia lie near the aortic valve and become partially occluded when the aortic valve opens during ventricular contraction or systole. However, when the aortic valve closes, the ostia are unobstructed, allowing blood to fill the coronary arteries. Because diastole is the time when the coronary arteries receive their blood supply, anything that shortens diastole, such as periods of increased heart rate or tachycardia, will also decrease coronary blood flow.

In addition, the left ventricle compresses intramuscular blood vessels during systole. During diastole, the cardiac muscle relaxes, and blood flow through the left ventricular capillaries is no longer obstructed.

Just like the other parts of the body, the heart has its own veins, which remove oxygen-depleted blood from the myocardium. About three quarters of the total coronary venous blood flow leaves the left ventricle by way of the coronary sinus, an enlarged vessel that returns blood to the right atrium. Most of the venous blood from the right ventricle flows directly into the right atrium through the small anterior cardiac veins, not by way of the coronary sinus. A small amount of coronary blood flows back into the heart through the thebesian veins, minute veins that empty directly into all chambers of the heart.

Heart valves

Valves in the heart keep blood flowing in only one direction through the heart, preventing blood from traveling the wrong way. Healthy valves open and close passively as a result of pressure changes within the four chambers.

The heart contains four valves: two AV valves (tricuspid and mitral) and two semilunar valves (aortic and pulmonic). Each valve consists of cusps, or leaflets, that open and close in response to pressure changes within the chambers they connect. The primary function of the valves is to keep blood flowing through the heart in a forward direction. When the valves close, they prevent backflow, or regurgitation, of blood from one chamber to another. Closure of the valves is associated with heart sounds.

The two AV valves are located between the atria and ventricles. The tricuspid valve, named for its three cusps, separates the right atrium from the right ventricle. The mitral valve, sometimes referred to as the *bicuspid valve* because of its two cusps, separates the left atrium from the left ventricle. Closure of the AV valves is associated with S_1, or the first heart sound.

The cusps, or leaflets, of these valves are anchored to the papillary muscles of the ventricles by small tendinous cords called chordae tendineae. The papillary muscles and chordae tendineae work together to prevent the cusps from bulging backward into the atria during ventricular contraction. (See *A look at the mitral valve*.) Disruption of either of these structures may prevent complete valve closure, allowing blood to flow backward into the atria. This backward blood flow may cause a heart murmur.

A LOOK AT THE MITRAL VALVE

These illustrations show the mitral valve and the attached papillary muscles and chordae tendineae. In the illustration on the left, the mitral valve is open, the papillary muscles are relaxed, and the chordae tendineae are slack. In the illustration on the right, the mitral valve is closed, the papillary muscles are contracted, and the chordae tendineae are tight to prevent the valve leaflets from entering the atria.

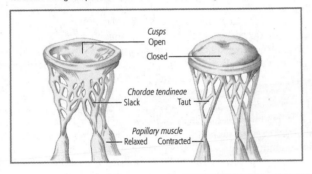

The semilunar valves are so called because their three cusps resemble half moons. The pulmonic valve, located where the pulmonary artery meets the right ventricle, permits blood to flow from the right ventricle to the pulmonary artery and prevents backflow into the right ventricle. The aortic valve, located where the left ventricle meets the aorta, allows blood to flow from the left ventricle to the aorta and prevents blood backflow into the left ventricle.

Increased pressure within the ventricles during ventricular systole causes the pulmonic and aortic valves to open, allowing ejection of blood into the pulmonary and systemic circulation. Loss of pressure as the ventricular chambers empty causes the valves to close. Closure of the semilunar valves is associated with S_2, or the second heart sound.

CARDIOVASCULAR PHYSIOLOGY

The ANS controls how the heart pumps by an electrical conduction system, which regulates myocardial contraction. This system includes the nerve fibers of the ANS and specialized nerves and fibers in the heart. The ANS involuntarily increases or decreases heart action to meet the individual's metabolic needs.

Both sympathetic and parasympathetic nerves participate in the control of cardiac function. With the body at rest, the parasympathetic nervous system controls the heart through branches of the vagus nerve (cranial nerve X). Heart rate and electrical impulse propagation slow down.

In times of activity or stress, the sympathetic nervous system takes control. It stimulates the heart's nerves and fibers to fire and conduct more rapidly and the ventricles to contract more forcefully.

Cardiac cycle

The cardiac cycle describes the period from the beginning of one heartbeat to the beginning of the next. During this cycle, electrical and mechanical events must occur in the proper order and to the proper degree to provide adequate blood flow to all body parts. Basically, the cardiac cycle has two phases: systole and diastole.

At the beginning of systole, the ventricles contract, increasing pressure and forcing the mitral and tricuspid valves to close. This valvular closing prevents blood backflow into the atria and coincides with the first heart sound (S_1), also known as the "lub" of "lub-dub." As the ventricles contract, ventricular pressure builds until it exceeds that in the pulmonary artery and the aorta. Then the aortic and pulmonary semilunar valves open, and the ventricles eject blood into the aorta and the pulmonary artery.

When the ventricles empty and relax, ventricular pressure falls below that in the pulmonary artery and the aorta. At the beginning of diastole, the semilunar valves close to prevent backflow into the ventricles. This coincides with the second heart sound, S_2, also known as the "dub" of "lub-dub."

As the ventricles relax, the mitral and tricuspid valves open and blood begins to flow into the ventricles from the atria. When the ventricles become full, near the end of diastole, the atria contract to send the remaining blood to the ventricles. A new cardiac cycle begins as the heart enters systole again. (See *Understanding the phases of the cardiac cycle.*)

Cardiac output and stroke volume

Cardiac output refers to the amount of blood the left ventricle pumps into the aorta in 1 minute. Cardiac output is measured by multiplying heart rate by stroke volume. Stroke volume refers to the amount of blood ejected with each ventricular contraction and is usually about 70 ml.

Normal cardiac output is 4 to 8 L per minute, depending on body size. The heart pumps only as much blood as the body requires,

UNDERSTANDING THE PHASES OF THE CARDIAC CYCLE

1. Isovolumetric ventricular contraction

In response to ventricular depolarization, tension in the ventricles increases. The rise in pressure within the ventricles leads to closure of the mitral and tricuspid valves. The pulmonic and aortic valves stay closed during the entire phase.

2. Ventricular ejection

When ventricular pressure exceeds aortic and pulmonary artery pressures, the aortic and pulmonic valves open and the ventricles eject blood.

3. Isovolumetric relaxation

When ventricular pressure falls below the pressures in the aorta and pulmonary artery, the aortic and pulmonic valves close. All valves are closed during this phase. Atrial diastole occurs as blood fills the atria.

4. Ventricular filling

Atrial pressure exceeds ventricular pressure, which causes the mitral and tricuspid valves to open. Blood then flows passively into the ventricles. About 70% of ventricular filling takes place during this phase.

5. Atrial systole

Known as the *atrial kick,* atrial systole (coinciding with late ventricular diastole) supplies the ventricles with the remaining 30% of the blood for each heartbeat.

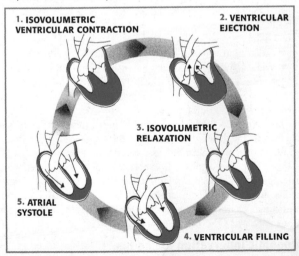

1. ISOVOLUMETRIC VENTRICULAR CONTRACTION

2. VENTRICULAR EJECTION

3. ISOVOLUMETRIC RELAXATION

5. ATRIAL SYSTOLE

4. VENTRICULAR FILLING

DEFINING PRELOAD AND AFTERLOAD

Preload refers to a passive stretching exerted by blood on the ventricular muscle fibers at the end of diastole. According to Starling's law, the more the cardiac muscles are stretched in diastole, the more forcefully they contract in systole.

Afterload refers to the pressure that the ventricles need to generate to overcome higher pressure in the aorta to eject blood into the systemic circulation. This systemic vascular resistance corresponds to the systemic systolic pressure.

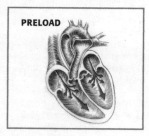

PRELOAD

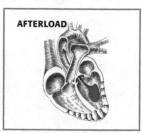

AFTERLOAD

based upon metabolic requirements. During exercise, for example, the heart increases cardiac output accordingly.

Three factors determine stroke volume:

- preload
- afterload
- myocardial contractility. (See *Defining preload and afterload*.)

Preload is the degree of stretch or tension on the muscle fibers when they begin to contract. It's usually considered to be the end-diastolic pressure when the ventricle has become filled.

Afterload is the load or amount of pressure the left ventricle must work against to eject blood during systole and corresponds to the systolic pressure: the greater this resistance, the greater the heart's workload. Afterload is also called the *systemic vascular resistance*.

Myocardial contractility is the ventricle's ability to contract, which is determined by the degree of muscle fiber stretch at the end of diastole. The more the muscle fibers stretch during ventricular filling, up to an optimal length, the more forceful the contraction. (See *Determining cardiac output*.)

Autonomic innervation of the heart

Nerves of the two branches of the ANS—the sympathetic (or *adrenergic*) and the parasympathetic (or *cholinergic*)—are abundant in the

DETERMINING CARDIAC OUTPUT

This illustration shows how preload, afterload, and contractility work together to determine cardiac output.

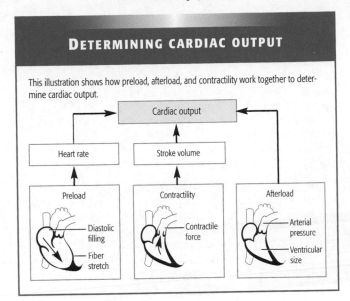

heart. Sympathetic fibers innervate all areas of the heart, whereas parasympathetic fibers primarily innervate the SA and AV nodes.

Sympathetic nerve stimulation causes the release of norepinephrine, which:

- increases the heart rate by increasing SA node discharge
- accelerates AV node conduction time
- increases the force of myocardial contraction and cardiac output.

Parasympathetic (vagal) stimulation causes the release of acetylcholine, which produces the opposite effects:

- decreases the rate of SA node discharge, thus slowing heart rate and conduction through the AV node
- reduces cardiac output.

Transmission of electrical impulses

For the heart to contract and pump blood to the rest of the body, an electrical stimulus needs to occur first. Generation and transmission of electrical impulses depend on the four key characteristics of cardiac cells:

- automaticity
- excitability
- conductivity
- contractility.

Automaticity refers to a cell's ability to spontaneously fire off an electrical impulse. Pacemaker cells usually possess this ability. Excitability results from ion shifts across the cell membrane and refers to the cell's ability to respond to an electrical stimulus. Conductivity is the ability of a cell to transmit an electrical impulse from one cell to another. Contractility refers to the cell's ability to contract after receiving a stimulus by shortening and lengthening its muscle fibers.

It's important to remember that the first three characteristics are electrical properties of the cells, while contractility represents a mechanical response to the electrical activity. Of the four characteristics, automaticity has the greatest effect on the start of cardiac rhythms.

Depolarization and repolarization

As impulses are transmitted, cardiac cells undergo cycles of depolarization and repolarization. (See *Understanding the depolarization-repolarization cycle.*) Cardiac cells at rest are considered polarized, meaning that no electrical activity takes place. Cell membranes separate different concentrations of ions, such as sodium and potassium, and create a more negative charge inside the cell. This is called the *resting potential*. After a stimulus occurs, ions cross the cell membrane and cause an action potential, or cell depolarization. When a cell is fully depolarized, it attempts to return to its resting state in a process called repolarization. Electrical charges in the cell reverse and return to normal.

A cycle of depolarization-repolarization consists of five phases—0 through 4. The action potential is represented by a curve that shows voltage changes during the five phases. (See *A look at action potential curves,* page 16.)

During phase 0 (or rapid depolarization), the cell receives a stimulus, usually from a neighboring cell. The cell becomes more permeable to sodium, the inside of the cell becomes less negative, the cell is depolarized, and myocardial contraction occurs. In phase 1 (or early repolarization), sodium stops flowing into the cell, and the transmembrane potential falls slightly. Phase 2 (the plateau phase) is a prolonged period of slow repolarization, when little change occurs in the cell's transmembrane potential.

During phases 1 and 2 and at the beginning of phase 3, the cardiac cell is said to be in its absolute refractory period. During that period, no stimulus, no matter how strong, can excite the cell.

Phase 3 (or rapid repolarization) occurs as the cell returns to its original state. During the last half of this phase, when the cell is in its relative refractory period, a very strong stimulus can depolarize it.

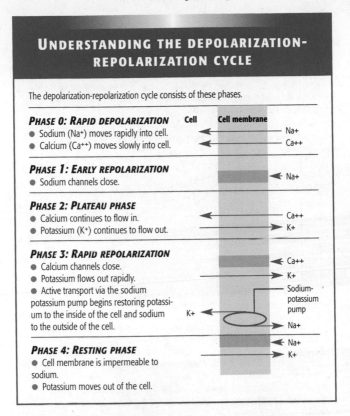

UNDERSTANDING THE DEPOLARIZATION-REPOLARIZATION CYCLE

The depolarization-repolarization cycle consists of these phases.

Cell   **Cell membrane**

PHASE 0: RAPID DEPOLARIZATION
- Sodium (Na+) moves rapidly into cell. ← Na+
- Calcium (Ca++) moves slowly into cell. ← Ca++

PHASE 1: EARLY REPOLARIZATION
- Sodium channels close. ← Na+

PHASE 2: PLATEAU PHASE
- Calcium continues to flow in. ← Ca++
- Potassium (K+) continues to flow out. → K+

PHASE 3: RAPID REPOLARIZATION
- Calcium channels close. ← Ca++
- Potassium flows out rapidly. → K+
- Active transport via the sodium potassium pump begins restoring potassium to the inside of the cell and sodium to the outside of the cell. K+ ← → Na+

Sodium-potassium pump

PHASE 4: RESTING PHASE
- Cell membrane is impermeable to sodium. ← Na+
- Potassium moves out of the cell. → K+

Phase 4 is the resting phase of the action potential. By the end of phase 4, the cell is ready for another stimulus.

The electrical activity of the heart is represented on an electrocardiogram (ECG). Keep in mind that the ECG represents electrical activity only, not the mechanical activity or actual pumping of the heart.

Electrical conduction system of the heart

After depolarization and repolarization occur, the resulting electrical impulse travels through the heart along a pathway called the conduction system. (See *Illustrating the cardiac conduction system*, page 17.)

Impulses travel out from the SA node and through the internodal tracts and Bachmann's bundle to the AV node. From there, they travel through the bundle of His, the bundle branches, and finally to the Purkinje fibers.

A LOOK AT ACTION POTENTIAL CURVES

An action potential curve shows the changes in a cell's electrical charge during the five phases of the depolarization-repolarization cycle. These graphs show electrical changes for nonpacemaker and pacemaker cells.

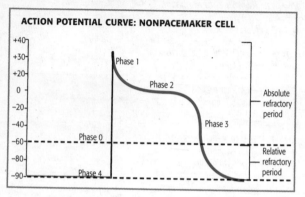

ACTION POTENTIAL CURVE: NONPACEMAKER CELL

As the graph below shows, the action potential curve for pacemaker cells, such as those in the sinoatrial node, differs from that of other myocardial cells. Pacemaker cells have a resting membrane potential of −60 mV (instead of −90 mV), and they begin to depolarize spontaneously. Called *diastolic depolarization*, this effect results mainly from calcium and sodium leaking into the cell.

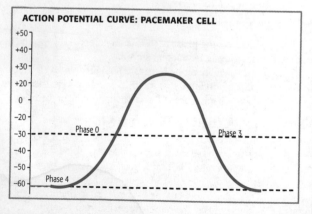

ACTION POTENTIAL CURVE: PACEMAKER CELL

ILLUSTRATING THE CARDIAC CONDUCTION SYSTEM

Specialized fibers propagate electrical impulses throughout the heart's cells, causing the heart to contract. This illustration shows the elements and the order of the cardiac conduction system.

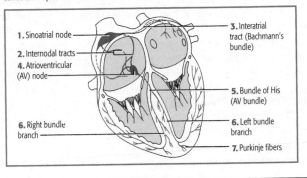

1. Sinoatrial node
2. Internodal tracts
4. Atrioventricular (AV) node
6. Right bundle branch

3. Interatrial tract (Bachmann's bundle)
5. Bundle of His (AV bundle)
6. Left bundle branch
7. Purkinje fibers

The SA node, located in the right atrium where the superior vena cava joins the atrial tissue mass, is the heart's main pacemaker. Under resting conditions, the SA node generates impulses 60 to 100 beats/minute. When initiated, the impulses follow a specific path through the heart. Electrical impulses usually don't travel in a backward or retrograde direction because the cells can't respond to a stimulus immediately after depolarization.

From the SA node, an impulse travels through the right and left atria. In the right atrium, the impulse is believed to be transmitted along three internodal tracts:

■ anterior
■ middle (or *Wenckebach's*)
■ posterior (or *Thorel's*).

The impulse travels through the left atrium via Bachmann's bundle, the interatrial tracts of tissue extending from the SA node to the left atrium. Impulse transmission through the right and left atria occurs so rapidly that the atria contract almost simultaneously.

The AV node is located in the inferior right atrium near the ostium of the coronary sinus. Although the AV node doesn't possess pacemaker cells, the tissue surrounding it, referred to as junctional tissue, contains pacemaker cells that can fire at a rate of 40 to 60 beats/minute. As the AV node conducts the atrial impulse to the ventricles, it causes a 0.04-second delay. This delay allows the ventricles to complete their filling phase as the atria contract. It also allows the cardiac muscle to stretch to its fullest for peak cardiac output.

Rapid conduction then resumes through the bundle of His, which divides into the right and left bundle branches and extends down either side of the interventricular septum. The right bundle branch extends down the right side of the interventricular septum and through the right ventricle. The left bundle branch extends down the left side of the interventricular septum and through the left ventricle. As a pacemaker site, the bundle of His has a firing rate between 40 and 60 beats/minute. The bundle of His usually fires when the SA node fails to generate an impulse at a normal rate or when the impulse fails to reach the AV junction.

The left bundle branch then splits into two branches, or fasciculations. The left anterior fasciculus extends through the anterior portion of the left ventricle. The left posterior fasciculus extends through the lateral and posterior portions of the left ventricle. Impulses travel much faster down the left bundle branch, which feeds the larger, thicker-walled left ventricle, than the right bundle branch, which feeds the smaller, thinner-walled right ventricle. The difference in the conduction speed allows both ventricles to contract simultaneously. The entire network of specialized nervous tissue that extends through the ventricles is known as the His-Purkinje system.

Purkinje fibers comprise a diffuse muscle fiber network beneath the endocardium that transmits impulses quicker than any other part of the conduction system. This pacemaker site usually doesn't fire unless the SA and AV nodes fail to generate an impulse or when the normal impulse is blocked in both bundle branches. The automatic firing rate of the Purkinje fibers ranges from 20 to 40 beats/minute.

ABNORMAL IMPULSE CONDUCTION
Causes of abnormal impulse conduction include:
- altered automaticity
- retrograde conduction of impulses
- reentry abnormalities
- ectopy.

Automaticity, a special characteristic of pacemaker cells, allows them to generate electrical impulses spontaneously. If a cell's automaticity is increased or decreased, an arrhythmia—or abnormality in the cardiac rhythm—can occur. Tachycardia and premature beats are commonly caused by an increase in the automaticity of pacemaker cells below the SA node. Likewise, a decrease in automaticity of cells in the SA node can cause the development of bradycardia or escape rhythms generated by lower pacemaker sites.

Impulses that begin below the AV node can be transmitted backward toward the atria. This backward, or retrograde, conduction usually takes longer than normal conduction and can cause the atria and ventricles to lose synchrony.

Reentry occurs when cardiac tissue is activated two or more times by the same impulse. This may happen when conduction speed is slowed or when the refractory periods for neighboring cells occur at different times. Impulses are delayed long enough that cells have time to repolarize. In those cases, the active impulse reenters the same area and produces another impulse.

Injured pacemaker (or nonpacemaker) cells may partially depolarize, rather than fully depolarizing. Partial depolarization can lead to spontaneous or secondary depolarization, repetitive ectopic firings called *triggered activity.*

The resultant depolarization is called *afterdepolarization.* Early afterdepolarization occurs before the cell is fully repolarized and can be caused by:
- hypokalemia
- slow pacing rates
- drug toxicity.

If it occurs after the cell has been fully repolarized, it's called delayed afterdepolarization, and tachycardia may result. This can be caused by:
- digoxin toxicity
- hypercalcemia
- increased catecholamine release.

Functions of the vascular system

About 60,000 miles of arteries, arterioles, capillaries, venules, and veins keep blood circulating to and from every functioning cell in the body. This network has two branches that include the pulmonary circulation and systemic circulation. (See *A look at the major blood vessels,* page 20, and *A look at the pulmonary and systemic circulation,* page 21.)

PULMONARY CIRCULATION

Pulmonary circulation refers to the movement of the blood as it travels back through the heart to the lungs to exchange carbon dioxide for

A LOOK AT THE MAJOR BLOOD VESSELS

This illustration shows the body's major arteries and veins.

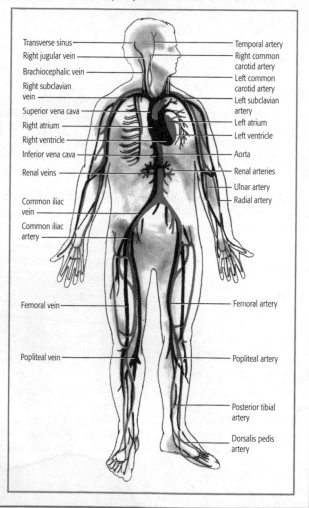

Transverse sinus

Right jugular vein

Brachiocephalic vein

Right subclavian vein

Superior vena cava

Right atrium

Right ventricle

Inferior vena cava

Renal veins

Common iliac vein

Common iliac artery

Femoral vein

Popliteal vein

Temporal artery

Right common carotid artery

Left common carotid artery

Left subclavian artery

Left atrium

Left ventricle

Aorta

Renal arteries

Ulnar artery

Radial artery

Femoral artery

Popliteal artery

Posterior tibial artery

Dorsalis pedis artery

A LOOK AT THE PULMONARY AND SYSTEMIC CIRCULATION

This illustration shows the relationship between the pulmonary and systemic circulation. The blood begins in the right ventricle (1), travels through the lungs to the left atrium (4) and ventricle (5), and enters the systemic circulation before returning to the right atrium (9).

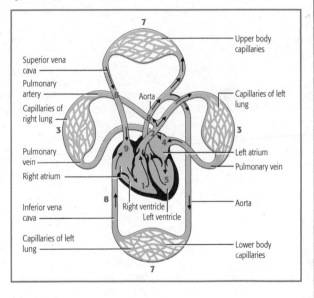

oxygen. Following are the actions that occur during pulmonary circulation:

- Deoxygenated blood travels from the right ventricle through the pulmonic valve into the pulmonary arteries.
- Blood passes through progressively smaller arteries and arterioles into the capillaries of the lungs.
- Blood reaches the alveoli and exchanges carbon dioxide for oxygen.
- The oxygenated blood then returns via venules and veins to the pulmonary veins, which carry it back to the left atrium of the heart.

SYSTEMIC CIRCULATION

Through the systemic circulation, blood carries oxygen and other nutrients to body cells and transports waste products for excretion. At specific sites, the pumping action of the heart that forces blood through the arteries becomes palpable. This regular expansion and contraction of the arteries is called the pulse.

The major artery—the aorta—branches into vessels that supply blood to specific organs and areas of the body. The left common carotid, left subclavian, and innominate arteries arise from the arch of the aorta and supply blood to the brain, arms, and upper chest. As the aorta descends through the thorax and abdomen, its branches supply blood to the GI and genitourinary organs, spinal column, and lower chest and abdominal muscles. Then the aorta divides into the iliac arteries, which further divide into femoral arteries.

As the arteries divide into smaller units, the number of vessels increases dramatically, thereby increasing the area of perfusion. Arteries are thick-walled because they transport blood under high pressure. Arterial walls contain a tough, elastic layer to help propel blood through the arterial system. At the end of the arterioles and the beginning of the capillaries, strong sphincters control blood flow into the tissues. These sphincters:

- dilate to permit more flow when needed
- close to shunt blood to other areas
- constrict to increase blood pressure.

Although the capillary bed contains the smallest vessels, it supplies blood to the largest area. Capillary pressure is extremely low to allow for the exchange of nutrients, oxygen, and carbon dioxide with body cells. From the capillaries, blood flows into venules and, eventually, into veins. Only about 5% of the circulating blood volume at any given moment is contained within the capillary network.

Nearly all veins carry oxygen-depleted blood, the sole exception being the pulmonary vein, which carries oxygenated blood from the lungs to the left atrium. Veins serve as a large reservoir for circulating blood. Valves in the veins prevent blood backflow, and the pumping action of skeletal muscles assists venous return. The wall of a vein is thinner and more pliable than the wall of an artery. That pliability allows the vein to accommodate variations in blood volume. The veins merge until they form two main branches—the superior and inferior venae cavae—that return blood to the right atrium.

LOCATING PULSE SITES

This illustration shows the locations of the major arterial pulses and the apical pulse.

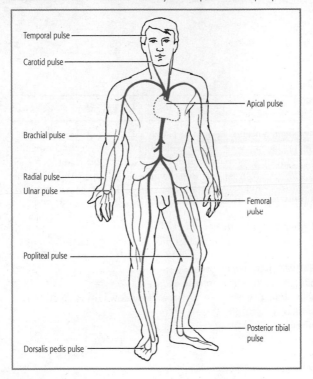

Temporal pulse

Carotid pulse

Apical pulse

Brachial pulse

Radial pulse

Ulnar pulse

Femoral pulse

Popliteal pulse

Posterior tibial pulse

Dorsalis pedis pulse

PULSES

Arterial pulses are pressure waves of blood generated by the pumping action of the heart. All vessels in the arterial system have pulsations, but the pulsations can be felt only where an artery lies near the skin. You can palpate for these peripheral pulses: temporal, carotid, brachial, radial, ulnar, femoral, popliteal, posterior tibial, and dorsalis pedis. (See *Locating pulse sites*.)

Assessment

HEALTH HISTORY

To obtain a health history of a patient's cardiovascular system, begin by introducing yourself and explaining what will occur during the health history interview and physical examination. To take an effective history, establish rapport with the patient. Ask open-ended questions and listen carefully to responses. Closely observe the patient's nonverbal behavior.

Chief complaint

A patient with a cardiovascular problem typically cites specific complaints, such as:
- chest pain
- irregular heartbeat or palpitations
- shortness of breath on exertion, lying down, or at night
- cough
- cyanosis or pallor
- weakness
- fatigue
- unexplained weight change
- swelling of the extremities
- dizziness
- headache
- high or low blood pressure
- peripheral skin changes, such as decreased hair distribution, skin color changes, or a thin, shiny appearance to the skin
- pain in the extremities, such as leg pain or cramps.

   Ask the patient how long he has had the problem, how it affects his daily routine, and when it began. Find out about any associated signs and symptoms. Ask about the location, radiation, intensity, and duration of any pain and any precipitating, exacerbating, or relieving factors. Ask him to rate the pain on a scale of 1 to 10, in which 1 means negligible and 10 means the worst pain imaginable.

Let the patient describe his problem in his own words. Avoid leading questions. Use expressions familiar to him rather than medical terms whenever possible. If the patient isn't in distress, ask questions that require more than a yes-or-no response. Try to obtain as accurate a description as possible of any chest pain.

AGE AWARE Even a child old enough to talk may have difficulty describing chest pain, so be alert for nonverbal clues, such as restlessness, facial grimaces, or holding of the painful area. Ask the child to point to the painful area and then to show you with his finger where the pain goes (to find out if it's radiating). Determine the pain's severity by asking the parents if the pain interferes with the child's normal activities and behavior. Because an elderly patient has a higher risk of developing life-threatening conditions, such as a myocardial infarction (MI), angina, and aortic dissection, carefully evaluate chest pain.

Current health history

In addition to checking for pain, ask the patient these questions:
- Are you ever short of breath? If so, what activities cause you to be short of breath?
- Do you feel dizzy or fatigued?
- Do your rings or shoes feel tight?
- Do your ankles swell?
- Have you noticed changes in the color or sensation in your legs? If so, what are those changes?
- If you have sores or ulcers, how quickly do they heal?
- Do you stand or sit in one place for long periods at work?
- How many pillows do you sleep on at night? (See *Key questions for assessing cardiac function,* page 26.)

Orthopnea or dyspnea that occurs when the patient is lying down and improves when he sits up suggests left ventricular heart failure or mitral stenosis. It can also accompany obstructive lung disease.

Pregnant women, especially those in the third trimester or those who stand for long periods of time, may report ankle edema. This is a common discomfort of pregnancy.

Past health history

Ask the patient about any history of cardiac-related disorders, such as hypertension, rheumatic fever, scarlet fever, diabetes mellitus, hyper-

KEY QUESTIONS FOR ASSESSING CARDIAC FUNCTION

These questions and statements will help you to assess your patient's cardiac function more accurately:

● Are you still in pain? Where's it located? Point to where you feel it.
● Describe what the pain feels like. (If the patient needs prompting, ask if he feels a burning, tightness, or squeezing sensation in his chest.)
● Does the pain radiate to any other part of your body? Your arm? Neck? Back? Jaw?
● When did the pain begin? What relieves it? What makes it feel worse?
● Tell me about any other feelings you're experiencing. (If the patient needs prompting, suggest nausea, dizziness, or sweating.)
● Tell me about any feelings of shortness of breath. Does a particular body position seem to bring this on? Which one? How long does the shortness of breath last? What relieves it?

● Has sudden breathing trouble ever awakened you from sleep? Tell me more about this.
● Do you ever wake up coughing? How often? Have you ever coughed up blood?
● Does your heart ever pound or skip a beat? If so, when does this happen?
● Do you ever get dizzy or faint? What seems to bring this on?
● Tell me about any swelling in your ankles or feet. At what time of day? Does anything relieve the swelling?
● Do you urinate more frequently at night?
● Tell me how you feel while you're doing your daily activities. Have you had to limit your activities or rest more often while doing them?

lipidemia, congenital heart defects, and syncope. Other questions to ask include:

■ Have you ever had severe fatigue not caused by exertion?
■ Are you taking any prescription, over-the-counter, or illicit drugs?
■ Are you allergic to any drugs, foods, or other products? If yes, describe the reaction you experienced.

In addition, ask a woman:

■ Have you begun menopause?
■ Do you use hormonal contraceptives or estrogen?
■ Have you experienced any medical problems during pregnancy? Have you ever had gestational hypertension?

Family history

Information about the patient's blood relatives may suggest a specific cardiac problem. Ask him if anyone in his family has ever had hypertension, MI, cardiomyopathy, diabetes mellitus, coronary artery disease (CAD), vascular disease, hyperlipidemia, or sudden death.

As you analyze a patient's problems, remember that age, gender, and race are essential considerations in identifying the risk for cardiovascular disorders. For example, CAD most commonly affects white men between ages 40 and 60. Hypertension occurs most commonly in blacks. Women are also vulnerable to heart disease, especially postmenopausal women and those with diabetes mellitus.

AGE AWARE Many elderly people have increased systolic blood pressure because aging increases the rigidity of blood vessel walls. Overall, elderly people have a higher incidence of cardiovascular disease than younger people.

Psychosocial history

Obtain information about your patient's occupation, educational background, living arrangements, daily activities, and family relationships.

Also obtain information about:

- stress and how he deals with it
- current health habits, such as smoking, alcohol intake, caffeine intake, exercise, and dietary intake of fat and sodium
- environmental or occupational considerations
- activities of daily living.

During the history-taking session, note the appropriateness of the patient's responses, his speech clarity, and his mood to aid in better identifying changes later.

PHYSICAL ASSESSMENT

Cardiovascular disease affects people of all ages and can take many forms. Using a consistent, methodical approach to your assessment will help you identify abnormalities. The key to accurate assessment is regular practice, which will help improve technique and efficiency.

Before assessing the patient's cardiovascular system, assess the factors that reflect cardiovascular function. These include vital signs, general appearance, and related body structures.

Wash your hands and gather the necessary equipment. Choose a private room. Adjust the thermostat, if necessary; cool temperatures may alter the patient's skin temperature and color, heart rate, and blood pressure. Make sure the room is quiet. If possible, close the door and windows and turn off radios and noisy equipment.

Combine parts of the physical assessment, as needed, to conserve time and the patient's energy. If a female patient feels embarrassed about exposing her chest, explain each assessment step beforehand, use drapes appropriately, and expose only the area being assessed. If the patient experiences cardiovascular difficulties, alter the order of the assessment as needed.

 RED FLAG If the patient develops chest pain and dyspnea, quickly check his vital signs and then auscultate the heart.

Vital sign assessment

Assessing vital signs includes measurement of temperature, blood pressure, pulse rate, and respiratory rate.

TEMPERATURE MEASUREMENT

Temperature is measured and documented in degrees Fahrenheit (° F) or degrees Celsius (° C). Choose the method of obtaining the patient's temperature (oral, tympanic, rectal, or axillary) based on the patient's age and condition. Normal body temperature ranges from 96.8° F to 99.5° F (36° C to 37.5° C).

If the patient has a fever, anticipate these possibilities:

- cardiovascular inflammation or infection
- heightened cardiac workload (Assess a febrile patient with heart disease for signs of increased cardiac workload such as tachycardia.)
- MI or acute pericarditis (mild to moderate fever usually occurs 2 to 5 days after an MI when the healing infarct passes through the inflammatory stage)
- infections, such as infective endocarditis, which causes fever spikes (high fever).

In patients with lower than normal body temperatures, findings include poor perfusion and certain metabolic disorders.

BLOOD PRESSURE MEASUREMENT

First, palpate and then auscultate the blood pressure in an arm or a leg. Wait 5 minutes between measurements. Normally, blood pressure readings are less than 120/80 mm Hg in a resting adult and 78/46 to 114/78 mm Hg in a young child. (See *Measuring blood pressure accurately*.)

Emotional stress caused by physical examination may elevate blood pressure. If the patient's blood pressure is high, allow him to relax for several minutes and then measure again to rule out stress.

When assessing a patient's blood pressure for the first time, take measurements in both arms.

 RED FLAG A difference of 10 mm Hg or more between the patient's arms can indicate thoracic outlet syndrome or another form of arterial obstruction.

MEASURING BLOOD PRESSURE ACCURATELY

When taking the patient's blood pressure, begin by applying the cuff properly, as shown below. Then be alert for these common problems to avoid recording an inaccurate blood pressure measurement.

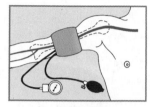

● *Wrong-sized cuff.* Select the appropriate-sized cuff for the patient. This ensures that adequate pressure is applied to compress the brachial artery during cuff inflation. If the cuff bladder is too narrow, a false-high reading will be obtained; too wide, a false-low reading. The cuff bladder width should be about 40% of the circumference of the midpoint of the limb; bladder length should be twice the width. If the arm circumference is less than 13″ (33 cm), select a regular-sized cuff; if it's between 13″ and 16″ (33 to 40.5 cm), a large-sized cuff; if it's more than 16″, a thigh cuff. Pediatric cuffs are also available.

● *Slow cuff deflation, causing venous congestion.* Don't deflate the cuff more slowly than 2 mm Hg/heartbeat; you'll get a false-high reading.

● *Cuff wrapped too loosely, reducing its effective width.* Tighten the cuff to avoid a false-high reading.

● *Mercury column not read at eye level.* Read the mercury column at eye level. If the column is below eye level, you may record a false-low reading; if it's above eye level, a false-high reading.

● *Poorly timed measurement.* Don't take the patient's blood pressure if he appears anxious or has just eaten or been ambulating; you'll get a false-high reading.

● *Incorrect position of the arm.* Keep the patient's arm level with his heart to avoid a false-low reading.

● *Failure to notice an auscultatory gap* (sound fades out for 10 to 15 mm Hg then returns). To avoid missing the top Korotkoff sounds, stimulate systolic pressure by palpation first.

● *Inaudibility of feeble sounds.* Before reinflating the cuff, have the patient raise his arm to reduce venous pressure and amplify low-volume sounds. After inflating the cuff, lower the patient's arm; then deflate the cuff and listen. Or, with the patient's arm positioned at heart level, inflate the cuff and have the patient make a fist. Have him rapidly open and close his hand 10 times before you begin to deflate the cuff; then listen. Be sure to document that the blood pressure reading was augmented.

If blood pressure is elevated in both arms, measure the pressure in the thigh. Wrap a large cuff around the patient's upper leg at least 1″ (2.5 cm) above the knee. Place the stethoscope over the popliteal artery, located on the posterior surface slightly above the knee joint. Listen for sounds when the bladder of the cuff is deflated.

High blood pressure in the patient's arms with normal or low pressure in the legs suggests aortic coarctation.

PULSE PRESSURE DETERMINATION

To calculate the patient's pulse pressure, subtract the diastolic pressure from the systolic pressure. This reflects arterial pressure during the resting phase of the cardiac cycle and normally ranges from 30 to 50 mm Hg.

Rising pulse pressure is seen with:

- increased stroke volume, which occurs with exercise, anxiety, and bradycardia
- declined peripheral vascular resistance or aortic distention, which occurs with anemia, hyperthyroidism, fever, hypertension, aortic coarctation, and aging.

Diminishing pulse pressure occurs with:

- mitral or aortic stenosis, which occurs with mechanical obstruction
- constricted peripheral vessels, which occurs with shock
- declined stroke volume, which occurs with heart failure, hypo-volemia, cardiac tamponade, or tachycardia.

RADIAL PULSE ASSESSMENT

If you suspect cardiac disease, palpate the radial pulse for 1 full minute to detect arrhythmias. Normally, an adult's pulse ranges from 60 to 100 beats/minute. Its rhythm should feel regular, except for a subtle slowing on expiration, caused by changes in intrathoracic pressure and vagal response. Note whether the pulse feels weak, normal, or bounding.

RESPIRATION EVALUATION

Observe for eupnea—a regular, unlabored, and bilaterally equal breathing pattern. In patients with irregular breathing, altered patterns may indicate:

- tachypnea with low cardiac output
- dyspnea, a possible indicator of heart failure (not evident at rest; however, pausing occurs after only a few words to take breaths)
- Cheyne-Stokes respirations, possibly accompanying severe heart failure (seen especially with coma)
- shallow breathing, possibly seen with acute pericarditis (deep respirations occur in an attempt to reduce the pain associated with deep respirations).

General appearance assessment

Begin by observing the patient's general appearance, particularly noting weight and muscle composition. Is he well developed, well nourished, alert, and energetic? Document any departures from normal. Does the patient appear older than his chronological age or seem unusually tired or slow-moving? Does the patient appear comfortable or does he seem anxious or in distress?

HEIGHT AND BODY WEIGHT MEASUREMENT

Accurately measure and record the patient's height and weight. These measurements will help:
- determine risk factors
- calculate hemodynamic indexes (such as cardiac index)
- guide treatment plans
- determine medication dosages
- assist with nutritional counseling
- detect fluid overload.

Fluctuations in weight may prove significant, especially when extreme.

RED FLAG Extreme weight fluctuation, for example, would occur if the patient with developing heart failure gains several pounds overnight.

Next, assess for cachexia—weakness and muscle wasting. Observe the amount of muscle bulk in the upper arms, thighs, and chest wall. For a more precise measurement, calculate the percentage of body fat. For men, this should be 12%; for women, it should be 18%. Loss of the body's energy stores slows healing and impairs immune function. A patient with chronic cardiac disease may develop cachexia. However, be aware that edema may mask these effects.

SKIN ASSESSMENT

Note the patient's skin color, temperature, turgor, and texture. Because normal skin color can vary widely among patients, ask him if his current skin tone is normal. Then inspect the skin color and note any cyanosis. Two types of cyanosis can occur in patients:
- central cyanosis, suggesting reduced oxygen intake or transport from the lungs to the bloodstream, which may occur with heart failure
- peripheral cyanosis, suggesting constriction of peripheral arterioles, a natural response to cold or anxiety or a result of hypovolemia, cardiogenic shock, or a vasoconstrictive disease.

Examine the underside of the tongue, buccal mucosa, and conjunctiva for signs of central cyanosis. Inspect the lips, tip of the nose, earlobes, and nail beds for signs of peripheral cyanosis. The color range for normal mucous membranes is narrower than that for the skin; therefore, it provides a more accurate assessment. In a dark-skinned patient, inspect the oral mucous membranes, such as the lips and gingivae, which normally appear pink and moist but would appear ashen if cyanotic.

When evaluating the patient's skin color, also observe for flushing, pallor, and rubor. Flushing of a patient's skin can result from:

- medications
- excess heat
- anxiety
- fear.

Pallor can result from anemia or increased peripheral vascular resistance caused by atherosclerosis. Dependent rubor may be a sign of chronic arterial insufficiency.

Next, assess the patient's perfusion by evaluating the arterial flow adequacy. With the patient lying down:

- Elevate one of the patient's legs 12″ (30.5 cm) above heart level for 60 seconds.
- Tell him to sit up and dangle both legs.
- Compare the color of both legs.

The leg that was elevated should show mild pallor compared with the other leg. Color should return to the pale leg in about 10 seconds, and the veins should refill in about 15 seconds. Suspect arterial insufficiency if the patient's foot shows marked pallor, delayed color return that ends with a mottled appearance, delayed venous filling, or marked redness.

Next, touch the patient's skin. It should feel warm and dry. If the patient's skin is cool and clammy, this is a sign of vasoconstriction, which occurs when cardiac output is low such as during shock. Warm, moist skin is a sign of vasodilation, which occurs when cardiac output is high such as during exercise.

Evaluate skin turgor by grasping and raising the skin between two fingers and then letting it go. Normally, the skin immediately returns to its original position. If the patient's skin is taut and shiny and can't be grasped, this may result from ascites or the marked edema that accompanies heart failure. Skin that doesn't immediately return to the original position exhibits tenting, a sign of decreased skin turgor, which may result from:

- dehydration, especially if the patient takes diuretics
- age

- malnutrition
- adverse reaction to corticosteroid treatment.

Observe the skin for signs of edema. Inspect the patient's arms and legs for symmetrical swelling. Because edema usually affects lower or dependent areas of the body first, be especially alert when assessing the arms, hands, legs, feet, and ankles of an ambulatory patient or the buttocks and sacrum of a bedridden patient. Determine the type of edema (pitting or nonpitting), its location, its extent, and its symmetry (unilateral or symmetrical). If the patient has pitting edema, assess the degree of pitting.

Edema can result from heart failure or venous insufficiency caused by varicosities or thrombophlebitis. Chronic right-sided heart failure may cause ascites, which leads to generalized edema and abdominal distention. Venous compression may result in localized edema along the path of the compressed vessel.

While inspecting the patient's skin, note the location, size, number, and appearance of any lesions. Dry, open lesions on the patient's lower extremities accompanied by pallor, cool skin, and lack of hair growth signify arterial insufficiency, possibly caused by arterial peripheral vascular disease. Wet, open lesions with red or purplish edges that appear on the patient's legs may result from the venous stasis associated with venous peripheral vascular disease.

EXTREMITY ASSESSMENT

Inspect the hair on the patient's arms and legs. Hair should be distributed symmetrically and should grow thicker on the anterior surface of the arms and legs. If the patient's hair isn't thicker on the anterior of the surface of the arms and legs, it may indicate diminished arterial blood flow to these extremities.

Note whether the length of the arms and legs is proportionate to the length of the trunk. A patient with long, thin arms and legs may have Marfan syndrome, a congenital disorder that causes cardiovascular problems, such as:

- aortic dissection
- aortic valve incompetence
- cardiomyopathy.

FINGERNAIL ASSESSMENT

Fingernails normally appear pinkish with no markings. A bluish color in the nail beds indicates peripheral cyanosis.

Estimate the rate of peripheral blood flow; assess the capillary refill in the patient's fingernails (or toenails) by applying pressure to the nail for 5 seconds, then assessing the time it takes for color to return.

CHECKING FOR CLUBBED FINGERS

To assess a patient for chronic tissue hypoxia, check his fingers for clubbing. Normally, the angle between the fingernail and the point where the nail enters the skin is about 160 degrees. Clubbing occurs when that angle increases to 180 degrees or more, as shown below.

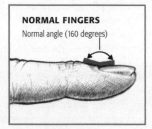

NORMAL FINGERS
Normal angle (160 degrees)

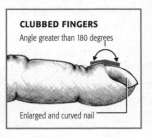

CLUBBED FINGERS
Angle greater than 180 degrees

Enlarged and curved nail

In a patient with a good arterial supply, color should return in less than 3 seconds.

Delayed capillary refill in the patient's fingernails suggests reduced circulation to that area, a sign of low cardiac output that may lead to arterial insufficiency.

Assess the angle between the nail and the cuticle. An angle of 180 degrees or greater indicates finger clubbing. Check for enlarged fingertips with spongy, slightly swollen nail bases. Normally, the nail bases feel firm; however, in early clubbing, they're spongy. Finger clubbing commonly indicates chronic tissue hypoxia. (See *Checking for clubbed fingers.*)

The shape of the patient's nails should be smooth and rounded. A concave depression in the middle of a thin nail indicates koilonychia (spoon nail), a sign of iron deficiency anemia or Raynaud's disease, whereas thick, ridged nails can result from arterial insufficiency.

Finally, check for splinter hemorrhages—small, thin, red or brown lines that run from the base to the tip of the nail. Splinter hemorrhages develop in patients with bacterial endocarditis.

EYE ASSESSMENT
Inspect the eyelids for xanthelasma—small, slightly raised, yellowish plaques that usually appear around the inner canthus. The plaques

that occur in xanthelasma result from lipid deposits and may signal severe hyperlipidemia, a risk factor of cardiovascular disease.

Next, observe the color of the patient's sclerae. Yellowish sclerae may be the first sign of jaundice, which occasionally results from liver congestion caused by right-sided heart failure.

Next, check for arcus senilis—a thin grayish ring around the edge of the cornea. A normal occurrence in elderly patients, arcus senilis can indicate hyperlipidemia in patients younger than age 65.

Using an ophthalmoscope, examine the retinal structures, including the retinal vessels and background. The retina is normally light yellow to orange, and the background should be free from hemorrhages and exudates. Structural changes, such as narrowing or blocking of a vein where an arteriole crosses over, indicate hypertension. Soft exudates may suggest hypertension or subacute bacterial endocarditis.

HEAD MOVEMENT ASSESSMENT

Assess the patient's head at rest and be alert for abnormal positioning or movements. Also check range of motion and rotation of the neck. A slight, rhythmic bobbing of the patient's head in time with his heartbeat (Musset's sign) may accompany the high backpressure caused by aortic insufficiency or aneurysm.

Heart assessment

Ask the patient to remove all clothing except his underwear and to put on an examination gown. Have the patient lie on his back, with the head of the examination table at a 30- to 45-degree angle. Stand on the patient's right side if you're right-handed or his left side if you're left-handed so you can auscultate more easily.

When assessing the heart, as with assessing other body systems, use the following steps:
- inspect
- palpate
- percuss
- auscultate.

INSPECTION

First, inspect the patient's chest and thorax. Expose the anterior chest and observe its general appearance. Normally, the lateral diameter is twice the anteroposterior diameter. Note any deviations from typical chest shape. (See *Identifying chest deformities,* page 36.)

IDENTIFYING CHEST DEFORMITIES

When inspecting the patient's chest, note deviations in size and shape. These illustrations show a normal adult chest, along with four common chest deformities.

NORMAL ADULT CHEST

No structural deformities or visible retractions

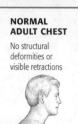

BARREL CHEST

Increased anteroposterior diameter

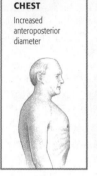

PIGEON CHEST

Anteriorly displaced sternum

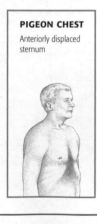

FUNNEL CHEST

Depressed lower sternum

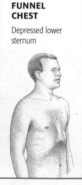

THORACIC KYPHO-SCOLIOSIS

Raised shoulder and scapula, thoracic convexity, and flared interspaces

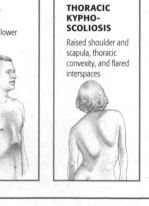

Note landmarks you can use to describe your findings as well as structures underlying the chest wall. (See *Identifying cardiovascular landmarks*.)

Look for pulsations, symmetry of movement, retractions, or heaves. A heave is a strong outward thrust of the chest wall and occurs during systole.

Position a light source, such as a flashlight or gooseneck lamp, so that it casts a shadow on the patient's chest. Note the location of the

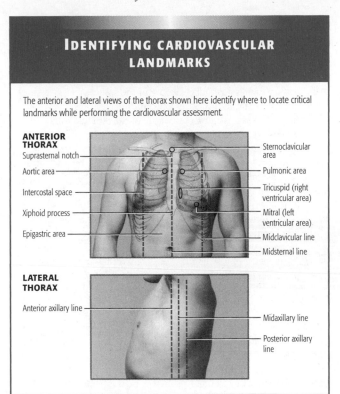

IDENTIFYING CARDIOVASCULAR LANDMARKS

The anterior and lateral views of the thorax shown here identify where to locate critical landmarks while performing the cardiovascular assessment.

ANTERIOR THORAX

- Suprasternal notch
- Aortic area
- Intercostal space
- Xiphoid process
- Epigastric area
- Sternoclavicular area
- Pulmonic area
- Tricuspid (right ventricular area)
- Mitral (left ventricular area)
- Midclavicular line
- Midsternal line

LATERAL THORAX

- Anterior axillary line
- Midaxillary line
- Posterior axillary line

apical impulse. This is typically also the point of maximum impulse (PMI) and should be located in the fifth intercostal space medial to the left midclavicular line. The apical impulse gives an indication of how well the left ventricle is working because it corresponds to the apex of the heart. The impulse can be seen in about one-half of all adults.

AGE AWARE In children and patients with thin chest walls, the apical impulse is noted more easily. In these patients, you may see slight sternal movement and pulsations over the pulmonary arteries or the aorta as well as visible pulsations in the epigastric area. To find the apical impulse in a woman with large breasts, move the breasts during the examination.

On inspection, irregularities in the patient's heart may be noted. Some of these findings can impair cardiac output by preventing chest expansion and inhibiting heart muscle movement, whereas others can indicate cardiac disease:

- barrel chest, indicated by a rounded thoracic cage caused by chronic obstructive pulmonary disease
- pectus excavatum, indicated by a depressed sternum
- scoliosis, which is a lateral curvature of the spine
- pectus carinatum, indicated by a protruding sternum
- kyphosis, which is a convex curvature of the thoracic spine
- retractions, indicated by visible indentations of the soft tissue covering the chest wall, or the use of accessory muscles to breathe, which typically results from a respiratory disorder, but may also indicate a congenital heart defect or heart failure
- visible pulsation to the right of the sternum, a possible indication of aortic aneurysm
- pulsation in the sternoclavicular or epigastric area, a possible indication of aortic aneurysm
- sustained, forceful apical impulse, a possible indication of left ventricular hypertrophy, which increases blood pressure and may cause cardiomyopathy and mitral insufficiency
- laterally displaced apical impulse, a possible sign of left ventricular hypertrophy.

PALPATION

Maintain a gentle touch when palpating so you won't obscure pulsations or similar findings. Follow a systematic palpation sequence covering the sternoclavicular, aortic, pulmonary, right ventricular, left ventricular (apical), and epigastric areas. Use the pads of the fingers to effectively assess large pulse sites. Finger pads prove especially sensitive to vibrations.

Start at the sternoclavicular area and move methodically through the palpation sequence down to the epigastric area. At the sternoclavicular area, you may feel pulsation of the aortic arch, especially in a thin or average-build patient. In a thin patient, you may palpate a pulsation in the abdominal aorta over the epigastric area.

Starting with the ball of your hand then using your fingertips, palpate over the precordium to find the apical impulse. Note heaves or thrills, fine vibrations that feel like the purring of a cat. (See *Palpating the apical impulse.*)

Keep in mind that the apical impulse may be difficult to palpate in obese patients, pregnant women, and patients with thick chest walls.

PALPATING THE APICAL IMPULSE

To find the apical impulse, use the ball of your hand, then your fingertips, to palpate over the precordium. Note heaves or thrills, fine vibrations that feel like the purring of a cat.

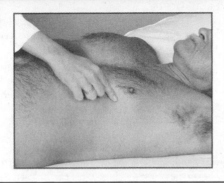

If it's difficult to palpate with the patient lying on his back, have him lie on his left side or sit upright. It may also be helpful to have the patient exhale completely and hold his breath for a few seconds.

Palpation of the patient's heart may reveal:

- apical impulse that exerts unusual force and lasts longer than one-third of the cardiac cycle—a possible indication of increased cardiac output
- displaced or diffuse impulse—a possible indication of left ventricular hypertrophy
- pulsation in the aortic, pulmonary, or right ventricular area—a sign of chamber enlargement or valvular disease
- pulsation in the sternoclavicular or epigastric area—a sign of aortic aneurysm
- palpable thrill or fine vibration—an indication of blood flow turbulence, usually related to valvular dysfunction (Determine how far the thrill radiates and make a mental note to listen for a murmur at this site during auscultation.)
- heave or a strong outward thrust during systole along the left sternal border—an indication of right ventricular hypertrophy
- heave over the left ventricular area—a sign of a ventricular aneurysm (A thin patient may experience a heave with exercise, fever, or anxiety because of increased cardiac output and more forceful contraction.)

- displaced PMI—a possible indication of left ventricular hypertrophy caused by volume overload from mitral or aortic stenosis, septal defect, acute MI, or other disorder.

PERCUSSION

Although percussion isn't as useful as other methods of assessment, this technique may help in locating cardiac borders. Begin percussing at the anterior axillary line, and percuss toward the sternum along the fifth intercostal space.

The sound changes from resonance to dullness over the left border of the heart, normally at the midclavicular line. If the cardiac border extends to the left of the midclavicular line, the patient's heart—and especially the left ventricle—may be enlarged.

The right border of the heart is usually aligned with the sternum and can't be percussed. In obese patients and women, percussion may be difficult because of the fat overlying the chest and because of breast tissue. In these cases, a chest X-ray can be used to provide information about the heart border.

AUSCULTATION

Auscultating for heart sounds provides a great deal of information about the heart. Cardiac auscultation requires a methodical approach and plenty of practice. Begin by warming the stethoscope in your hands, and then identify the sites where you'll auscultate: over the four cardiac valves and at Erb's point, the third intercostal space at the left sternal border. Use the bell to hear low-pitched sounds and the diaphragm to hear high-pitched sounds. (See *Using auscultation sites.*)

Auscultate for heart sounds with the patient in three positions:
- lying on his back with the head of the bed raised 30 to 45 degrees
- sitting up
- lying on his left side.

Use a zigzag pattern over the precordium, either auscultating from the base to the apex or the apex to the base. Whichever approach you use, be consistent.

Use the diaphragm of the stethoscope to listen as you go in one direction; use the bell as you come back in the other direction. Be sure to listen over the entire precordium, not just over the valves. Note the heart rate and rhythm.

Always identify the first heart sound (S_1) and the second heart sound (S_2), and then listen for adventitious sounds, such as third (S_3) and fourth heart sounds (S_4), murmurs, and rubs.

USING AUSCULTATION SITES

When auscultating for heart sounds, place the stethoscope over four different sites. Follow the same auscultation sequence during every cardiovascular assessment:

● Place the stethoscope in the second intercostal space along the right sternal border, as shown. In the aortic area, blood moves from the left ventricle during systole, crossing the aortic valve and flowing through the aortic arch.

● Move to the pulmonic area, located in the second intercostal space at the left sternal border. In the pulmonic area, blood ejected from the right ventricle during systole crosses the pulmonic valve

and flows through the main pulmonary artery.

● In the third auscultation site, assess the tricuspid area, which lies in the fifth intercostal space along the left sternal border. In the tricuspid area, sounds reflect blood movement from the right atrium across the tricuspid valve, filling the right ventricle during diastole.

● Finally, listen in the mitral area, located in the fifth intercostal space near the midclavicular line. (If the patient's heart is enlarged, the mitral area may be closer to the anterior axillary line.) In the mitral (apical) area, sounds represent blood flow across the mitral valve and left ventricular filling during diastole.

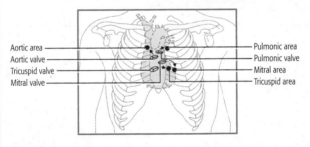

Aortic area — Aortic valve — Tricuspid valve — Mitral valve — — Pulmonic area — Pulmonic valve — Mitral area — Tricuspid area

Normal heart sounds

Start auscultating at the aortic area where S_2 is loudest. S_2 is best heard at the base of the heart at the end of ventricular systole. This sound corresponds to closure of the pulmonic and aortic valves and is generally described as sounding like "dub." It's a shorter, higher-pitched, louder sound than S_1. When the pulmonic valve closes later than the aortic valve during inspiration, you'll hear a split S_2.

From the base of the heart, move to the pulmonic area and down to the tricuspid area. Then move to the mitral area, where S_1 is the loudest. S_1 is best heard at the apex of the heart. This sound corresponds to closure of the mitral and tricuspid valves and is generally

QUICK GUIDE TO EXTRA HEART SOUNDS

This chart lists some common extra heart sounds along with their characteristics.

SOUND	LOCATION	PITCH
S₃	Apex	Low
S₄	Mitral or tricuspid area (with bell of stethoscope)	Low
Summation gallop	Apex	Low
Quadruple rhythm	Apex	Low
Click	Apex or lower left sternal border	High
Snap	Apex along lower left sternal border	High
Rub	Third left intercostal space at the lower left sternal border	High

described as sounding like "lub." It's low-pitched and dull. S_1 occurs at the beginning of ventricular systole. It may be split if the mitral valve closes just before the tricuspid.

Auscultation may detect S_1 and S_2 that are accentuated, diminished, or inaudible. These abnormalities may result from:
- pressure changes
- valvular dysfunctions
- conduction defects.

A prolonged, persistent, or reversed split sound may result from a mechanical or electrical problem.

Abnormal heart sounds

Auscultation may reveal an S_3, an S_4, or both. Other abnormal sounds include a summation gallop, click, opening snap, rubs, and murmur. (See *Quick guide to extra heart sounds*.)

TIMING	PATIENT POSITION	CAUSE
Early to middiastole	Supine or left lateral	Noncompliant ventricle
Late diastole	Supine	Atrial contraction into a noncompliant ventricle
Middiastole	Left lateral	S_3 and S_4 occurring together to produce one heart sound
Throughout cardiac cycle	Left lateral	Hearing S_1, S_2, S_3, and S_4
Mid to late systole	Sitting or standing	Tensing of the chordae tendineae and mitral valve cusps
Mid to late diastole	Left lateral	Stenotic valve attempting to open
Throughout systole, diastole, or both	Leaning forward	Pericarditis

S_3

Also known as a *ventricular gallop*, S_3 is a low-pitched noise that's best heard by placing the bell of the stethoscope at the apex of the heart. Its rhythm resembles a horse galloping, and its tempo resembles the word "Ken-tuc-ky" (lub-dub-by). Listen for S_3 with the patient in a supine or left-lateral decubitus position.

S_3 usually occurs during early diastole to middiastole, at the end of the passive-filling phase of either ventricle. Listen for this sound immediately after S_2. It may signify that the ventricle isn't compliant enough to accept the filling volume without additional force. If the right ventricle is noncompliant, the sound will occur in the tricuspid area; if the left ventricle is noncompliant, in the mitral area. A heave may be palpable when the sound occurs.

AGE AWARE In a child or young adult, S_3 may occur normally. It may also occur during the last trimester of pregnancy. In a patient over age 30, it usually indicates a disorder, such as right-sided heart failure, left-sided heart failure, pulmonary congestion, intracardiac shunting of blood, MI, anemia, or thyrotoxicosis.

S_4

S_4 is an abnormal heart sound that occurs late in diastole, just before the pulse upstroke. It immediately precedes the S_1 of the next cycle and is associated with acceleration and deceleration of blood entering a chamber that resists additional filling. Known as the *atrial* or *presystolic gallop*, it occurs during atrial contraction.

S_4 shares the same tempo as the word "Ten-nes-see" (le-lub-dub). Heard best with the bell of the stethoscope and with the patient in a supine position, S_4 may occur in the tricuspid or mitral area, depending on which ventricle is dysfunctional.

AGE AWARE In elderly patients, S_4 commonly appears with age-related systolic hypertension and aortic stenosis.

Although rare, S_4 may occur normally in a young patient with a thin chest wall. More commonly, it indicates cardiovascular disease, such as:

- acute MI
- hypertension
- CAD
- cardiomyopathy
- angina
- anemia
- elevated left ventricular pressure
- aortic stenosis.

If the sound persists, it may indicate impaired ventricular compliance or volume overload.

Summation gallop

Occasionally, a patient may have both S_3 and S_4. Auscultation may reveal two separate abnormal heart sounds and two normal sounds. Usually, the patient has tachycardia and diastole is shortened. S_3 and S_4 occur so close together that they appear to be one sound—a summation gallop.

Clicks

Clicks are high-pitched abnormal heart sounds that result from tensing of the chordae tendineae structures and mitral valve cusps. Initially, the mitral valve closes securely, but a large cusp prolapses into the left atrium. The click usually precedes a late systolic murmur caused by regurgitation of a little blood from the left ventricle into the left atrium. Clicks occur in 5% to 10% of young adults and affect more women than men.

To detect the high-pitched click of mitral valve prolapse in the patient, place the stethoscope diaphragm at the apex and listen during midsystole to late systole. To enhance the sound, change the patient's position to sitting or standing, and listen along the lower left sternal border.

Snaps

Upon placing the stethoscope diaphragm at the apex along the lower left sternal border, you may detect an opening snap immediately after S_2. The snap resembles the normal S_1 and S_2 in quality; its high pitch helps differentiate it from an S_3. Because the opening snap may accompany mitral or tricuspid stenosis, it usually precedes a middiastolic to late diastolic murmur—a classic sign of stenosis. It results from the stenotic valve attempting to open.

Rubs

To detect a pericardial friction rub, use the diaphragm of the stethoscope to auscultate in the third left intercostal space along the lower left sternal border. Listen for a harsh, scratchy, scraping, or squeaking sound that occurs throughout systole, diastole, or both. To enhance the sound, have the patient sit upright and lean forward or exhale. A rub usually indicates pericarditis.

Murmurs

Longer than a heart sound, a murmur occurs as a vibrating, blowing, or rumbling noise. Just as turbulent water in a stream babbles as it passes through a narrow point, turbulent blood flow produces a murmur.

If you detect a murmur, identify where it's loudest, pinpoint the time it occurs during the cardiac cycle, and describe its pitch, pattern, quality, intensity, and implications.

Location and timing

Murmurs may occur in any cardiac auscultatory site and may radiate from one site to another. To identify the radiation area, auscultate from the site where the murmur seems loudest to the farthest site it's still heard. Note the anatomic landmark of this farthest site.

Determine if the murmur occurs during systole (between S_1 and S_2) or diastole (between S_2 and the next S_1). Pinpoint when in the cardiac cycle the murmur occurs—for example, during middiastole or

IDENTIFYING MURMUR PATTERNS

To help classify a murmur, begin by identifying its configuration (pattern). Shown here are four basic patterns of murmurs.

CRESCENDO/DECRESCENDO
(diamond-shaped)
● Begins softly, peaks sharply, and then fades
● Examples: Pulmonic stenosis, aortic stenosis, mitral valve prolapse, mitral stenosis

DECRESCENDO
● Starts loudly and then gradually diminishes
● Examples: Aortic insufficiency, pulmonic insufficiency

PANSYSTOLIC
(holosystolic or plateau-shaped)
● Is uniform from beginning to end
● Examples: Mitral or tricuspid regurgitation

CRESCENDO
● Begins softly and then gradually increases
● Examples: Tricuspid stenosis, mitral valve prolapse

late systole. A murmur that's heard throughout systole is called *holosystolic* or *pansystolic*, whereas a murmur heard throughout diastole is called a *pandiastolic* murmur. Occasionally murmurs occur during both portions of the cycle, known as *continuous murmur.*

Pitch
Depending on rate and pressure of blood flow, pitch may be high, medium, or low. You can best hear a low-pitched murmur with the bell of the stethoscope, a high-pitched murmur with the diaphragm, and a medium-pitched murmur with both.

Pattern
Crescendo occurs when the velocity of blood flow increases and the murmur becomes louder. Decrescendo occurs when velocity decreases and the murmur becomes quieter. A crescendo-decrescendo pattern

GRADING MURMURS

Use the system outlined here to grade the intensity of a murmur. When recording your findings, use Roman numerals as part of a fraction, always with VI as the denominator. For example, a grade III murmur would be recorded as "grade III/VI."

- Grade I is barely audible.
- Grade II is audible but quiet and soft.
- Grade III is moderately loud, without a thrust or thrill.
- Grade IV is loud, with a thrill.
- Grade V is very loud, with a thrust or a thrill.
- Grade VI is loud enough to be heard before the stethoscope comes into contact with the patient's chest.

describes a murmur with increasing loudness followed by increasing softness. (See *Identifying murmur patterns*.)

Quality
The volume of blood flow, the force of the contraction, and the degree of valve damage all contribute to murmur quality. Terms used to describe quality include:

- musical
- blowing
- harsh
- rasping
- rumbling
- machinelike.

Intensity
Use a standard, six-level grading scale to describe the intensity of the murmur. (See *Grading murmurs*.)

Implications
An innocent or functional murmur may appear in a patient without heart disease. Best heard in the pulmonic area, it occurs early in systole and seldom exceeds grade II in intensity. When the patient changes from a supine to a sitting position, the murmur may disappear. If fever, exercise, anemia, anxiety, pregnancy, or other factors increase cardiac output, the murmur may increase in intensity.

AGE AWARE Innocent murmurs affect up to one-fourth of children but usually disappear by adolescence. Similarly, elderly patients who experience changes in the aortic valve structures and the aorta also experi-

POSITIONING THE PATIENT FOR AUSCULTATION

Forward-leaning position

The forward-leaning position is best suited for hearing high-pitched sounds related to semilunar valve problems, such as aortic and pulmonic valve murmurs. To auscultate for these sounds, place the diaphragm of the stethoscope over the aortic and pulmonic areas in the right and left second intercostal spaces, as shown.

Left lateral recumbent position

The left lateral recumbent position is best suited for hearing low-pitched sounds, such as mitral valve murmurs and extra heart sounds. To hear these sounds, place the bell of the stethoscope over the apical area, as shown.

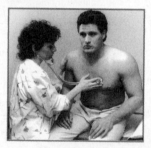

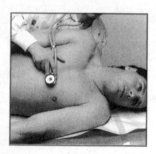

ence a nonpathologic murmur. This murmur occurs as a short systolic murmur, best heard at the left sternal border.

Pathologic murmurs in a patient may occur during systole or diastole and may affect any heart valve. These murmurs may result from:

- valvular stenosis (inability of the heart valves to open properly)
- valvular insufficiency (inability of the heart valves to close properly, allowing regurgitation of blood
- a septal defect (a defect in the septal wall separating two heart chambers).

The best way to hear murmurs is with the patient sitting up and leaning forward. You can also have him lie on his left side. (See *Positioning the patient for auscultation*, and *Differentiating murmurs*.)

DIFFERENTIATING MURMURS

WHAT YOU'LL HEAR	WHERE YOU'LL HEAR IT	WHAT CAUSES IT
• Medium pitch • Harsh quality • Possibly musical at apex • Crescendo-decrescendo • Loudest with expiration • Variable-grade intensity	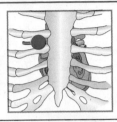	Aortic stenosis
• High pitch • Blowing quality • Grade I to III intensity • Decrescendo	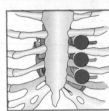	Aortic insufficiency
• Medium to high pitch • Blowing quality • Holosystolic • Soft to loud grade intensity	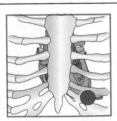	Mitral insufficiency
• Medium to high pitch • Blowing quality • Holosystolic • Variable intensity	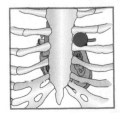	Tricuspid insufficiency

Key

 Diaphragm

(continued)

DIFFERENTIATING MURMURS *(continued)*

WHAT YOU'LL HEAR	WHERE YOU'LL HEAR IT	WHAT CAUSES IT
• Low pitch • Rumbling quality • Crescendo-decrescendo • Grade I to III intensity **Key** ● Bell		Mitral stenosis

Vascular assessment

Assessment of the vascular system is an important part of a full cardio-vascular assessment. Examination of the patient's arms and legs can reveal arterial or venous disorders. Examine the patient's arms when you take his vital signs. Check the legs later during the physical examination, when the patient is lying on his back. Remember to evaluate leg veins when the patient is standing.

INSPECTION

Start the vascular assessment in the same way as starting the cardiac assessment—by making general observations. Are the patient's arms equal in size? Are the legs symmetrical?

Inspect the patient's skin color. Note how body hair is distributed. Note lesions, scars, clubbing, and edema of the extremities. If the patient is bedridden, check the sacrum for swelling. Examine the fingernails and toenails for abnormalities.

Upon inspection of the patient's vascular system, note these irregularities, including:

- cyanosis, pallor, or cool or cold skin, indicating poor cardiac output and tissue perfusion
- warm skin caused by fever or increased cardiac output
- absence of body hair on the patient's arms or legs, indicating diminished arterial blood flow to those areas (see *Differentiating arterial and chronic venous insufficiency*)
- swelling or edema, indicating heart failure or venous insufficiency, or varicosities or thrombophlebitis

DIFFERENTIATING ARTERIAL AND CHRONIC VENOUS INSUFFICIENCY

Assessment findings differ in patients with arterial insufficiency and those with chronic venous insufficiency. These illustrations show those differences.

Arterial insufficiency

In a patient with arterial insufficiency, pulses may be decreased or absent. His skin will be cool, pale, and shiny, and he may have pain in his legs and feet. Ulcerations typically occur in the area around the toes, and the foot usually turns deep red when dependent. Nails may be thick and ridged.

Chronic venous insufficiency

In a patient with chronic venous insufficiency, check for ulcerations around the ankle. Pulses are present but may be difficult to find because of edema. The foot may become cyanotic when dependent.

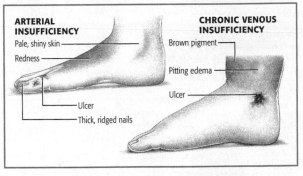

ARTERIAL INSUFFICIENCY
Pale, shiny skin
Redness
Ulcer
Thick, ridged nails

CHRONIC VENOUS INSUFFICIENCY
Brown pigment
Pitting edema
Ulcer

- ascites and generalized edema suggesting chronic right-sided heart failure
- localized swelling due to compressed veins
- lower leg swelling indicating right-sided heart failure.

Observe the vessels in the patient's neck. The carotid artery should appear as a brisk, localized pulsation. The internal jugular vein has a softer, undulating pulsation. The carotid pulsation doesn't decrease when the patient is upright, when he inhales, or when you palpate the carotid artery. The internal jugular pulsation, on the other hand, changes in response to position, breathing, and palpation.

EVALUATING JUGULAR VEIN DISTENTION

With the patient in a supine position, position him so that you can see his jugular vein with pulsations reflected from the right atrium.

● Elevate the head of the bed 45 to 50 degrees. (In the normal patient, veins distend only when the patient lies flat.)

● Locate the angle of Louis (sternal notch)—the reference point for measuring venous pressure. To do so, palpate the clavicles where they join the sternum (the suprasternal notch). Place your first two fingers on the suprasternal notch. Then, without lifting them from the skin, slide them down the sternum until you feel a bony protuberance—this is the angle of Louis.

● Find the internal jugular vein, which indicates venous pressure more reliably than the external jugular vein.

● Shine a penlight across the patient's neck to create shadows that highlight his venous pulse.

● Distinguish jugular vein pulsations from carotid artery pulsations. One way to do this is to palpate the vessel: Arterial pulsations continue, but venous pulsations disappear with light finger pressure. Also, venous pulsations increase or decrease with changes in body position; arterial pulsations remain constant.

● Locate the highest point along the vein where you can see pulsations.

● Using a centimeter ruler, measure the distance between the highest point and the sternal notch. Record this finding as well as the angle at which the patient was lying. A finding greater than 1¼″ to 1½″ (3 to 4 cm) above the sternal notch, with the head of the bed at a 45-degree angle, indicates jugular vein distention.

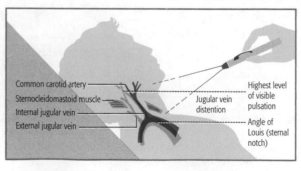

Common carotid artery
Sternocleidomastoid muscle
Internal jugular vein
External jugular vein
Jugular vein distention
Highest level of visible pulsation
Angle of Louis (sternal notch)

Check carotid artery pulsations. Are they weak or bounding? Inspect the jugular veins. Inspection of these vessels can provide information about blood volume and pressure in the right side of the heart.

To check jugular pulsation, have the patient lie on his back. Elevate the head of the bed 30 to 45 degrees, and turn the patient's head

EDEMA: PITTING OR NONPITTING?

To differentiate pitting from nonpitting edema, press your finger against a swollen area for 5 seconds, then quickly remove it.

With pitting edema, pressure forces fluid into the underlying tissues, causing an indentation that slowly fills. To determine the severity of pitting edema, estimate the indentation's depth in centimeters: 1+ (1 cm), 2+ (2 cm), 3+ (3 cm), or 4+ (4 cm).

With nonpitting edema, pressure leaves no indentation because fluid has coagulated in the tissues. Typically, the skin feels unusually tight and firm.

PITTING EDEMA (4+)	NONPITTING EDEMA
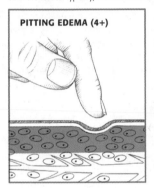	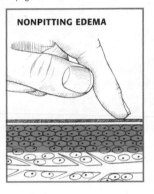

slightly away from you. Normally, the highest pulsation occurs no more than 1½″ (3.8 cm) above the sternal notch.

If the patient's pulsations appear higher, this indicates elevation in central venous pressure and jugular vein distention. Characterize this distention as mild, moderate, or severe. Determine the level of distention in fingerbreadths above the clavicle or in relation to the jaw or clavicle. Also note the amount of distention in relation to head elevation. (See *Evaluating jugular vein distention.*)

PALPATION

The first step in palpating the vascular system is to assess skin temperature, texture, and turgor. Then check capillary refill time by assessing the nail beds on the fingers and toes. Refill time should be no more than 3 seconds, or long enough to say "capillary refill."

Palpate the patient's arms and legs for temperature and edema. Edema is graded on a four-point scale. (See *Edema: Pitting or nonpitting?*)

Palpate for arterial pulses by gently pressing with the pads of your index and middle fingers. Start at the top of the patient's body at the temporal artery, and work your way down. Check the carotid, brachial, radial, femoral, popliteal, posterior tibial, and dorsalis pedis pulses. Palpate for the pulse on each side, comparing pulse volume and symmetry.

RED FLAG Don't palpate both carotid arteries at the same time or press too firmly. If you do, the patient may faint or become brady-cardic.

Put on gloves for the examination when you palpate the femoral arteries.

All pulses should be regular in rhythm and equal in strength. Pulses are graded on the following scale: 4+ is bounding, 3+ is in-creased, 2+ is normal, 1+ is weak, and 0 is absent. (See *Assessing arterial pulses.*)

A weak arterial pulse may indicate decreased cardiac output or increased peripheral vascular resistance, both of which point to arterial atherosclerotic disease.

Strong or bounding pulsations usually occur in a patient with a condition that causes increased cardiac output, such as hypertension, hypoxia, anemia, exercise, or anxiety. (See *Identifying pulse waveforms,* pages 56 and 57.)

AUSCULTATION

After you palpate, use the bell of the stethoscope to begin auscultating the vascular system; then follow the palpation sequence and listen over each artery. You shouldn't hear sounds over the carotid arteries. A hum, or bruit, sounds like buzzing or blowing and could indicate ar-teriosclerotic plaque formation.

Assess the upper abdomen for abnormal pulsations, which could indicate the presence of an abdominal aortic aneurysm. Finally, aus-cultate the femoral and popliteal pulses, checking for bruits or other abnormal sounds. (See *Locating abdominal auscultation points,* page 56.)

If you hear a bruit during arterial auscultation, the patient may have occlusive arterial disease or an arteriovenous fistula. Various high cardiac output conditions, such as anemia, hyperthyroidism, and pheochromocytoma, may also cause bruits.

ASSESSING ARTERIAL PULSES

To assess arterial pulses, apply pressure with your index and middle fingers. These illustrations show where to position your fingers when palpating for various arterial pulses.

Carotid pulse

Lightly place your fingers just medial to the trachea and below the jaw angle. Never palpate both carotid arteries at the same time.

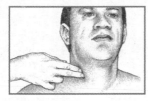

Brachial pulse

Position your fingers medial to the biceps tendon.

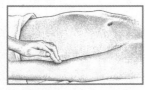

Radial pulse

Apply gentle pressure to the medial and ventral side of the wrist, just below the base of the thumb.

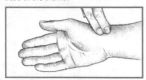

Femoral pulse

Press relatively hard at a point inferior to the inguinal ligament. For an obese patient, palpate in the crease of the groin, halfway between the pubic bone and the hip bone.

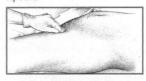

Popliteal pulse

Press firmly in the popliteal fossa at the back of the knee.

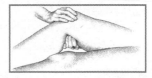

Posterior tibial pulse

Apply pressure behind and slightly below the malleolus of the ankle.

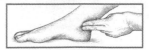

Dorsalis pedis pulse

Place your fingers on the medial dorsum of the foot while the patient points his toes down. (*Note:* The pulse is difficult to detect here and may be nonpalpable in healthy patients.)

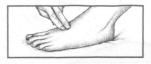

IDENTIFYING PULSE WAVEFORMS

To identify abnormal arterial pulses, check the waveforms below and see which one matches the patient's peripheral pulse.

Weak pulse

A weak pulse has decreased amplitude with a slower upstroke and downstroke. Possible causes of a weak pulse include increased peripheral vascular resistance (from cold weather or severe heart failure) and decreased stroke volume (from hypovolemia or aortic stenosis).

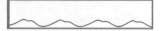

Bounding pulse

A bounding pulse has a sharp upstroke and downstroke with a pointed peak. The amplitude is elevated. Possible causes of a bounding pulse include increased stroke volume, as with aortic insufficiency; or stiffness of arterial walls, as with aging.

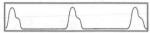

Pulsus alternans

Pulsus alternans has a regular, alternating pattern of a weak and a strong pulse. This pulse is associated with left-sided heart failure.

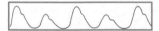

LOCATING ABDOMINAL AUSCULTATION POINTS

If the patient has hypertension, you may hear a bruit—a vascular sound similar to a heart murmur that's caused by turbulent blood flow through a narrowed artery. Occasionally, you may hear a bruit limited to systole in the epigastric region of a healthy person.

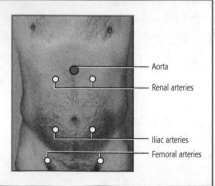

Aorta

Renal arteries

Iliac arteries

Femoral arteries

Pulsus bigeminus

Pulsus bigeminus is similar to alternating pulse but occurs at irregular intervals. This pulse is caused by premature atrial or ventricular beats.

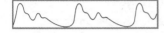

Pulsus paradoxus

Pulsus paradoxus has increases and decreases in amplitude associated with the respiratory cycle. Marked decreases occur when the patient inhales. Pulsus paradoxus is associated with pericardial tamponade, advanced heart failure, and constrictive pericarditis.

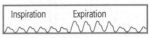

Inspiration   Expiration

Pulsus biferiens

Pulsus biferiens shows an initial upstroke, a subsequent downstroke, and then another upstroke during systole. Pulsus biferiens is caused by aortic stenosis and aortic insufficiency.

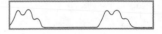

ABNORMAL FINDINGS

A patient's chief complaint may be due to any of the signs and symptoms related to the cardiovascular system. Common findings include:

- decreased or increased blood pressure
- bruits
- increased capillary refill time
- chest pain
- fatigue
- atrial or ventricular gallop
- intermittent claudication
- jugular vein distention
- palpitations
- absent or weak pulse
- peripheral edema.

The following history, physical assessment, and analysis summaries will help you interpret each finding quickly and accurately. (See *Interpreting your findings,* pages 58 to 66.)

(Text continues on page 67.)

INTERPRETING YOUR FINDINGS

After you assess the patient, a group of findings may lead you to a particular disorder of the cardiovascular system. This chart shows some common groups of findings for major signs and symptoms related to the cardiovascular assessment, along with their probable causes.

SIGN OR SYMPTOM AND FINDINGS	PROBABLE CAUSE
BLOOD PRESSURE, DECREASED	
● Orthostatic hypotension ● Fatigue ● Weakness ● Nausea, vomiting ● Abdominal discomfort ● Weight loss ● Fever ● Tachycardia ● Hyperpigmentation of fingers, nails, nipples, scars, and body folds	Adrenal insufficiency, acute
● Fall in systolic pressure to less than 80 mm Hg or to 30mm Hg less than baseline ● Tachycardia ● Narrowed pulse pressure ● Diminished Korotkoff sounds ● Peripheral cyanosis ● Pale, cool clammy skin ● Restlessness and anxiety	Cardiogenic shock

SIGN OR SYMPTOM AND FINDINGS	PROBABLE CAUSE
BLOOD PRESSURE, DECREASED *(continued)*	
● Fall in systolic pressure to less than 80 mm Hg or to 30mm Hg less than baseline ● Diminished Korotkoff sounds ● Narrowed pulse pressure ● Rapid, weak irregular pulse ● Cyanosis of extremities ● Pale, cool clammy skin	Hypovolemic shock
● Fever ● Chills ● Low blood pressure ● Tachycardia and tachypnea (early) ● Increasingly severe low blood pressure as condition progresses with narrowed pulse pressure	Septic shock

INTERPRETING YOUR FINDINGS *(continued)*

SIGN OR SYMPTOM AND FINDINGS	PROBABLE CAUSE	SIGN OR SYMPTOM AND FINDINGS	PROBABLE CAUSE
BLOOD PRESSURE, ELEVATED		**BRUITS**	
● Elevated diastolic pressure with orthostatic hypotension ● Constipation ● Muscle weakness ● Polyuria ● Polydipsia ● Personality changes	Aldosteronism, primary	● Pulsatile abdominal mass ● Systolic bruit over aorta ● Rigid tender abdomen ● Mottled skin ● Diminished peripheral pulses ● Claudication	Aortic aneurysm, abdominal
● Elevated pressure with widened pulse pressure ● Truncal obesity ● Moon face	Cushing's syndrome	● Systolic bruits over one or both carotid arteries ● Dizziness ● Vertigo ● Headache ● Syncope ● Aphasia ● Dysarthria ● Sudden vision loss ● Hemiparesis or hemiparalysis signaling transient ischemic attack	Carotid artery stenosis
● Elevated pressure; possibly produces no symptoms ● Suboccipital headache ● Light-headedness ● Tinnitus ● Fatigue	Hypertension		

(continued)

INTERPRETING YOUR FINDINGS *(continued)*

SIGN OR SYMPTOM AND FINDINGS	PROBABLE CAUSE
BRUITS *(continued)*	
● Bruits over femoral arteries and other arteries in the legs ● Diminished, absent femoral, popliteal, or pedal pulses ● Intermittent claudication ● Numbness, weakness, pain, and cramping in legs ● Cool, shiny skin and hair loss on affected extremity	Peripheral vascular disease
CAPILLARY REFILL TIME, INCREASED	
● Increased refill time with absent pulses distal to obstruction ● Affected limb cool and pale or cyanotic ● Intermittent claudication ● Moderate to severe pain, numbness, paresthesia, or paralysis of affected limb	Arterial occlusion, acute

SIGN OR SYMPTOM AND FINDINGS	PROBABLE CAUSE
CAPILLARY REFILL TIME, INCREASED *(continued)*	
● Increased refill time as a compensatory mechanism ● Shivering ● Fatigue ● Weakness ● Decreased level of consciousness ● Slurred speech ● Ataxia ● Muscle stiffness	Hypothermia
● Refill time prolonged in fingers ● Blanching of fingers followed by cyanosis, then erythema before fingers return to normal	Raynaud's disease
CHEST PAIN	
● A feeling of tightness or pressure in the chest described as pain or a sensation of indigestion or expansion	Angina

INTERPRETING YOUR FINDINGS *(continued)*

SIGN OR SYMPTOM AND FINDINGS	PROBABLE CAUSE	SIGN OR SYMPTOM AND FINDINGS	PROBABLE CAUSE
CHEST PAIN *(continued)*		**CHEST PAIN** *(continued)*	
● Pain may radiate to the neck, jaw, and arms, classically to the inner aspect of the left arm ● Pain begins gradually, reaches a maximum, then slowly subsides ● Pain is provoked by exertion, emotional stress, or a heavy meal ● Pain typically lasts 2 to 10 minutes (usually no more than 20 minutes) ● Dyspnea ● Nausea and vomiting ● Tachycardia ● Dizziness ● Diaphoresis	Angina	● Crushing substernal pain, unrelieved by rest or nitroglycerin ● Pain that may radiate to the left arm, jaw, neck, or shoulder blades ● Pain that lasts from 15 minutes to hours ● Pallor ● Clammy skin ● Dyspnea ● Diaphoresis ● Feeling of impending doom	Myocardial infarction
		● Sharp, severe pain aggravated by inspiration, coughing, or pressure ● Shallow, splinted breaths ● Dyspnea ● Cough ● Local tenderness and edema	Rib fracture
		FATIGUE	
		● Fatigue following mild activity ● Pallor ● Tachycardia ● Dyspnea	Anemia

(continued)

INTERPRETING YOUR FINDINGS *(continued)*

SIGN OR SYMPTOM AND FINDINGS	PROBABLE CAUSE	SIGN OR SYMPTOM AND FINDINGS	PROBABLE CAUSE
FATIGUE *(continued)*		**GALLOP, ATRIAL** *(continued)*	
● Persistent fatigue unrelated to exertion ● Headache ● Anorexia ● Constipation ● Sexual dysfunction ● Loss of concentration ● Irritability	Depression	● Atrial gallop accompanied by soft short diastolic murmur on left sternal border ● Possible soft, short midsystolic murmur ● Tachycardia ● Dyspnea ● Jugular vein distention ● Crackles ● Possible angina	Aortic insufficiency
● Progressive fatigue ● Cardiac murmur ● Exertional dyspnea ● Cough ● Hemoptysis	Valvular heart disease	● Atrial gallop occurring early in the onset of disease ● Possibly produces no symptoms ● Headache ● Weakness ● Dizziness ● Fatigue ● Epistaxis ● Tinnitus	Hypertension
GALLOP, ATRIAL			
● Intermittent gallop during attack, disappearing when attack is over ● Possible paradoxical S_2 or new murmur ● Chest tightness, pressure, or achiness that radiates	Angina		

INTERPRETING YOUR FINDINGS *(continued)*

SIGN OR SYMPTOM AND FINDINGS	PROBABLE CAUSE	SIGN OR SYMPTOM AND FINDINGS	PROBABLE CAUSE
GALLOP, VENTRICULAR		**GALLOP, VENTRICULAR** *(continued)*	
● S_3 with atrial gallop and soft short diastolic murmur over left sternal border ● S_2 possibly soft or absent ● Tachycardia ● Dyspnea ● Jugular vein distention ● Crackles	Aortic insufficiency	● Ventricular gallop with early or holosystolic decrescendo murmur at apex ● Atrial gallop ● Widely split S_2 ● Sinus tachycardia ● Tachypnea ● Orthopnea ● Crackles ● Fatigue ● Jugular vein distention	Mitral insufficiency
● Ventricular gallop accompanied by alternating pulse and altered S_1 and S_2 ● Fatigue ● Dyspnea ● Orthopnea ● Chest pain ● Palpitations ● Crackles ● Peripheral edema ● Atrial gallop	Cardiomyopathy	**INTERMITTENT CLAUDICATION**	
		● Pain in lower extremities along the femoral and popliteal arteries ● Diminished or absent popliteal and pedal pulses ● Coolness of affected limb; pallor on elevation ● Numbness, tingling, paresthesia ● Ulceration and possible gangrene	Arteriosclerosis obliterans

(continued)

INTERPRETING YOUR FINDINGS *(continued)*

SIGN OR SYMPTOM AND FINDINGS	PROBABLE CAUSE	SIGN OR SYMPTOM AND FINDINGS	PROBABLE CAUSE

INTERMITTENT CLAUDICATION *(continued)*

● Pain in the instep ● Erythema along extremity blood vessels ● Feet becoming cold, cyanotic, and numb on exposure to cold; then becoming reddened, hot, and tingling ● Impaired peripheral pulses	Buerger's disease

JUGULAR VEIN DISTENTION

● Distention with anxiety, restlessness ● Cyanosis ● Chest pain ● Dyspnea ● Hypotension ● Clammy skin ● Tachycardia ● Muffled heart sounds ● Pericardial friction rub ● Pulsus paradoxus	Cardiac tamponade

JUGULAR VEIN DISTENTION *(continued)*

● Sudden or gradual distention ● Weakness ● Anxiety ● Cyanosis ● Dependent edema of legs and sacrum ● Steady weight gain ● Confusion ● Hepatomegaly ● Nausea and vomiting ● Abdominal discomfort ● Anorexia	Heart failure
● Vein distention more prominent on inspiration ● Chest pain ● Fluid retention and dependent edema ● Hepatomegaly ● Ascites ● Pericardial friction rub	Pericarditis, chronic constrictive

INTERPRETING YOUR FINDINGS *(continued)*

SIGN OR SYMPTOM AND FINDINGS	PROBABLE CAUSE	SIGN OR SYMPTOM AND FINDINGS	PROBABLE CAUSE
PALPITATIONS		**PERIPHERAL EDEMA**	
● Paroxysmal palpitations ● Diaphoresis ● Facial flushing ● Trembling ● Impending sense of doom ● Hyperventilation ● Dizziness	Acute anxiety attack	● Headache ● Bilateral leg edema with pitting ankle edema ● Weight gain despite anorexia ● Nausea ● Chest tightness ● Hypotension ● Pallor ● Palpitations ● Inspiratory crackles	Heart failure
● Paroxysmal or sustained palpitations ● Dizziness ● Weakness ● Fatigue ● Irregular, rapid, or slow pulse rate ● Decreased blood pressure ● Confusion ● Diaphoresis	Arrhythmias	● Bilateral arm edema with facial and neck edema ● Edematous areas marked by dilated veins ● Headache ● Vertigo ● Vision disturbances	Superior vena cava syndrome
● Sustained palpitations ● Fatigue ● Irritability ● Hunger ● Cold sweats ● Tremors ● Anxiety	Hypoglycemia	● Moderate to severe, unilateral or bilateral leg edema ● Darkened skin ● Stasis ulcers around the ankle	Venous insufficiency

(continued)

INTERPRETING YOUR FINDINGS *(continued)*

SIGN OR SYMPTOM AND FINDINGS	PROBABLE CAUSE	SIGN OR SYMPTOM AND FINDINGS	PROBABLE CAUSE
PULSE, ABSENT OR WEAK		**PULSE, ABSENT OR WEAK** *(continued)*	
● Weak or absent pulse distal to affected area ● Sudden tearing pain in chest and neck radiating to upper and lower back and abdomen ● Syncope ● Loss of consciousness ● Weakness or transient paralysis of legs or arms ● Diastolic murmur ● Systemic hypotension ● Mottled skin below the waist	Aortic aneurysm, dissecting	● Absence of pulses distal to obstruction; usually unilaterally weak and then absent ● Cool, pale, cyanotic affected limb ● Increased capillary refill time ● Moderate to severe pain and paresthesia ● Line of color and temperature demarcating the level of obstruction	Arterial occlusion
		● Weakening and loss of peripheral pulses ● Aching pain distal to occlusion that worsens with exercise and abates with rest ● Cool skin with decreased hair growth ● Possible impotence in male	Peripheral vascular disease

Blood pressure, decreased

Normal blood pressure varies considerably; what qualifies as low blood pressure for one person may be perfectly normal for another. Consequently, every blood pressure reading must be compared against the patient's baseline. Typically, a reading below 90/60 mm Hg, or a drop of 30 mm Hg from the baseline, is considered low blood pressure, which could result in an inadequate intravascular pressure to maintain the oxygen requirements of the body's tissues.

HISTORY

If the patient is conscious, ask him about associated symptoms. For example, find out if he feels unusually weak or fatigued; if he has had nausea, vomiting, or dark or bloody stools; if his vision is blurred; or if his gait is unsteady. Ask him if he has palpitations or chest or abdominal pain or difficulty breathing. Then ask if he has had episodes of dizziness or fainting. Find out if these episodes occur when he stands up suddenly. If so, take the patient's blood pressure while he's lying down, sitting, and then standing; compare readings. A drop in systolic or diastolic pressure of 10 to 20 mm Hg or more and an increase in heart rate of more than 15 beats/minute between position changes suggest orthostatic hypotension.

PHYSICAL ASSESSMENT

Next, continue with a physical examination. Inspect the skin for pallor, sweating, and clamminess. Palpate peripheral pulses. Note paradoxical pulse, an accentuated fall in systolic pressure during inspiration, which suggests pericardial tamponade. Then auscultate for abnormal heart sounds, such as gallops and murmurs; heart rate, signaling bradycardia or tachycardia; and heart rhythm. Auscultate the lungs for abnormal breath sounds, such as diminished sounds, crackles, wheezing; breath rate, signaling bradypnea or tachypnea; and breath rhythm, such as agonal or Cheyne-Stokes respirations. Look for signs of hemorrhage, including:
- visible bleeding
- palpable masses
- bruising
- tenderness.

Assess the patient for abdominal rigidity and rebound tenderness; auscultate for abnormal bowel sounds. Carefully assess the patient for possible sources of infection such as open wounds.

ANALYSIS

Although commonly linked to shock, decreased blood pressure may also result from a cardiovascular, respiratory, neurologic, or metabolic disorder. Hypoperfusion states especially affect the kidneys, brain, and heart, and may lead to renal failure, change in level of consciousness (LOC), or myocardial ischemia. Low blood pressure may be drug-induced or may accompany diagnostic tests—typically those using contrast media. It may stem from stress or change of position—specifically, rising abruptly from a supine or sitting position to a standing position (orthostatic hypotension). Low blood pressure can reflect an expanded intravascular space, as in severe infections, allergic reactions, or adrenal insufficiency; reduced intravascular volume, as in dehydration and hemorrhage; or decreased cardiac output, as in impaired cardiac muscle contractility. Because the body's pressure-regulating mechanisms are complex and interrelated, a combination of these factors usually contributes to low blood pressure.

⬤ **AGE AWARE** In children, normal blood pressure is lower than blood pressure in adults. Because accidents occur frequently in children, suspect trauma or shock first as a possible cause of low blood pressure. Remember that low blood pressure typically doesn't accompany head injury in adults because intracranial hemorrhage is insufficient to cause hypovolemia. However, it does accompany head injury in infants and young children because their expandable cranial vaults allow significant blood loss into the cranial space, resulting in hypovolemia. Another common cause of low blood pressure in children is dehydration, which results from failure to thrive or from persistent diarrhea or vomiting occurring for as few as 24 hours.

In elderly patients, low blood pressure commonly results from the use of multiple drugs with hypotension as a potential adverse effect. Orthostatic hypotension due to autonomic dysfunction is another common cause.

Blood pressure, elevated

Elevated blood pressure—an intermittent or sustained increase in blood pressure exceeding 140/90 mm Hg—strikes more men than women and twice as many Blacks as Whites. By itself, this common sign is easily ignored by the patient because he can't see or feel it. However, its causes can be life-threatening.

Hypertension has been reported to be two to three times more common in women taking hormonal contraceptives than those not taking them. Women age 35 and older who smoke cigarettes should be strongly encouraged to stop. If they continue to smoke, they should be discouraged from using hormonal contraceptives.

HISTORY

If you detect sharply elevated blood pressure, act quickly to rule out possible life-threatening causes. After ruling out life-threatening causes, complete a more leisurely history and physical examination. Determine if the patient has a history of diabetes or cardiovascular, cerebrovascular, or renal disease. Ask about a family history of high blood pressure—a likely finding with essential hypertension, pheochromocytoma, and polycystic kidney disease. Then ask about its onset and if the high blood pressure appeared abruptly. Ask the patient's age. Sudden onset of high blood pressure in middle-aged or elderly patients suggests renovascular stenosis. Although essential hypertension may begin in childhood, it typically isn't diagnosed until near age 35.

Note headache, palpitations, blurred vision, and sweating. Ask about wine-colored urine and decreased urine output; these signs suggest glomerulonephritis, which can cause elevated blood pressure.

Obtain a drug history, including past and present prescriptions, herbal preparations, and over-the-counter drugs especially decongestants.

RED FLAG Ephedra (ma huang), ginseng, and licorice may cause high blood pressure or irregular heartbeat. St. John's wort can also raise blood pressure, especially when taken with substances that antagonize hypericin, such as amphetamines, cold and hay fever medications, nasal decongestants, pickled foods, beer, coffee, wine, and chocolate.

If the patient is already taking an antihypertensive, determine how well he complies with the regimen. Ask about his perception of the elevated blood pressure. Find out how serious he believes it is and if he expects drug therapy will help. Explore psychosocial or environmental factors that may impact blood pressure control.

PHYSICAL ASSESSMENT

Obtain vital signs and check for orthostatic hypotension. Take the patient's blood pressure with him laying down, sitting, and then standing. Normally, systolic pressure falls and diastolic pressure rises on standing. With orthostatic hypotension, both pressures fall.

Using a funduscope, check for intraocular hemorrhage, exudate, and papilledema, which characterize severe hypertension. Perform a thorough cardiovascular assessment. Check for carotid bruits and jugular vein distention. Assess skin color, temperature, and turgor. Palpate peripheral pulses. Auscultate for abnormal heart sounds, including gallops, louder S_2, and murmurs; heart rate, including bradycardia and tachycardia; and heart rhythm. Then auscultate for abnormal breath sounds, such as crackles and wheezing; abnormal respiratory rate, such as bradypnea and tachypnea; and breath rhythm.

Palpate the abdomen for tenderness, masses, and liver enlargement. Auscultate for abdominal bruits. Renal artery stenosis produces bruits over the upper abdomen or in the costovertebral angles. Easily palpable, enlarged kidneys and a large, tender liver suggest polycystic kidney disease. Obtain a urine sample to check for microscopic hematuria.

ANALYSIS

Elevated blood pressure may develop suddenly or gradually. A sudden, severe rise in pressure (exceeding 180/110 mm Hg) may indicate life-threatening hypertensive crisis. However, even a less dramatic rise may be equally significant if it heralds a dissecting aortic aneurysm, increased intracranial pressure, MI, eclampsia, or thyrotoxicosis.

Usually associated with essential hypertension, elevated blood pressure may also result from a renal or endocrine disorder, a drug's adverse effect, or a treatment that affects fluid status, such as dialysis. Ingestion of large amounts of certain foods, such as black licorice and cheddar cheese, may temporarily elevate blood pressure.

Sometimes elevated blood pressure may simply reflect inaccurate blood pressure measurement. However, careful measurement alone doesn't ensure a useful reading. To be useful, each blood pressure reading must be compared with the patient's baseline. Also, serial readings may be needed to establish elevated blood pressure.

The patient may experience elevated blood pressure in a health care provider's office (known as *"white-coat hypertension"*). In such cases, 24-hour blood pressure monitoring is indicated to confirm elevated readings in other settings. In addition, other risk factors for CAD, such as smoking and elevated cholesterol levels, need to be addressed.

AGE AWARE Normally, blood pressure in children is lower than it is in adults. In children, elevated blood pressure may result from lead or mercury poisoning, essential hypertension, renovascular stenosis, chronic pyelonephritis, coarctation of the aorta, patent ductus arteriosus, glomerulonephritis, adrenogenital syndrome, or neuroblastoma. In elderly patients, atherosclerosis commonly produces isolated systolic hypertension.

Bruits

Typically an indicator of life- or limb-threatening vascular disease, bruits are swishing sounds caused by turbulent blood flow. They're characterized by location, duration, intensity, pitch, and time of onset in the cardiac cycle. Loud bruits produce intense vibration and a palpable thrill. A thrill, however, doesn't provide any further clue to the causative disorder or to its severity.

HISTORY

If you detect a bruit, be sure to check for further vascular damage and perform a thorough cardiac assessment.

PHYSICAL ASSESSMENT

If you detect bruits over the abdominal aorta, check for a pulsating mass or a bluish discoloration around the umbilicus (Cullen's sign). Either of these signs—or severe, tearing pain in the abdomen, flank, or lower back—may signal life-threatening dissection of an aortic aneurysm. Also check peripheral pulses, comparing intensity in the arms versus the legs.

If you detect bruits over the thyroid gland, ask the patient if he has a history of hyperthyroidism or signs and symptoms, such as nervousness, tremors, weight loss, palpitations, heat intolerance, and (in women) amenorrhea.

RED FLAG Watch for signs and symptoms of life-threatening thyroid storm, such as tremors, restlessness, diarrhea, abdominal pain, and hepatomegaly.

If you detect carotid artery bruits, be alert for signs and symptoms of a transient ischemic attack, including dizziness, diplopia, slurred speech, flashing lights, and syncope. These findings may indicate impending stroke. Evaluate the patient frequently for changes in LOC and muscle function.

If you detect bruits over the femoral, popliteal, or subclavian artery, watch for signs and symptoms of decreased or absent peripheral circulation—edema, weakness, and paresthesia. Ask the patient if he has a history of intermittent claudication. Frequently check distal pulses and skin color and temperature. Also watch for the sudden absence of pulse, pallor, or coolness, which may indicate a threat to the affected limb.

ANALYSIS

Bruits are most significant when heard over the abdominal aorta; the renal, carotid, femoral, popliteal, or subclavian artery; or the thyroid gland. They're also significant when heard consistently despite changes in patient position and when heard during diastole.

AGE AWARE In young children, bruits are common but are usually of little significance—for example, cranial bruits are normal until age 4. However, certain bruits may be significant. Because birthmarks commonly accompany congenital arteriovenous fistulas, carefully auscultate for bruits in a child with port-wine spots or cavernous or diffuse hemangioma.

Elderly people with atherosclerosis may experience bruits over several arteries. Bruits related to carotid artery stenosis are particularly important because of the high incidence of associated stroke.

Capillary refill time, increased

Capillary refill time is the duration required for color to return to the nail bed of a finger or toe after application of slight pressure, which causes blanching. This duration reflects the quality of peripheral vasomotor function. Normal capillary refill time is less than 3 seconds.

Capillary refill time is typically tested during a routine cardiovascular assessment. It isn't tested with suspected life-threatening disorders because other, more characteristic signs and symptoms appear earlier.

HISTORY

Take a brief medical history, especially noting previous peripheral vascular disease. Find out which drugs the patient is taking.

PHYSICAL EXAMINATION

If you detect increased capillary refill time, take the patient's vital signs and check pulses in the affected limb. Does the limb feel cold or look cyanotic? Ask the patient about pain or any unusual sensations in his fingers or toes, especially after exposure to cold.

ANALYSIS

Increased refill time isn't diagnostic of any disorder but must be evaluated along with other signs and symptoms. However, this sign usually signals obstructive peripheral arterial disease or decreased cardiac output.

Chest pain

Chest pain can arise suddenly or gradually, and its cause may be difficult to ascertain initially. The pain can radiate to the arms, neck, jaw, or back. It can be steady or intermittent and mild or acute. It can range from a sharp shooting sensation to a feeling of heaviness, fullness, or even indigestion. It can be provoked or aggravated by stress, anxiety, exertion, deep breathing, or eating certain foods.

HISTORY

If the patient's chest pain isn't severe, proceed with the health history. Ask if the patient feels diffuse pain or can point to the painful area. Sometimes a patient won't perceive the sensation he's feeling as pain, so ask whether he has any discomfort radiating to the neck, jaw, arms, or back. If he does, ask him to describe it, such as a dull, aching, pressure-like sensation or a sharp, stabbing, knifelike pain. Find out if he feels it on the surface or deep inside.

Next, find out whether the pain is constant or intermittent. If it's intermittent, ask him how long it lasts. Ask if movement, exertion, breathing, position changes, or the eating of certain foods worsens or helps relieve the pain. Find out what in particular seems to bring on the pain.

Review the patient's history for cardiac or pulmonary disease, chest trauma, intestinal disease, or sickle cell anemia. Find out what medication he's taking, if any, and ask about recent dosage or schedule changes.

PHYSICAL ASSESSMENT

When taking the patient's vital signs, note the presence of tachycardia, paradoxical pulse, and hypertension or hypotension. Also look for jugular vein distention and peripheral edema. Observe the patient's breathing pattern, and inspect his chest for asymmetrical expansion. Auscultate his lungs for pleural friction rub, crackles, rhonchi, wheezing, and diminished or absent breath sounds. Next, auscultate for murmurs, clicks, gallops, and pericardial friction rubs. Palpate for lifts, heaves, thrills, gallops, tactile fremitus, and abdominal mass or tenderness.

ANALYSIS

Chest pain usually results from disorders that affect thoracic or abdominal organs, such as the heart, pleurae, lungs, esophagus, rib cage, gallbladder, pancreas, or stomach. An important indicator of several acute and life-threatening cardiopulmonary and GI disorders, chest pain can also result from musculoskeletal and hematologic disorders, anxiety, and drug therapy.

Keep in mind that cardiac-related pain may not always occur in the chest. Pain originating in the heart is transmitted through the thoracic region via the upper five thoracic spinal cord segments. Thus, it may be referred to areas served by the cervical or lower thoracic segments, such as the neck and arms. (See *Understanding chest pain,* pages 74 and 75.)

Fatigue

Fatigue is a feeling of excessive tiredness, lack of energy, or exhaustion, accompanied by a strong desire to rest or sleep. This common
(Text continues on page 76.)

UNDERSTANDING CHEST PAIN

This table outlines the different types of chest pain including location, exacerbating factors, causes, and alleviating measures. Use it to accurately assess your patients with chest pain.

DESCRIPTION	LOCATION
Aching, squeezing, pressure, heaviness, burning pain, tightness; usually subsides within 10 minutes	Substernal; may radiate to jaw, neck, arms, and back
Tightness or pressure; burning, aching pain; possible dyspnea, diaphoresis, weakness, anxiety, or nausea; sudden onset; lasts ½ to 2 hours	Substernal; may radiate to jaw, neck, arms, or back
Sharp and continuous; may be accompanied by friction rub; sudden onset; increased with inspiration	Substernal; may radiate to neck, arm, or back
Excruciating, tearing pain; may be accompanied by blood pressure difference between right and left arms; sudden onset	Retrosternal, upper abdominal, or epigastric; may radiate to back, neck, or shoulders
Sudden, stabbing pain, pressure, deep ache; may be accompanied by cyanosis, dyspnea, or cough with hemoptysis	Substernal; lateral chest; may radiate to neck or shoulders
Sudden and severe pain; possible dyspnea, increased pulse rate, decreased breath sounds, or deviated trachea	Lateral thorax; may radiate to back, shoulders, or arms
Dull, pressurelike, squeezing pain	Substernal, epigastric areas
Sharp, severe pain; usually occurs shortly after eating	Lower chest or upper abdomen
Burning feeling after eating; possible hematemesis or tarry stools; sudden onset that generally subsides within 15 to 20 minutes	Epigastric
Gripping, sharp pain; possible nausea and vomiting	Right epigastric or abdominal areas; possible radiation to shoulders
Continuous or intermittent sharp pain; possible tenderness to touch; gradual or sudden onset	Anywhere in chest
Dull or stabbing pain usually with hyperventilation or breathlessness; sudden onset; lasting less than 1 minute or as long as several days	Anywhere in chest

EXACERBATING FACTORS	CAUSES	ALLEVIATING MEASURES
Eating, physical effort, smoking, cold weather, stress, anger, hunger	Angina pectoris	Rest, nitroglycerin, oxygen (*Note:* Unstable angina appears even at rest.)
Exertion, anxiety	Acute myocardial infarction (MI)	Opioid analgesics such as morphine
Deep breathing; lying in a supine position	Pericarditis	Sitting up, leaning forward, anti-inflammatory drugs
Hypertension	Dissecting aortic aneurysm	Analgesics, surgery
Inspiration; venous status	Pulmonary embolus	Analgesics, high Fowler's position
Coughing	Pneumothorax	Analgesics, chest tube insertion
Food, cold liquids, exercise	Esophageal spasm	Nitroglycerin, calcium channel blockers
Eating a heavy meal, bending, lying down	Hiatal hernia	Antacids, walking, semi-Fowler's position
Lack of food or highly acidic foods	Peptic ulcer	Food, antacids
Eating fatty foods, lying down	Cholecystitis	Rest and analgesics, surgery
Movement, palpation	Chest-wall syndrome	Time, analgesics, heat applications
Increased respiratory rate, stress or anxiety	Acute anxiety	Slowing of respiratory rate, stress relief

symptom is distinct from weakness, which involves the muscles, but may occur with it.

HISTORY

Obtain a history to identify the patient's fatigue pattern. Ask about related symptoms and any recent viral illness or stressful changes in lifestyle.

Explore nutritional habits and appetite or weight changes. Carefully review the patient's medical and psychiatric history for chronic disorders that commonly produce fatigue. Ask about a family history of such disorders.

PHYSICAL ASSESSMENT

Observe the patient's general appearance for overt signs of depression or organic illness. Is he unkempt or expressionless? Does he appear tired or sickly, or have a slumped posture? If warranted, evaluate his mental status, noting especially mental clouding, attention deficits, agitation, or psychomotor retardation.

ANALYSIS

Fatigue that worsens with activity and improves with rest generally indicates a physical disorder; the opposite pattern, a psychological disorder. Fatigue lasting longer than 4 months, constant fatigue that's unrelieved by rest, and transient exhaustion that quickly gives way to bursts of energy are other findings associated with psychological disorders.

Fatigue is a normal and important response to physical overexertion, prolonged emotional stress, and sleep deprivation. However, it can also be a nonspecific symptom of a psychological or physiologic disorder, especially viral infection and endocrine, cardiovascular, or neurologic disease.

Fatigue reflects hypermetabolic and hypometabolic states in which nutrients needed for cellular energy and growth are lacking because of overly rapid depletion, impaired replacement mechanisms, insufficient hormone production, or inadequate nutrient intake or metabolism. Cardiac causes include heart failure, MI, and valvular heart disease.

AGE AWARE When evaluating a child for fatigue, ask his parents if they've noticed any change in his activity level. Fatigue without an organic cause occurs normally during accelerated growth phases in preschool age and prepubescent children. However, psychological causes of fatigue must be considered—for example, a depressed child may try to escape problems at home or school by taking refuge in sleep. In the pubescent child, consider the possibility of drug abuse, particularly of hypnotics and tranquilizers. Always ask elderly patients about fatigue because this symptom may be insidious and mask more serious underlying conditions in this age-group.

Gallop, atrial

An atrial or presystolic gallop is an extra heart sound (known as S_4) that's heard or often palpated immediately before S_1, late in diastole, as described in "Abnormal heart sounds," page 42.

HISTORY

When the patient's condition permits, ask about a history of hypertension, angina, valvular stenosis, or cardiomyopathy. If appropriate, have him describe the frequency and severity of anginal attacks.

PHYSICAL ASSESSMENT

Carefully auscultate the chest for S_4. Use the bell of the stethoscope. Note any murmurs or abnormalities in S_1 and S_2. Then listen for pulmonary crackles. Next, assess peripheral pulses, noting an alternating strong and weak pulse. Finally, palpate the liver to detect enlargement or tenderness, and assess for jugular vein distention and peripheral edema.

ANALYSIS

An atrial S_4 gallop typically results from hypertension, conduction defects, valvular disorders, or other problems such as ischemia. Occasionally, it helps differentiate angina from other causes of chest pain. It results from abnormal forceful atrial contraction caused by augmented ventricular filling or by decreased left ventricular compliance. An atrial gallop usually originates from left atrial contraction, is heard at the apex, and doesn't vary with inspiration. A left-sided S_4 can occur in hypertensive heart disease, coronary artery disease, aortic stenosis, and cardiomyopathy. It may also originate from right atrial contraction. A right-sided S_4 is indicative of pulmonary hypertension and pulmonary stenosis. If so, it's heard best at the lower left sternal border and intensifies with inspiration.

An atrial gallop seldom occurs in normal hearts; however, it may occur in athletes with physiologic hypertrophy of the left ventricle.

AGE AWARE In children, an atrial gallop may occur normally, especially after exercise. However, it may also result from congenital heart diseases, such as atrial septal defect, ventricular septal defect, patent ductus arteriosus, and severe pulmonary valvular stenosis.

Because the absolute intensity of an atrial gallop doesn't decrease with age, as it does with an S_1, the relative intensity of S_4 increases compared with S_1. This explains the increased frequency of an audible S_4 in elderly patients and why this sound may be considered a normal finding in older patients.

Gallop, ventricular

A ventricular gallop is a heart sound known as S_3, associated with rapid ventricular filling in early diastole. Usually palpable, this low-frequency sound occurs about 0.15 second after S_2. It may originate in either the left or right ventricle. A right-sided gallop usually sounds louder on inspiration and is heard best along the lower left sternal border or over the xiphoid region. A left-sided gallop usually sounds louder on expiration and is heard best at the apex.

HISTORY

Focus the history on the cardiovascular system. Begin the history by asking the patient if he has had any chest pain. If so, have him describe its character, location, frequency, duration, and any alleviating or aggravating factors. Also ask about palpitations, dizziness, or syncope. Find out if the patient has difficulty breathing after exertion, while lying down, or at rest. Ask the patient if he has a cough. Also ask about a history of cardiac disorders. Find out if the patient is currently receiving any treatment for heart failure. If so, find out which medications he's taking.

PHYSICAL ASSESSMENT

During the physical examination, carefully auscultate for murmurs or abnormalities in S_1 and S_2. Then listen for pulmonary crackles. Next, assess peripheral pulses, noting an alternating strong and weak pulse. Finally, palpate the liver to detect enlargement or tenderness, and assess for jugular vein distention and peripheral edema.

ANALYSIS

Ventricular gallops are easily overlooked because they're usually faint. Fortunately, certain techniques make their detection more likely. These include auscultating in a quiet environment; examining the patient in the supine, left lateral, and semi-Fowler's positions; and having the patient cough or raise his legs to augment the sound.

AGE AWARE A physiologic ventricular gallop normally occurs in children and adults younger than age 40; however, most people lose this S_3 by age 40. Ventricular gallop may also occur during the third trimester of pregnancy. Abnormal S_3 (in adults older than age 40) can be a sign of decreased myocardial contractility, myocardial failure, and volume overload of the ventricle, as in mitral and tricuspid valve regurgitation.

Although the physiologic S$_3$ has the same timing as the pathologic S$_3$, its intensity waxes and wanes with respiration. It's also heard more faintly if the patient is sitting or standing.

A pathologic ventricular gallop may be one of the earliest signs of ventricular failure. It may result from one of two mechanisms: rapid deceleration of blood entering a stiff, noncompliant ventricle, or rapid acceleration of blood associated with increased flow into the ventricle. A gallop that persists despite therapy indicates a poor prognosis.

Patients with cardiomyopathy or heart failure may develop both a ventricular gallop and an atrial gallop—a condition known as a *summation gallop.*

Intermittent claudication

Typically occurring in the legs, intermittent claudication is cramping limb pain brought on by exercise and relieved by 1 to 2 minutes of rest. This pain may be acute or chronic. Without treatment, it may progress to pain at rest.

HISTORY

If the patient has chronic intermittent claudication, gather history data first. Ask how far he can walk before pain occurs and how long he must rest before it subsides. Find out if he can walk less further now than before, or if he needs to rest longer. Next, ask if the pain-rest pattern varies and if this symptom has affected his lifestyle.

RED FLAG If the patient has sudden intermittent claudication with severe or aching leg pain at rest, check the leg's temperature and color and palpate femoral, popliteal, posterior tibial, and dorsalis pedis pulses. Ask about numbness and tingling. Suspect acute arterial occlusion if pulses are absent; if the leg feels cold and looks pale, cyanotic, or mottled; and if paresthesia and pain are present. Mark the area of pallor, cyanosis, or mottling, and reassess it frequently, noting an increase in the area.

Obtain a history of risk factors for atherosclerosis, such as smoking, diabetes, hypertension, and hyperlipidemia. Next, ask about associated signs and symptoms, such as paresthesia in the affected limb and visible changes in the color of the fingers (white to blue to pink) when he's smoking, exposed to cold, or under stress. If the patient is male, ask if he experiences impotence.

PHYSICAL ASSESSMENT

Focus the physical examination on the cardiovascular system. Palpate for femoral, popliteal, dorsalis pedis, and posterior tibial pulses. Note character, amplitude, and bilateral equality. Note diminished or absent popliteal and pedal pulses with the femoral pulse present.

Listen for bruits over the major arteries. Note color and temperature differences between his legs or compared with his arms; also note where on his leg the changes in temperature and color occur. Elevate the affected leg for 60 seconds; if it becomes pale or white, blood flow is severely decreased. When the leg hangs down, how long does it take for color to return? (30 seconds or longer indicates severe disease.) If possible, check the patient's deep tendon reflexes after exercise; note if they're diminished in his lower extremities.

Examine his feet, toes, and fingers for ulceration, and inspect his hands and lower legs for small, tender nodules and erythema along blood vessels. Note the quality of his nails and the amount of hair on his fingers and toes. Physical findings include pallor on elevation, rubor on dependency (especially the toes and soles), loss of hair on the toes, and diminished arterial pulses.

If the patient has arm pain, inspect his arms for a change in color (to white) on elevation. Next, palpate for changes in temperature, muscle wasting, and a pulsating mass in the subclavian area. Palpate and compare the radial, ulnar, brachial, axillary, and subclavian pulses to identify obstructed areas.

ANALYSIS

When acute, this pain may signal acute arterial occlusion. Intermittent claudication is most common in men ages 50 to 60 with a history of diabetes mellitus, hyperlipidemia, hypertension, or tobacco use. With chronic arterial occlusion, limb loss is uncommon because collateral circulation usually develops.

With occlusive artery disease, intermittent claudication results from an inadequate blood supply. Pain in the calf (the most common area) or foot indicates disease of the femoral or popliteal arteries; pain in the buttocks and upper thigh, disease of the aortoiliac arteries. During exercise, the pain typically results from the release of lactic acid due to anaerobic metabolism in the ischemic segment, secondary to obstruction. When exercise stops, the lactic acid clears and the pain subsides. Diminished femoral and distal pulses may indicate disease of the terminal aorta or iliac branches. Absent pedal and popliteal pulses with normal femoral pulses may suggest atherosclerotic disease of the femoral artery. Absent pedal pulses with normal femoral and popliteal pulses may indicate Buerger's disease.

Intermittent claudication may also have a neurologic cause: narrowing of the vertebral column at the level of the cauda equina. This condition creates pressure on the nerve roots to the lower extremities.

Walking stimulates circulation to the cauda equina, causing increased pressure on those nerves and resultant pain.

AGE AWARE In children, intermittent claudication rarely occurs. Although it sometimes develops in patients with coarctation of aorta, extensive compensatory collateral circulation typically prevents manifestation of this sign. Muscle cramps from exercise and growing pains may be mistaken for intermittent claudication in children.

Jugular vein distention

Jugular vein distention is the abnormal fullness and height of the pulse waves in the internal or external jugular veins. For a patient in a supine position with his head elevated 45 degrees, a pulse wave height greater than 1¼″ to 1½″ (3 to 4 cm) above the angle of Louis indicates distention.

HISTORY

If the patient isn't in severe distress, obtain a personal history. Find out if he has recently gained weight, has difficulty putting on his shoes, and if his ankles are swollen. Ask about chest pain, shortness of breath, paroxysmal nocturnal dyspnea, anorexia, nausea or vomiting, and a history of cancer or cardiac, pulmonary, hepatic, or renal disease. Obtain a drug history noting diuretic use and dosage. Find out if the patient is taking drugs as prescribed. Ask the patient about his regular diet patterns, noting a high sodium intake.

PHYSICAL ASSESSMENT

Next, perform a physical examination, beginning with vital signs. Tachycardia, tachypnea, and increased blood pressure indicate fluid overload that's stressing the heart. Inspect and palpate the patient's extremities and face for edema. Then weigh the patient and compare that weight to his baseline.

Auscultate his lungs for crackles and his heart for gallops, a pericardial friction rub, and muffled heart sounds. Inspect his abdomen for distention, and palpate and percuss for an enlarged liver. Finally, monitor urine output and note any decrease.

ANALYSIS

Engorged, distended veins reflect increased venous pressure in the right side of the heart, which in turn, indicates an increased central venous pressure. This common sign characteristically occurs in heart failure and other cardiovascular disorders, such as constrictive pericarditis, tricuspid stenosis, and obstruction of the superior vena cava.

AGE AWARE In most infants and toddlers, jugular vein distention is difficult (sometimes impossible) to evaluate because of their short, thick necks. Even in school-age children, measurement of jugular vein distention can be unreliable because the sternal angle may not be the same distance (2″ to 2¾″ [5 to 7 cm]) above the right atrium as it is in adults.

Palpitations

Defined as a conscious awareness of one's heartbeat, palpitations are usually felt over the precordium or in the throat or neck. The patient may describe them as pounding, jumping, turning, fluttering, or flopping, or as missing or skipping beats. Palpitations may be regular or irregular, fast or slow, paroxysmal or sustained.

HISTORY

If the patient isn't in distress, obtain a complete cardiac history. Ask about cardiovascular or pulmonary disorders, which may produce arrhythmias. Find out if the patient has a history of hypertension or hypoglycemia.

Obtain a drug history. Ask the patient if he has recently started digoxin (Lanoxin) therapy. In addition, ask about caffeine, tobacco, and alcohol consumption. Ask about associated symptoms, such as weakness, fatigue, and angina.

To help characterize the palpitations, ask the patient to simulate their rhythm by tapping his finger on a hard surface. An irregular "skipped beat" rhythm points to premature ventricular contractions, whereas an episodic racing rhythm that ends abruptly suggests paroxysmal atrial tachycardia.

PHYSICAL ASSESSMENT

If the patient isn't in distress, perform a complete physical assessment of the cardiovascular system. Auscultate for gallops, murmurs, and abnormal breath sounds.

ANALYSIS

Although frequently insignificant, palpitations are a common chief complaint that may result from a cardiac or metabolic disorder or from the adverse effects of certain drugs. Nonpathologic palpitations may occur with a newly implanted prosthetic valve because the valve's clicking sound heightens the patient's awareness of his heartbeat. Transient palpitations may accompany emotional stress, such as fright, anger, and anxiety, or physical stress, such as exercise and fever. They can also accompany the use of stimulants, such as tobacco and caffeine.

AGE AWARE In children, palpitations commonly result from fever and congenital heart defects, such as patent ductus arteriosus and septal defects. Because many children have difficulty describing this symptom, focus your attention on objective measurements, such as cardiac monitoring, physical examination, and laboratory test results.

Peripheral edema

The result of excess interstitial fluid in the arms or legs, peripheral edema may be unilateral or bilateral, slight or dramatic, or pitting or nonpitting.

HISTORY

Begin by asking how long the patient has had the edema and if it developed suddenly or gradually. Find out if the edema decreases if the patient elevates his arms or legs, if it's worse in the mornings, and if it gets progressively worse during the day.

Find out if the patient recently injured the affected extremities or had surgery or an illness that may have immobilized him. Ask about a history of cardiovascular disease. Find out what medication he's taking and which drugs he has taken in the past.

PHYSICAL ASSESSMENT

Begin the assessment by examining each extremity for pitting edema. In pitting edema, pressure forces fluid into the underlying tissues, causing an indentation that slowly fills. In nonpitting edema, pressure leaves no indentation in the skin, but the skin may feel unusually firm. Because edema may compromise arterial blood flow, palpate peripheral pulses to detect insufficiency. Observe the color of the extremity and look for unusual vein patterns. Then palpate for warmth, tenderness, and cords and gently squeeze the muscle against the bone to check for deep pain. Finally, note any skin thickening or ulceration in the edematous areas.

ANALYSIS

Peripheral edema signals a localized fluid imbalance between the vascular and interstitial spaces. It may result from trauma, a venous disorder, or a bone or cardiac disorder.

Cardiovascular causes of arm edema are superior vena cava syndrome, which leads to slowly progressing arm edema accompanied by facial and neck edema with dilated veins marking these edematous areas, and thrombophlebitis, which may cause arm edema, pain, and warmth.

Leg edema is an early sign of right-sided heart failure. It can also signal thrombophlebitis and chronic venous insufficiency.

AGE AWARE Uncommon in children, arm edema can result from trauma. Leg edema, also uncommon, can result from osteomyelitis, leg trauma or, rarely, heart failure.

Pulse, absent or weak

An absent or weak pulse may be generalized or affect only one extremity.

HISTORY

When time allows, obtain a complete cardiovascular history from the patient. Note any history of trauma, MI, heart failure, recent cardiac surgery, infection, venous problems, or allergy.

RED FLAG If you detect an absent or weak pulse, quickly palpate the remaining arterial pulses to distinguish between localized or generalized loss or weakness. Then quickly check other vital signs and evaluate cardiopulmonary status, obtain a brief history, and intervene accordingly.

PHYSICAL ASSESSMENT

Carefully check the rate, amplitude, and symmetry of all pulses. Note any confusion or restlessness, hypotension, and cool, pale clammy skin.

ANALYSIS

When generalized, absent or weak pulse is an important indicator of such life-threatening conditions as shock and arrhythmia. Localized loss or weakness of a pulse that's normally present and strong may indicate acute arterial occlusion, which could require emergency surgery. However, the pressure of palpation may temporarily diminish or obliterate superficial pulses, such as the posterior tibial or the dorsalis pedis. Thus, bilateral weakness or absence of these pulses doesn't necessarily indicate an underlying disorder.

AGE AWARE In infants and small children, radial, dorsalis pedis, and posterior tibial pulses aren't easily palpable, so be careful not to mistake these normally hard-to-find pulses for weak or absent pulses. Instead, palpate the brachial, popliteal, or femoral pulses to evaluate arterial circulation to the extremities. In children and young adults, weak or absent femoral and more distal pulses may indicate coarctation of the aorta.

Diagnostic tests and procedures

Advances in diagnostic testing allow for earlier and easier diagnosis and treatment of cardiovascular disorders. For example, in some patients, echocardiography, a noninvasive and risk-free test, can provide as much diagnostic information about valvular heart disease as cardiac catheterization, an invasive and high-risk test. Monitoring and testing also help guide and evaluate treatment and identify complications. Before the patient undergoes testing, explain the procedure in terms he can easily understand. Make sure an informed consent form is signed, if necessary. Because these diagnostic tests may cause anxiety, be sure to provide emotional support.

Cardiac tests range from a relatively simple test that analyzes the patient's blood for cardiac enzymes, proteins, and clotting time to very sophisticated imaging and radiographic tests that reveal a detailed image of the heart. Other cardiovascular tests include various forms of electrocardiography, ultrasound, and hemodynamic monitoring.

CARDIAC ENZYMES AND PROTEINS

Analyzing cardiac enzymes and proteins (markers) is an important step in diagnosing acute myocardial infarction (MI) and in evaluating other cardiac disorders. After an MI, damaged cardiac tissue releases significant amounts of enzymes and proteins into the blood. Specific blood tests help reveal the extent of cardiac damage and help monitor healing progress.

Creatine kinase and isoforms

Creatine kinase (CK) is present in heart muscle, skeletal muscle, and brain tissue. Its isoenzymes, CK-MB, is found specifically in the heart muscle. Elevated levels of CK-MB reliably indicate acute MI. Generally, CK-MB levels rise 4 to 8 hours after the onset of an acute MI, peak after 20 hours, and may remain elevated for up to 72 hours. (See *Cardiac enzyme and protein patterns.*) Normal CK levels are 55 to 170 units/L for men and 30 to 135 units/L for women. CK-MB levels are normally less than 5% for men and women.

NURSING CONSIDERATIONS

- Explain to the patient that the test will help confirm or rule out MI.
- Inform the patient that blood samples will be drawn at timed intervals.
- Muscle trauma caused by I.M. injections, cardioversion, or cardiopulmonary resuscitation can raise CK levels.
- Patients who are muscular may have significantly higher CK levels.
- Handle the collection tube gently to prevent hemolysis, and send the sample to the laboratory immediately after collection.
- If a hematoma develops at the venipuncture site, apply warm soaks to help ease discomfort.

Myoglobin

Myoglobin, which is normally found in skeletal and cardiac muscle, functions as an oxygen-bonding muscle protein. It's released into the bloodstream when ischemia, trauma, and inflammation of the muscle occur. Normal myoglobin values are 0 to 0.09 mcg/ml.

Rising myoglobin levels are one of the first markers of cardiac injury after an acute MI. Levels may rise within 2 hours, peak within 4 hours, and return to baseline by 24 hours. However, because skeletal muscle damage may also cause myoglobin levels to rise, other tests (such as CK-MB or troponin) may be required to determine myocardial injury.

NURSING CONSIDERATIONS

- I.M. injections, recent angina, or cardioversion can cause elevated myoglobin levels.
- Handle the collection tube gently to prevent hemolysis, and send the sample to the laboratory immediately after collection.
- If a hematoma develops at the venipuncture site, apply warm soaks to help ease discomfort.

Troponin I and troponin T

Troponin is a protein found in skeletal and cardiac muscles. Two isotypes of troponin, troponin I and troponin T, are found in the myocardium. When injury occurs to the myocardial tissue, these proteins are released into the bloodstream. Troponin T can also be found in

CARDIAC ENZYME AND PROTEIN PATTERNS

Because they're released by damaged tissue, serum proteins and isoenzymes (catalytic proteins that vary in concentration in specific organs) can help identify the compromised organ and assess the extent of damage. After acute myocardial infarction, cardiac enzymes and proteins rise and fall in a characteristic pattern, as shown in this graph.

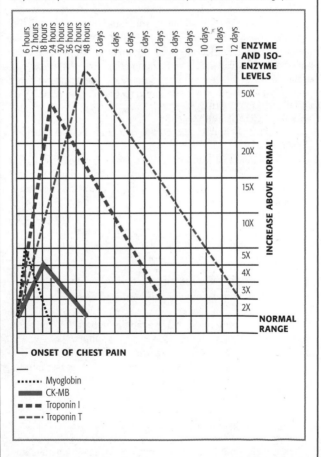

.... Myoglobin
━━━ CK-MB
■ ■ ■ Troponin I
– – – Troponin T

skeletal muscle. Troponin I, however, is found only in the myocardium. In fact, it's more specific to myocardial damage than CK, CK-MB isoenzymes, and myoglobin. Because troponin T levels can occur in certain muscle disorders or renal failure, they're less specific for myocardial injury than troponin I levels.

Normal troponin I levels are less than 0.35 mcg/L and normal troponin T levels are less than 0.1 mcg/L. Troponin I levels greater than 2 mcg/L suggest cardiac injury.

Troponin levels rise within 3 to 6 hours after myocardial damage. Troponin I peaks in 14 to 20 hours, with a return to baseline in 5 to 7 days, and troponin T peaks in 12 to 24 hours, with a return to baseline in 10 to 15 days. Because troponin levels stay elevated for a prolonged time, they can detect an infarction that occurred several days earlier. Troponin T levels can be determined at the bedside in minutes, making them a useful tool for determining treatment in acute MI.

NURSING CONSIDERATIONS

- Inform the patient that he need not restrict food or fluids before the test.
- Tell the patient that multiple blood samples may be drawn.
- Sustained vigorous exercise, cardiotoxic drugs such as doxorubicin, renal disease, and certain surgical procedures can cause elevated troponin T levels.
- Handle the collection tube gently to prevent hemolysis, and send the sample to the laboratory immediately after collection.
- If a hematoma develops at the venipuncture site, apply warm soaks to help ease discomfort.

Ischemia modified albumin

The ischemia modified albumin (IMA) test measures the changes in human serum albumin when it comes in contact with ischemic tissue. When ischemia occurs, IMA will rise rapidly. In over 80% of patients with acute coronary syndrome, IMA has been found to be elevated. However, IMA doesn't rise in tissue necrosis.

Normally, there's no IMA found in the blood. Increases in IMA are seen within 15 minutes of the onset of ischemia. This is significantly earlier than any other cardiac marker. When the ischemic event is resolved, IMA levels return to normal within several hours. The IMA test is used in conjunction with other cardiac markers, such as troponin, and an electrocardiogram (ECG). If the IMA test is negative and the troponin and ECG are negative, cardiac involvement is ruled out.

NURSING CONSIDERATIONS

- Inform the patient that he need not restrict food or fluids before the test.
- Tell the patient that other tests will be performed along with the IMA test.
- Handle the collection tube gently to prevent hemolysis, and send the sample to the laboratory immediately after collection.
- If a hematoma develops at the venipuncture site, apply warm soaks to help ease discomfort.

Homocysteine

Homocysteine is an amino acid that's produced by the body. High homocysteine levels can irritate blood vessels, leading to arteriosclerosis. High levels can also raise low-density lipoprotein levels and make blood clot more easily, increasing the risk of blood vessel blockages. In patients with type 2 diabetes, high homocysteine levels are seen when the patient has a decrease in renal function. Normal homocysteine levels are 4 to 17 μmol/L.

NURSING CONSIDERATIONS

- Perform a venipuncture; collect the sample in a 5-ml tube containing EDTA.
- Send the specimen to the laboratory immediately after collection in a plastic vial on ice.
- If a hematoma develops at the venipuncture site, apply warm soaks to help ease discomfort.

C-reactive protein

C-reactive protein (CRP) is a substance produced by the liver. A high CRP level indicates that inflammation exists at some location in the body. Other diagnostic tests are needed to determine the location of the inflammation and its cause. Elevated CRP levels can indicate such conditions as:

- MI
- angina
- systemic lupus erythematosus
- postoperative infection
- trauma
- heatstroke.

CRP appears in the blood 18 to 24 hours after the onset of tissue damage, and then declines rapidly when the inflammatory process regresses. Some studies have shown a correlation between increased CRP levels and coronary artery disease. Normally, CRP isn't present in the blood; however, levels less than 0.8 mg/dl may be reported as normal.

NURSING CONSIDERATIONS
- Have the patient withhold fluids, except water, for 8 hours before the test.
- Perform a venipuncture and collect the sample in a 5-ml nonanticoagulated tube.
- Handle the collection tube gently to prevent hemolysis, and send the sample to the laboratory immediately after collection.
- If a hematoma develops at the venipuncture site, apply warm soaks to help ease discomfort.

B-type natriuretic peptide

B-type natriuretic peptide (BNP) is a hormone polypeptide secreted by ventricular tissues in the heart. The substance is secreted as a response to the increased ventricular volume and pressure that occurs when a patient is in heart failure. It's an excellent hormonal marker of ventricular systolic and diastolic dysfunction.

The normal BNP level in the blood is less than 100 pg/ml. Blood concentrations greater than 100 pg/ml are an accurate predictor of heart failure. The level of BNP in the blood is relative to the severity of heart failure. The higher the level, the worse the symptoms of heart failure. (See *Linking BNP levels to heart failure symptom severity*.)

NURSING CONSIDERATIONS
- Perform a venipuncture, and collect the sample in a 5-ml tube containing EDTA.
- Handle the collection tube gently to prevent hemolysis, and send the sample to the laboratory immediately after collection.
- If a hematoma develops at the venipuncture site, apply warm soaks to help ease discomfort.

Atrial natriuretic peptide

Atrial natriuretic peptide (ANP) is a neurohormone similar to BNP that's released by the atria in response to increased atrial pressure. ANP helps:
- promote sodium excretion
- inhibit the renin-angiotensin system's effects on aldosterone secretion
- decrease venous return to the atria, thereby reducing blood pressure and volume.

LINKING BNP LEVELS TO HEART FAILURE SYMPTOM SEVERITY

This table shows the level of B-type natriuretic peptide (BNP) levels and the correlation with symptoms of heart failure. The higher the level of BNP, the more severe the symptoms.

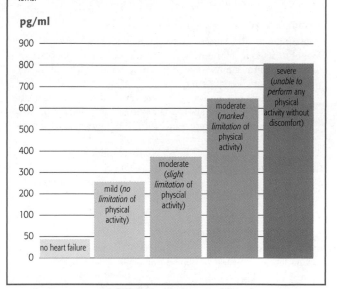

Normal levels of ANP are 20 to 77 pg/ml. A patient with overt heart failure will have highly elevated levels of ANP. A patient with cardiovascular disease and elevated cardiac filling pressure but no heart failure will also have increased ANP levels.

NURSING CONSIDERATIONS
- The patient must fast for 12 hours before the test.
- Withhold drugs that may interfere with the test, such as beta-adrenergic blockers, diuretics, vasodilators, and cardiac glycosides.
- Perform a venipuncture and collect the blood in a prechilled potassium-EDTA tube.
- Handle the collection tube gently to prevent hemolysis, and send the sample to the laboratory immediately after collection.

- If a hematoma develops at the venipuncture site, apply warm soaks to help ease discomfort.

LIPID STUDIES

Lipid studies include triglycerides, total cholesterol, and lipoprotein fractionation. They measure lipid levels in the body and help evaluate the risk of coronary artery disease.

Triglycerides

Triglycerides are the main storage form of lipids and constitute about 95% of fatty tissue. Monitoring triglyceride levels in the blood helps with early identification of hyperlipidemia and identification of patients at risk for coronary artery disease (CAD).

Triglyceride values are age- and gender-related, and some controversy exists over the most appropriate normal ranges. The most widely accepted normal values are 44 to 180 mg/dl for men and 10 to 190 mg/dl for women.

Triglyceride levels above or below these values suggest a clinical abnormality; for a definitive diagnosis, you'll need additional tests. For example, measuring cholesterol levels may also be necessary, because cholesterol and triglyceride levels vary independently. If both triglyceride and cholesterol levels are high, the patient is at risk for CAD.

NURSING CONSIDERATIONS

- Because triglycerides are highly affected by a fat-containing meal, with levels rising and peaking 4 hours after ingesting a meal, tell the patient that he should abstain from food for 10 to 14 hours before the test and from alcohol for 24 hours before the test. The patient may drink water.
- Perform a venipuncture, collect a sample in a 7-ml tube containing EDTA, and send the sample to the laboratory immediately after collection.
- Avoid prolonged venous occlusion. Remove the tourniquet within 1 minute of application.

Total cholesterol

The total serum cholesterol test measures the circulating levels of the two forms in which cholesterol appears in the body—free cholesterol and cholesterol esters.

For adults, desirable cholesterol levels are less than 200 mg/dl. Levels are considered borderline high up to 240 mg/dl, and high if they're greater than 240 mg/dl. High serum cholesterol levels may be associated with an increased risk for CAD.

NURSING CONSIDERATIONS

- Fasting isn't needed for isolated cholesterol checks or screening, but fasting is required if total cholesterol is part of a lipid profile. If fasting is required, instruct the patient to abstain from food and drink for 12 hours before the test.
- Perform a venipuncture, and collect the sample in a 7-ml tube containing EDTA. The patient should be in a sitting position for 5 minutes before the blood is drawn. Fingersticks can also be used for initial screening when using an automated analyzer.
- Document the drugs the patient is taking.
- Handle the collection tube gently to prevent hemolysis, and send the sample to the laboratory immediately after collection.
- If a hematoma develops at the venipuncture site, apply warm soaks to help ease discomfort.

Lipoprotein fractionation

Lipoprotein fractionation tests are used to isolate and measure the two types of cholesterol in blood: high-density lipoproteins (HDLs) and low-density lipoproteins (LDLs).

The HDL level is inversely related to the risk of CAD—that is, the higher the HDL level, the lower the incidence of CAD. For men, HDL values range from 37 to 70 mg/dl; in women, from 40 to 85 mg/dl.

Conversely, the higher the LDL level, the higher the incidence of CAD. In individuals who don't have CAD, desirable LDL levels are less than 130 mg/dl, borderline high levels are in the range of 130 to 159 mg/dl, and high levels are more than 160 mg/dl.

The American College of Cardiology recommends:

- HDL levels of 40 mg/dl or higher for men
- HDL levels of at least 45 mg/dl for women. (HDL levels greater than 60 mg/dl are considered heart healthy for all.)
- LDL levels of less than 100 mg/dl (Levels of 60 mg/dl or more are considered high.)

Increased HDL levels can occur as a result of long-term aerobic and vigorous exercise. Rarely, a sharp rise (to as high as 100 mg/dl) in a second type of HDL (alpha$_2$-HDL) may signal CAD. (See *Predicting CAD with the PLAC test,* page 94.)

NURSING CONSIDERATIONS

- Tell the patient to maintain a normal diet for 2 weeks before the test.

PREDICTING CAD WITH THE PLAC TEST

The PLAC test, a blood test that can help determine who might be at risk for coronary artery disease (CAD), has been approved by the Food and Drug Administration (FDA). The FDA's decision was based on a study of more than 1,300 patients, which was a part of a large multicenter study sponsored by the National Heart, Lung, and Blood Institute.

The PLAC test works by measuring lipoprotein-associated phospholipase A2, an enzyme produced by macrophages, a type of white blood cell. When heart disease is present, macrophages increase production of the enzyme. According to the FDA, an elevated PLAC test result, in conjunction with a low-density-lipoprotein (LDL) cholesterol level of less than 130 mg/dl, generally indicates that a patient has two to three times the risk of coronary heart disease compared to similar patients with lower PLAC test results. The study also found that those people with the highest PLAC test results and LDL cholesterol levels lower than 130mg/dL had the greatest risk of heart disease.

- Tell him to abstain from alcohol for 24 hours before the test.
- Tell the patient to stop the use of thyroid hormone, hormonal contraceptives, and antilipemics until after the test because they alter results.
- Perform a venipuncture, and collect the sample in a 7-ml tube containing EDTA.
- Send the sample to the laboratory immediately after collection to avoid spontaneous redistributions among the lipoproteins. If the sample can't be transported immediately, refrigerate it but don't allow it to freeze.
- If a hematoma develops at the venipuncture site, apply warm soaks to help ease discomfort.

COAGULATION TESTS

Partial thromboplastin time, prothrombin time, international normalized ratio, and activated clotting time are tests that measure clotting time. They're used to measure response to treatment and to screen for clotting disorders.

Partial thromboplastin time

The partial thromboplastin time (PTT) test evaluates all of the clotting factors of the intrinsic pathway except platelets. The test measures the time it takes a clot to form after adding calcium and phospholipid emulsion to a plasma sample. Normally a clot forms 21 to 35 seconds after the reagents are added.

The PTT test also helps monitor a patient's response to heparin therapy. For a patient on anticoagulant therapy, check with the practitioner to find out what PTT results to expect.

NURSING CONSIDERATIONS

- Tell the patient receiving heparin therapy that this test may be repeated at regular intervals to assess response to treatment.
- Perform a venipuncture, and collect the sample in a 7-ml tube containing sodium citrate.
- Completely fill the collection tube, invert it gently several times, and send it to the laboratory on ice.
- For a patient on anticoagulant therapy, additional pressure may be needed at the venipuncture site to control bleeding.

Prothrombin time

Prothrombin, or factor II, is a plasma protein produced by the liver. The prothrombin time (PT) test (also known as *pro time*) measures the time required for a clot to form in a citrated plasma sample after the addition of calcium ions and tissue thromboplastin (factor III).

The PT test is an excellent screening procedure for overall evaluation of extrinsic coagulation factors V, VII, and X and of prothrombin and fibrinogen. It's also the test of choice for monitoring oral anticoagulant therapy.

Normally PT ranges from 10 to 14 seconds. In a patient receiving warfarin therapy, the goal of treatment is to attain a PT level 1 to 2.5 times the normal control value.

NURSING CONSIDERATIONS

- Check the patient's history for use of drugs that may affect test results, such as vitamin K or antibiotics.
- Perform a venipuncture, and collect the sample in a 7-ml siliconized tube.
- Completely fill the collection tube, and invert it gently several times to adequately mix the sample and anticoagulant. If the tube isn't filled to the correct volume, an excess of citrate appears in the sample.

International normalized ratio

The international normalized ratio (INR) system is viewed as the best means of standardizing measurement of prothrombin time to monitor

oral anticoagulant therapy. It isn't used as a screening test for coagu-
lopathies.

A normal INR in patients receiving warfarin therapy is 2.0 to 3.0.
For patients with mechanical prosthetic heart valves, an INR of 2.5 to
3.5 is suggested. Increased INR values may indicate disseminated intravascular coagulation, cirrhosis, hepatitis, vitamin K deficiency, salicylate intoxication, uncontrolled oral anticoagulation, or massive
blood transfusion.

NURSING CONSIDERATIONS

- Tell the patient that the test may be repeated at regular intervals
  until he reaches his target INR level.
- Perform a venipuncture and collect the sample in a tube with sodium citrate added.
- Completely fill the collection tube, and invert it gently several
  times to adequately mix the sample and anticoagulant. If the tube
  isn't filled to the correct volume, an excess of citrate appears in the
  sample.
- Place the sample on ice and send it to the laboratory immediately
  after collection.

Activated clotting time

Activated clotting time, or automated coagulation time, measures the
time it takes whole blood to clot.

This test is commonly performed during procedures that require
extracorporeal circulation, such as:
- cardiopulmonary bypass
- ultrafiltration
- hemodialysis
- extracorporeal membrane oxygenation (ECMO).

In a nonanticoagulated patient, the normal activated clotting time
is 107 seconds. During cardiopulmonary bypass, heparin is titrated to
maintain an activated clotting time between 400 and 600 seconds.
During ECMO, heparin is titrated to maintain the activated clotting
time between 220 and 260 seconds.

NURSING CONSIDERATIONS

- Explain to the patient that the test requires a blood sample that's
  usually drawn from an existing vascular access site; therefore, no
  venipuncture is necessary.
- Explain that two samples will be drawn. The first one will be dis-
  carded so that heparin in the tubing doesn't interfere with the results.

- If the sample is drawn from a line with a continuous infusion, stop the infusion before drawing the sample.
- Withdraw 5 to 10 ml of blood from the line and discard it.
- Withdraw a clean sample of blood into the special tube containing the celite provided with the activated clotting time unit.
- Turn on the activated clotting time unit, and wait for the signal to insert the tube.
- Flush the vacular access site according to your facility's protocol.

ELECTROCARDIOGRAPHY

The heart's electrical conduction system can be recorded by using a number of different tests. The most common tests used are a 12-lead electrocardiogram, continuous cardiac monitoring, exercise electrocardiography, Holter monitoring, and signal-averaged electrocardiography.

12-lead electrocardiogram

The 12-lead electrocardiogram (ECG) measures the heart's electrical activity and records it as waveforms. It's one of the most valuable and commonly used diagnostic tools.

The standard 12-lead ECG uses a series of electrodes placed on the patient's extremities and chest wall to assess the heart from 12 different views (leads). The 12 leads include:

- three bipolar limb leads (I, II, and III)
- three unipolar augmented limb leads (aV_R, aV_L, and aV_F)
- six unipolar precordial leads (V_1 to V_6).

The limb leads and augmented leads show the heart from the frontal plane. The precordial leads show the heart from the horizontal plane. (See *Understanding ECG leads,* page 98.)

ECG can be used to identify myocardial ischemia and infarction, rhythm and conduction disturbances, chamber enlargement, electrolyte imbalances, and drug toxicity.

NURSING CONSIDERATIONS

- Use a systematic approach to interpret the ECG recording. (See *Visualizing normal ECG waveforms,* pages 99 and 100.) Compare the patient's previous ECG with the current one, if available. This will help you identify changes.
- P waves should be upright; however they may be inverted in lead aV_R or biphasic or inverted in leads III, aV_L, and V_1.

UNDERSTANDING ECG LEADS

Each of the leads on a 12-lead ECG views the heart from a different angle. These illustrations show the direction of electrical activity (depolarization) monitored by each lead and the 12 views of the heart.

VIEWS REFLECTED ON A 12-LEAD ECG	LEAD	VIEW OF THE HEART
	STANDARD LIMB LEADS (BIPOLAR)	
	I	lateral wall
	II	inferior wall
	III	inferior wall
	AUGMENTED LIMB LEADS (UNIPOLAR)	
	aV_R	no specific view
	aV_L	lateral wall
	aV_F	inferior wall
	PRECORDIAL, OR CHEST, LEADS (UNIPOLAR)	
	V_1	septal wall
	V_2	septal wall
	V_3	anterior wall
	V_4	anterior wall
	V_5	lateral wall
	V_6	lateral wall

- PR intervals should always be constant, like QRS-complex durations.
- QRS-complex deflections vary in different leads.
- ST segments should be isoelectric or have minimal deviation.
- ST-segment elevation greater than 1 mm above the baseline and ST-segment depression greater than 0.5 mm below the baseline are considered abnormal. Leads facing toward an injured area have

VISUALIZING NORMAL ECG WAVEFORMS

Each of the 12 standard leads of an electrocardiogram (ECG) takes a different view of heart activity, and each generates its own characteristic tracing. The tracings shown here represent a normal heart rhythm viewed from each of the 12 leads. Keep in mind:

● An upward (positive) deflection indicates that the wave of depolarization flows toward the positive electrode.

● A downward (negative) deflection indicates that the wave of depolarization flows away from the positive electrode.

● An equally positive and negative (biphasic) deflection indicates that the wave of depolarization flows perpendicularly to the positive electrode.

Each lead represents a picture of a different anatomic area; when you find abnormal tracings, compare information from the different leads to pinpoint areas of cardiac damage.

LEAD I

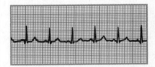

LEAD II

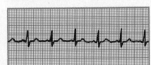

LEAD III

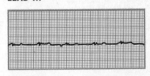

LEAD aV$_R$

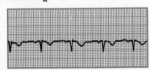

LEAD aV$_L$

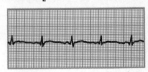

LEAD aV$_F$

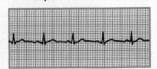

LEAD V$_1$

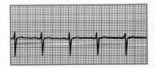

LEAD V$_2$

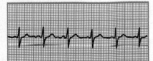

(continued)

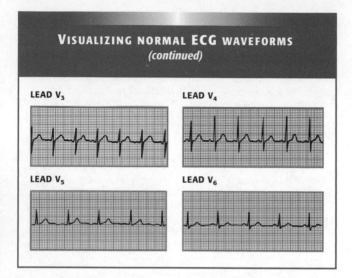

VISUALIZING NORMAL ECG WAVEFORMS
(continued)

LEAD V₃

LEAD V₄

LEAD V₅

LEAD V₆

ST-segment elevations, and leads facing away show ST-segment depressions.

- The T wave normally deflects upward in leads I, II, and V_3 through V_6. It's inverted in lead aV_R and variable in the other leads. T-wave changes have many causes and aren't always a reason for alarm. Excessively tall, flat, or inverted T waves occurring with such symptoms as chest pain may indicate ischemia.

- A normal Q wave generally has a duration of less than 0.04 second. An abnormal Q wave has a duration of 0.04 second or more, a depth greater than 4 mm, or a height one-fourth of the R wave. Abnormal Q waves indicate myocardial necrosis, developing when depolarization can't follow its normal path because of damaged tissue in the area.

- Remember that aV_R normally has a large Q wave, so disregard this lead when searching for abnormal Q waves.

- The R wave in lead II should be taller than in lead I. The R wave in lead III should be a smaller version of the R wave in lead I. Normally, the R waves get progressively taller from lead V_1 to V_5 and get slightly smaller in lead V_6. (See *R-wave progression*.)

Continuous cardiac monitoring

Because it allows continuous observation of the heart's electrical activity, cardiac monitoring is used in patients at risk for life-threatening ar-

R-WAVE PROGRESSION

R waves should progress normally through the precordial leads. Note that the R wave shown here is the first positive deflection in the QRS complex. Also note that the S wave gets smaller, or regresses, from lead V_1 to V_6 until it finally disappears.

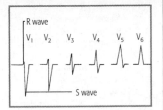

rhythmias. Like other forms of electrocardiography, cardiac monitoring uses electrodes placed on the patient's chest to transmit electrical signals that are converted into a cardiac rhythm tracing on an oscilloscope. (See *Positioning monitor leads,* pages 102 and 103.)

Two types of monitoring may be performed: *hardwire* or *telemetry*. In hardwire monitoring, the patient is connected to a monitor at the bedside. The rhythm display appears at the bedside, or it may be transmitted to a console at a remote location. Telemetry uses a small transmitter connected to the ambulatory patient to send electrical signals to another location, where they're displayed on a monitor screen. Regardless of the type, cardiac monitors can display the patient's heart rate and rhythm, produce a printed record of cardiac rhythm, and sound an alarm if the heart rate exceeds or falls below specified limits. Monitors also recognize and count abnormal heartbeats as well as changes. (See *Identifying cardiac monitor problems,* page 104.)

NURSING CONSIDERATIONS

- Make sure that all electrical equipment and outlets are grounded to avoid electrical shock and interference (artifacts). Also ensure that the patient is clean and dry to prevent electric shock.
- If the patient's skin is very oily, scaly, or diaphoretic, rub the electrode site with a dry 4″ × 4″ gauze pad before applying the electrode, to help reduce interference in the tracing.
- Assess skin integrity and reposition the electrodes every 24 hours or as necessary.
- Document a rhythm strip at least every 8 hours and with any change in the patient's condition (or as stated by your facility's policy).

POSITIONING MONITOR LEADS

This chart shows the correct electrode positions for some of the leads you'll use most often—the five-leadwire, three-leadwire, and telemetry systems. The chart uses the abbreviations RA for the right arm, LA for the left arm, RL for the right leg, LL for the left leg, C for the chest, and G for the ground.

Electrode positions

In the three- and five-leadwire systems, electrode positions for one lead may be identical to those for another lead. When that happens, change the lead selector switch to the setting that corresponds to the lead you want. In some cases, you'll need to reposition the electrodes.

Telemetry

In a telemetry monitoring system, you can create the same leads as the other systems with just two electrodes and a ground wire.

FIVE-LEADWIRE SYSTEM	THREE-LEADWIRE SYSTEM	TELEMETRY SYSTEM

LEAD I

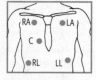 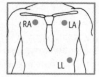

LEAD II

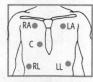 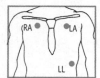 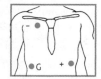

LEAD III

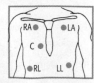 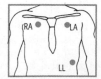 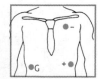

POSITIONING MONITOR LEADS *(continued)*

FIVE-LEADWIRE SYSTEM	THREE-LEADWIRE SYSTEM	TELEMETRY SYSTEM

LEAD MCL₁

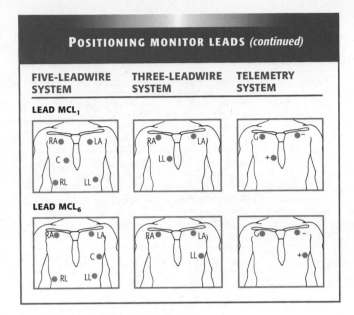

LEAD MCL₆

Exercise electrocardiography

Exercise electrocardiography is a noninvasive test that helps the practitioner assess cardiovascular response to an increased workload. Commonly known as a *stress test,* it provides diagnostic information that can't be obtained from a resting electrocardiogram (ECG). This test may also assess response to treatment.

An ECG and blood pressure readings are taken while the patient walks on a treadmill or pedals a stationary bicycle, and his response to a constant or increasing workload is observed. Unless complications develop, the test continues until the patient reaches the target heart rate (determined by an established protocol) or experiences chest pain or fatigue.

Stop the test if the patient experiences chest pain, fatigue, or other signs and symptoms that reflect exercise intolerance. These may include:
- severe dyspnea
- claudication
- weakness
- dizziness
- hypotension

IDENTIFYING CARDIAC MONITOR PROBLEMS

PROBLEM	POSSIBLE CAUSES	SOLUTIONS
FALSE–HIGH-RATE ALARM	● Monitor interpreting large T waves as QRS complexes, which doubles the rate	● Reposition electrodes to lead where QRS complexes are taller than T waves.
	● Skeletal muscle activity	● Place electrodes away from major muscle masses.
FALSE–LOW-RATE ALARM	● Shift in electrical axis from patient movement, making QRS complexes too small to register	● Reapply electrodes. Set gain so height of complex is greater than 1 mV.
	● Low amplitude of QRS	● Increase gain.
	● Poor contact between electrode and skin	● Reapply electrodes.
ARTIFACT (WAVEFORM INTERFERENCE)	● Patient having seizures, chills, or anxiety	● Notify the practitioner and treat the patient as indicated. Keep the patient warm and reassure him.
	● Patient movement	● Help the patient relax.
	● Electrodes applied improperly	● Check electrodes and reapply, if necessary.
	● Static electricity	● Make sure cables don't have exposed connectors. Change static-causing bedclothes.
	● Electrical short circuit in leadwires or cable	● Replace broken equipment. Use stress loops when applying leadwires.
	● Interference from decreased room humidity	● Regulate humidity to 40%.

- pallor
- vasoconstriction
- disorientation
- ataxia
- ischemic ECG changes (with or without pain)
- rhythm disturbances
- heart block
- ventricular conduction abnormalities.

Because exercise electrocardiography places considerable stress on the heart, it may be contraindicated in the patient with ventricular aneurysm, dissecting aortic aneurysm, uncontrolled arrhythmias, pericarditis, myocarditis, severe anemia, uncontrolled hypertension, unstable angina, or heart failure.

If the patient can't perform physical exercise, a stress test can be performed by I.V. injection of a coronary vasodilator, such as dipyridamole or adenosine. Other methods of stressing the heart include dobutamine administration and pacing (in the patient with a pacemaker).

In normal exercise electrocardiography, the P and T waves, the QRS complex, and the ST segment change minimally; a slight ST-segment depression occurs in some cases, especially in women. The heart rate rises in direct proportion to the workload and metabolic oxygen demand; blood pressure also rises as workload increases. The patient should attain the endurance level predicted by his age and appropriate exercise protocol.

NURSING CONSIDERATIONS

- Tell the patient not to eat, drink caffeinated beverages, or smoke cigarettes for 4 hours before the test.
- Explain that he should wear loose, lightweight clothing and snug-fitting, but comfortable shoes, and emphasize that he should immediately report any chest pain, leg discomfort, breathlessness, or fatigue.
- Check with the practitioner to determine which cardiac drugs should be given or withheld before the test. A beta-adrenergic receptor/blocker, for example, can limit the patient's ability to raise his heart rate.
- Inform the patient that he may receive an injection of thallium during the test so that the physician can evaluate coronary blood flow. Reassure him that the injection involves negligible radiation exposure.

- Tell the patient that, after the test, his blood pressure and ECG will be monitored for 10 to 15 minutes.
- Explain that he should wait at least 2 hours before showering and that he should then use warm water.

Signal-averaged electrocardiography

Although a standard 12-lead electrocardiogram (ECG) is obtained on most patients, some may benefit from obtaining a signal-averaged ECG. This simple, noninvasive test helps identify patients at risk for sudden death from sustained ventricular tachycardia.

The test uses a computer to identify late electrical potentials, which are tiny impulses that follow normal depolarization. A standard 12-lead ECG doesn't detect late electrical potentials. Patients who are prone to ventricular tachycardia, or who have had a recent myocardial infarction or unexplained syncope, are good candidates for signal-averaged electrocardiography.

A signal-averaged ECG is a noise-free, surface ECG recording taken from three specialized leads for several hundred heartbeats. (See *Placing electrodes for a signal-averaged ECG.*) The machine's computer detects late electrical potentials and then enlarges them so they're recognizable.

NURSING CONSIDERATIONS

- The test is performed by a technician who's specially trained to operate the recording and computer equipment used in analyzing the signal-averaged ECG.
- Tell the patient to lie as still as possible to avoid distorting the signal.
- Although the predictive accuracy of a positive signal-averaged ECG is relatively low, it's advocated as a screening test for the patient who should undergo electrophysiologic testing.

Holter monitoring

Also called *ambulatory electrocardiography,* Holter monitoring allows recording of heart activity as the patient follows his normal routine. Like an exercise electrocardiography, it can provide considerable more diagnostic information than a standard resting electrocardiogram. In addition, Holter monitoring can record intermittent arrhythmias.

This test usually lasts about 24 hours (about 100,000 cardiac cycles). The patient wears a small tape recorder connected to bipolar electrodes placed on his chest and keeps a diary of his activities and associated symptoms.

PLACING ELECTRODES FOR A SIGNAL-AVERAGED ECG

Positioning electrodes for a signal-averaged ECG is much different than for a 12-lead ECG. Here's one method:

1. Place the positive X electrode at the left fourth intercostal space, midaxillary line.

2. Place the negative X electrode at the right fourth intercostal space, midaxillary line.

3. Place the positive Y electrode at the left iliac crest.

4. Place the negative Y electrode at the superior aspect of the manubrium of the sternum.

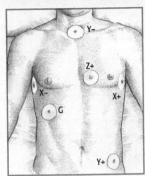

5. Place the positive Z electrode at the fourth intercostal space, left of the sternum.

6. Place the ground (G) on the lower right at the eighth rib.

7. Reposition the patient on his side, or have him sit forward. Then place the negative Z electrode on his back (not shown), directly posterior to the positive Z electrode.

8. Attach all the leads to the electrodes, being careful not to dislodge the posterior lead. Now, you can obtain the tracing.

NURSING CONSIDERATIONS

- Urge the patient not to tamper with the monitor or disconnect leadwires or electrodes. Demonstrate how to check the recorder for proper function.
- Tell the patient that he can't bathe or shower while wearing the monitor. He also needs to avoid electrical appliances, which can interfere with the monitor's recording.
- Emphasize to the patient the importance of keeping track of his activities, regardless of symptoms.
- Evaluation of the recordings will guide further treatment.

HEMODYNAMIC MONITORING

Hemodynamic monitoring is used to assess cardiac function and determine the effectiveness of therapy by measuring:

- cardiac output

USING HEMODYNAMIC MONITORING

Hemodynamic monitoring provides information on intracardiac pressures, arterial pressure, and cardiac output. To understand intracardiac pressures, picture the heart and vascular system as a continuous loop with constantly changing pressure gradients that keep the blood moving. Hemodynamic monitoring records the gradients within the vessels and heart chambers. Cardiac output indicates the amount of blood ejected by the heart each minute.

PRESSURE AND DESCRIPTION	NORMAL VALUES
CENTRAL VENOUS PRESSURE OR RIGHT ATRIAL PRESSURE The central venous pressure (CVP) or right atrial pressure (RAP) shows right ventricular function and end-diastolic pressure.	Normal mean pressure ranges from 1 to 6 mm Hg (1.34 to 8 cm H_2O).
RIGHT VENTRICULAR PRESSURE Typically, the physician measures right ventricular pressure only when initially inserting a pulmonary artery catheter. Right ventricular systolic pressure normally equals pulmonary artery systolic pressure; right ventricular end-diastolic pressure, which reflects right ventricular function, equals RAP.	Normal systolic pressure ranges from 20 to 30 mm Hg; normal diastolic pressure, from 0 to 5 mm Hg.
PULMONARY ARTERY PRESSURE Pulmonary artery systolic pressure shows right ventricular function and pulmonary circulation pressures. Pulmonary artery diastolic pressure reflects left ventricular pressures, specifically left ventricular end-diastolic pressure, in a patient without significant pulmonary disease.	Systolic pressure normally ranges from 20 to 30 mm Hg. The mean pressure usually ranges from 10 to 15 mm Hg.
PULMONARY ARTERY WEDGE PRESSURE Pulmonary artery wedge pressure (PAWP) reflects left atrial and left ventricular pressures, unless the patient has mitral stenosis. Changes in PAWP reflect changes in left ventricular filling pressure.	The mean pressure normally ranges from 6 to 12 mm Hg.

- mixed venous blood
- oxygen saturation
- intracardiac pressures
- blood pressure (See *Using hemodynamic monitoring*.)

CAUSES OF INCREASED PRESSURE	CAUSES OF DECREASED PRESSURE
● Right-sided heart failure ● Volume overload ● Tricuspid valve stenosis or insufficiency ● Constrictive pericarditis ● Pulmonary hypertension ● Cardiac tamponade ● Right ventricular infarction	● Reduced circulating blood volume
● Mitral stenosis or insufficiency ● Pulmonary disease ● Hypoxemia ● Constrictive pericarditis ● Chronic heart failure ● Atrial and ventricular septal defects ● Patent ductus arteriosus	● Reduced circulating blood volume
● Left-sided heart failure ● Increased pulmonary blood flow (left or right shunting, as in atrial or ventricular septal defects) ● Any condition causing increased pulmonary arteriolar resistance (such as pulmonary hypertension, volume overload, mitral stenosis, or hypoxia)	● Reduced circulating blood volume
● Left-sided heart failure ● Mitral stenosis or insufficiency ● Pericardial tamponade	● Reduced circulating blood volume

Follow your facility's procedure for setting up, zero referencing, calibrating, maintaining, and troubleshooting equipment. Common uses of hemodynamic monitoring include arterial blood pressure monitoring, central venous pressure monitoring, and pulmonary artery pressure monitoring.

Arterial blood pressure monitoring

In arterial blood pressure monitoring, the practitioner inserts a catheter into the radial or femoral artery to measure blood pressure or obtain samples of arterial blood for diagnostic tests such as arterial blood gas (ABG) studies.

A transducer transforms the flow of blood during systole and diastole into a waveform that appears on an oscilloscope. The waveform has five distinct components. (See *Types of normal arterial waveforms.*)

NURSING CONSIDERATIONS

- Explain the procedure to the patient and his family, including the purpose of arterial pressure monitoring.
- After catheter insertion, observe the pressure waveform to assess arterial pressure. (See *Recognizing abnormal arterial waveforms,* pages 112 and 113.)
- Assess the insertion site for signs of infection, such as redness and swelling. Notify the practitioner immediately if these signs appear.
- Maintain 300 mm Hg pressure in the pressure bag to permit a flush flow of 3 to 6 ml/hour.
- Document the date and time of catheter insertion, catheter insertion type, type of flush solution used, type of dressing applied, and the patient's tolerance of the procedure.

Central venous pressure monitoring

In central venous pressure (CVP) monitoring, the physician inserts a catheter through a vein and advances it until its tip lies in or near the right atrium. Because no major valves lie at the junction of the vena cava and right atrium, pressure at end diastole reflects back to the catheter. When connected to the transducer or manometer, the catheter measures CVP, an index of right ventricular function.

NURSING CONSIDERATIONS

- Explain the procedure to the patient and his family, including the purpose of CVP monitoring.
- After insertion, observe the waveform to assess CVP. (See *Differentiating normal from abnormal waveforms,* page 114.)
- Monitor the patient for complications, such as infection, pneumothorax, air embolism, and thrombosis. Notify the practitioner immediately if you notice such complications.

TYPES OF NORMAL ARTERIAL WAVEFORMS

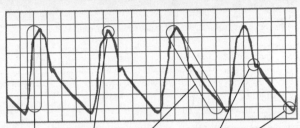

ANACROTIC LIMB

The *anacrotic limb* marks the waveform's initial upstroke, which occurs as blood is rapidly ejected from the ventricle through the open aortic valve into the aorta.

SYSTOLIC PEAK

Arterial pressure then rises sharply, resulting in the *systolic peak* — the waveform's highest point.

DICROTIC LIMB

As blood continues into the peripheral vessels, arterial pressure falls and the waveform begins a downward trend, called the *dicrotic limb*. Arterial pressure usually keeps falling until pressure in the ventricle is less than pressure in the aortic root.

DICROTIC NOTCH

When ventricular pressure is lower than aortic root pressure, the aortic valve closes. This event appears as a small notch on the waveform's downside, called the *dicrotic notch*.

END DIASTOLE

When the aortic valve closes, diastole begins, progressing until aortic root pressure gradually falls to its lowest point. On the waveform, this is known as *end diastole*.

- Adhere to your facility's policy for dressing, tubing, catheter, and flush changes.
- Document the date and time of catheter insertion, catheter insertion site, type of flush solution used, type of dressing applied, and the patient's tolerance of the procedure.
- Document the CVP readings according to your facility's policy.

RECOGNIZING ABNORMAL ARTERIAL WAVEFORMS

Use this chart to help you recognize and resolve waveform abnormalities.

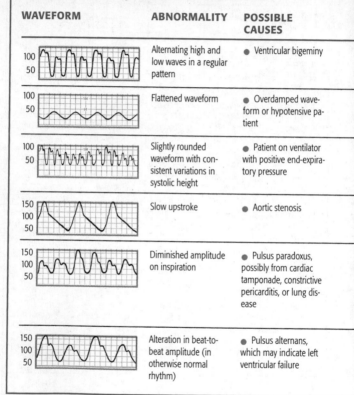

WAVEFORM	ABNORMALITY	POSSIBLE CAUSES
100 / 50	Alternating high and low waves in a regular pattern	● Ventricular bigeminy
100 / 50	Flattened waveform	● Overdamped waveform or hypotensive patient
100 / 50	Slightly rounded waveform with consistent variations in systolic height	● Patient on ventilator with positive end-expiratory pressure
150 / 100 / 50	Slow upstroke	● Aortic stenosis
150 / 100 / 50	Diminished amplitude on inspiration	● Pulsus paradoxus, possibly from cardiac tamponade, constrictive pericarditis, or lung disease
150 / 100 / 50	Alteration in beat-to-beat amplitude (in otherwise normal rhythm)	● Pulsus alternans, which may indicate left ventricular failure

Pulmonary artery pressure monitoring

Continuous pulmonary artery pressure (PAP) and intermittent pulmonary artery wedge pressure (PAWP) measurements provide important information about left ventricular function and preload. (See *Understanding pulmonary artery pressures,* page 115.) Use this information for monitoring and for aiding diagnosis, refining assessment, guiding interventions, and projecting patient outcomes.

NURSING INTERVENTIONS

● Check the patient's ECG to confirm ventricular bigeminy. The tracing should reflect premature ventricular contractions every second beat.

● Check the patient's blood pressure with a sphygmomanometer. If you obtain a higher reading, suspect overdamping. Correct the problem by trying to aspirate the arterial line. If you succeed, flush the line. If the reading is very low or absent, suspect hypotension.

● Check the patient's systolic blood pressure regularly. The difference between the highest and lowest systolic pressure reading should be less than 10 mm Hg. If the difference exceeds that amount, suspect pulsus paradoxus, possibly from cardiac tamponade.

● Check the patient's heart sounds for signs of aortic stenosis. Also notify the practitioner, who will document suspected aortic stenosis in his notes.

● Note systolic pressure during inspiration and expiration. If inspiratory pressure is at least 10 mm Hg less than expiratory pressure, call the practitioner.
● If you're also monitoring pulmonary artery pressure, observe for a diastolic plateau. This abnormality occurs when the mean central venous pressure (right atrial pressure), mean pulmonary artery pressure, and mean pulmonary artery wedge pressure (pulmonary artery obstructive pressure) are within 5 mm Hg of one another.

● Observe the patient's ECG, noting any deviation in the waveform.
● Notify the practitioner if this is a new and sudden abnormality.

PAP monitoring is indicated for patients who:
■ are hemodynamically unstable
■ need fluid management or continuous cardiopulmonary assessment
■ are receiving multiple or frequently administered cardioactive drugs.

DIFFERENTIATING NORMAL FROM ABNORMAL CVP WAVEFORMS

These illustrations show a normal central venous pressure (CVP) waveform and abnormal CVP waveforms, along with possible causes of abnormal waveforms.

Normal waveforms

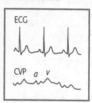

Elevated *a* wave

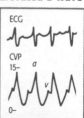

Physiologic causes
- Increased resistance to ventricular filling
- Increased atrial contraction

Associated conditions
- Heart failure
- Tricuspid stenosis

- Pulmonary hypertension

Elevated *v* wave

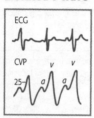

Physiologic cause
- Regurgitating flow

Associated conditions
- Tricuspid insufficiency
- Inadequate closure of the tricuspid valve due to heart failure

Absent *a* wave

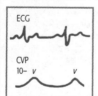

Physiologic cause
- Decreased or absent atrial contraction

Associated conditions
- Atrial fibrillation

- Junctional arrhythmias
- Ventricular pacing

Elevated *a* and *v* waves

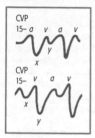

Physiologic causes
- Increased resistance to ventricular filling, which causes an elevated *a* wave
- Functional regurgitation, which causes an elevated *v* wave

Associated conditions
- Cardiac tamponade (smaller *y* descent than *x* descent)
- Constrictive pericardial disease (*y* descent exceeds *x* descent)
- Heart failure
- Hypervolemia
- Atrial hypertrophy

UNDERSTANDING PULMONARY ARTERY PRESSURES

PA systolic pressure

Pulmonary artery (PA) systolic pressure measures right ventricular systolic ejection or, simply put, the amount of pressure needed to open the pulmonic valve and eject blood into the pulmonary circulation. When the pulmonic valve is open, PA systolic pressure should be the same as right ventricular pressure.

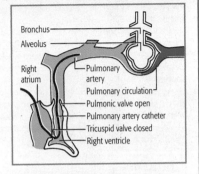

Bronchus
Alveolus
Right atrium
Pulmonary artery
Pulmonary circulation
Pulmonic valve open
Pulmonary artery catheter
Tricuspid valve closed
Right ventricle

PA diastolic pressure

PA diastolic pressure represents the resistance of the pulmonary vascular bed as measured when the pulmonic valve is closed and the tricuspid valve is open. To a limited degree (under absolutely normal conditions), PA diastolic pressure also reflects left ventricular end-diastolic pressure.

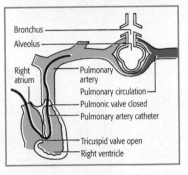

Bronchus
Alveolus
Right atrium
Pulmonary artery
Pulmonary circulation
Pulmonic valve closed
Pulmonary artery catheter
Tricuspid valve open
Right ventricle

PAP monitoring is also crucial for patients experiencing shock, trauma, pulmonary or cardiac disease, or multiple organ dysfunction syndrome.

A pulmonary artery (PA) catheter has up to six lumens that gather hemodynamic information. In addition to distal and proximal lumens used to measure CVP and PAP, a PA catheter has a balloon inflation lumen that inflates the balloon for PAWP measurement and a thermistor connector lumen that allows cardiac output measurement.

DIFFERENTIATING PULMONARY ARTERY CATHETER PORTS

A pulmonary artery (PA) catheter contains several lumen ports to allow various catheter functions:

- The balloon inflation lumen inflates the balloon at the distal tip of the catheter for pulmonary artery wedge pressure (PAWP) measurement.
- A distal lumen measures PA pressure when connected to a transducer and measures PAWP during balloon inflation. It also permits drawing of mixed venous blood samples.
- A proximal lumen measures right atrial pressure (central venous pressure).
- The thermistor connector lumen contains temperature-sensitive wires, which feed information into a computer for cardiac output calculation.
- Another lumen may provide a port for pacemaker electrodes or measurement of mixed venous oxygen saturation ($S\overline{v}O_2$).

FIVE-LUMEN PA CATHETER

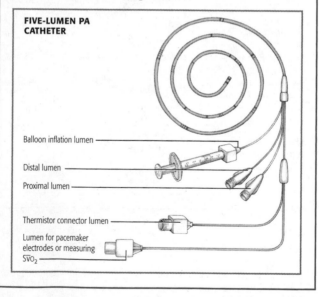

Balloon inflation lumen

Distal lumen

Proximal lumen

Thermistor connector lumen

Lumen for pacemaker electrodes or measuring $S\overline{v}O_2$

Some catheters also have a pacemaker wire lumen that provides a port for pacemaker electrodes and measures continuous mixed venous oxygen saturation. (See *Differentiating pulmonary artery catheter ports.*)

The physician inserts the balloon-tipped, multilumen catheter into the patient's internal jugular or subclavian vein. When the catheter reaches the right atrium, the balloon is inflated to float the catheter through the right ventricle into the pulmonary artery. This permits PAWP measurement through an opening at the catheter's tip.

The deflated catheter rests in the pulmonary artery, allowing diastolic and systolic PAP readings. The balloon should be totally deflated except when taking a PAWP reading because prolonged wedging can cause pulmonary infarction. (See *Observing pulmonary artery waveforms,* page 118.)

NURSING CONSIDERATIONS

- Inform the patient that he'll be conscious during catheterization, and that he may feel temporary local discomfort from the administration of the local anesthetic. Catheter insertion takes about 15 to 30 minutes.
- After catheter insertion, you may inflate the balloon with a syringe to take PAWP readings. Be careful not to inflate the balloon with more than 1.5 cc of air. Overinflation could distend the pulmonary artery causing vessel rupture. Don't leave the balloon wedged for a prolonged period because this could lead to a pulmonary infarction.
- After each PAWP reading, flush the line; if you encounter difficulty, notify the practitioner.
- Maintain 300 mm Hg pressure in the pressure bag to permit a flush flow of 3 to 6 ml/hour.
- If fever develops when the catheter is in place, inform the practitioner. He may remove the catheter and send its tip to the laboratory for culture.
- Make sure stopcocks are properly positioned and connections are secure. Loose connections may introduce air into the system or cause blood backup, leakage of deoxygenated blood, or inaccurate pressure readings. Also make sure the lumen hubs are properly identified to serve the appropriate catheter ports. (See *Identifying hemodynamic pressure monitoring problems,* pages 119 and 120.)
- Because the catheter can slip back into the right ventricle and irritate it, check the monitor for a right ventricular waveform to detect this problem promptly. Running a continuous infusion through the distal lumen will interfere with your ability to monitor this waveform for changes.
- To minimize vascular trauma, make sure the balloon is deflated whenever the catheter is withdrawn from the pulmonary artery to the right ventricle or from the right ventricle to the right atrium.

(Text continues on page 120.)

OBSERVING PULMONARY ARTERY WAVEFORMS

During pulmonary artery catheter insertion, the waveforms on the monitor change as the catheter advances through the heart.

Right atrium

When the catheter tip enters the right atrium, the first heart chamber on its route, a waveform like the one shown below appears on the monitor. Note the two small upright waves. The *a* waves represent the right ventricular end-diastolic pressure; the *v* waves, right atrial filling.

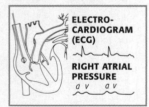

Right ventricle

As the catheter tip reaches the right ventricle, you'll see a waveform with sharp systolic upstrokes and lower diastolic dips, as shown below.

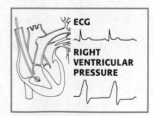

Pulmonary artery

The catheter then floats into the pulmonary artery, causing a pulmonary artery pressure (PAP) waveform such as the one shown below. Note that the upstroke is smoother than on the right ventricle waveform. The dicrotic notch indicates pulmonic valve closure.

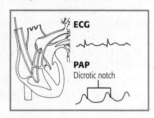

PAWP

Floating into a distal branch of the pulmonary artery, the balloon wedges where the vessel becomes too narrow for it to pass. The monitor now shows a pulmonary artery wedge pressure (PAWP) waveform, with two small upright waves, as shown below. The *a* wave represents left ventricular end-diastolic pressure; the *v* wave, left atrial filling. The balloon is then deflated, and the catheter is left in the pulmonary artery.

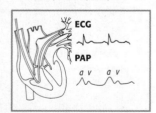

IDENTIFYING HEMODYNAMIC PRESSURE MONITORING PROBLEMS

This table reviews common hemodynamic pressure monitoring problems, their possible causes, and appropriate interventions.

PROBLEM	POSSIBLE CAUSES	INTERVENTIONS
LINE FAILS TO FLUSH	● Stopcocks positioned incorrectly	● Make sure the stopcocks are positioned correctly.
	● Inadequate pressure from pressure bag	● Make sure the pressure bag gauge reads 300 mm Hg.
	● Kink in pressure tubing	● Check the pressure tubing for kinks.
	● Blood clot in catheter	● Try to aspirate the clot with a syringe. If the line still won't flush, notify the practitioner and prepare to replace the line. *Important:* Never use a syringe to flush a hemodynamic line.
DAMPED WAVEFORM	● Air bubbles	● Secure all connections. ● Remove air from the lines and the transducer. ● Check for and replace cracked equipment.
	● Blood clot in catheter	● Refer to "Line fails to flush" (above).
	● Blood flashback in line	● Make sure stopcock positions are correct; tighten loose connections and replace cracked equipment; flush the line with the fast-flush valve; replace the transducer dome if blood backs up into it.
	● Incorrect transducer position	● Make sure the transducer is kept at the level of the right atrium at all times. Improper levels give false-high or false-low pressure readings.

(continued)

IDENTIFYING HEMODYNAMIC PRESSURE MONITORING PROBLEMS *(continued)*

PROBLEM	POSSIBLE CAUSES	INTERVENTIONS
DAMPED WAVEFORM *(continued)*	● Arterial catheter out of blood vessel or pressed against vessel wall	● Reposition the catheter if it's against the vessel wall. ● Try to aspirate blood to confirm proper placement in the vessel. If you can't aspirate blood, notify the practitioner and prepare to replace the line. *Note:* Bloody drainage at the insertion site may indicate catheter displacement. Notify the practitioner immediately.
PULMONARY ARTERY WEDGE PRESSURE TRACING UNOBTAINABLE	● Ruptured balloon	● If you feel no resistance when injecting air or if you see blood leaking from the balloon inflation lumen, stop injecting air and notify the practitioner. If the catheter is left in, label the inflation lumen with a warning not to inflate.
	● Incorrect amount of air in balloon ● Catheter malpositioned	● Deflate the balloon. Check the label on the catheter for correct volume. Reinflate slowly with the correct amount. To avoid rupturing the balloon, never use more than the stated volume. ● Notify the practitioner. Obtain a chest X-ray.

- Adhere to your facility's policy for dressing, tubing, catheter, and flush changes.
- Document the date and time of catheter insertion, the physician who performed the procedure, the catheter insertion site, pressure waveforms and values for the various heart chambers, balloon inflation volume required to obtain a wedge tracing, arrhythmias that occurred during or after the procedure, type of flush solution used and its heparin concentration (if any), type of dressing applied, and the patient's tolerance of the procedure.

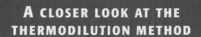

A CLOSER LOOK AT THE THERMODILUTION METHOD

This illustration shows the path of the injectate solution through the heart during thermodilution cardiac output monitoring.

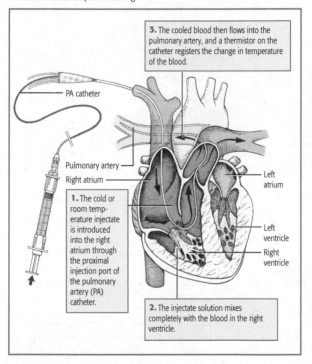

3. The cooled blood then flows into the pulmonary artery, and a thermistor on the catheter registers the change in temperature of the blood.

PA catheter

Pulmonary artery

Right atrium

Left atrium

Left ventricle

Right ventricle

1. The cold or room temperature injectate is introduced into the right atrium through the proximal injection port of the pulmonary artery (PA) catheter.

2. The injectate solution mixes completely with the blood in the right ventricle.

Cardiac output monitoring

Cardiac output, the amount of blood ejected by the heart in 1 minute, is monitored to evaluate cardiac function. The normal range for cardiac output is 4 to 8 L/minute.

The most widely used method for monitoring cardiac output is the bolus thermodilution technique. (See *A closer look at the thermodilution method*.) Other methods include the Fick method and the dye

CALCULATING CARDIAC OUTPUT

One way to calculate cardiac output is by using the Fick method. In this method, the blood's oxygen content is measured before and after it passes through the lungs. First, blood is removed from the pulmonary and brachial arteries and analyzed for oxygen content. Next, a spirometer is used to measure oxygen consumption (the amount of air entering the lungs each minute).

Use this formula to calculate cardiac output:

$$\text{cardiac output (L/minute)} = \frac{\text{oxygen consumption (ml/minute)}}{\text{arterial oxygen content} - \text{venous oxygen content (ml/minute)}}$$

dilution test. (See *Calculating cardiac output*.) To measure cardiac output, a solution is injected into the right atrium through a port on a PA catheter. Iced or room-temperature injectant may be used depending on your facility's policy and on the patient's status.

This indicator solution mixes with the blood as it travels through the right ventricle into the pulmonary artery, and a thermistor on the catheter registers the change in temperature of the flowing blood. A computer then plots the temperature change over time as a curve and calculates flow based on the area under the curve. (See *Analyzing thermodilution curves*.)

Some PA catheters contain a filament that permits continuous cardiac output monitoring. When using such a device, an average cardiac output value is determined over a 3-minute span; the value is updated every 30 to 60 seconds. This type of monitoring allows close scrutiny of the patient's hemodynamic status and prompt intervention in case problems arise.

Cardiac output is better assessed by calculating cardiac index, which takes body size into account. To calculate the patient's cardiac index, divide his cardiac output by his body surface area, a function of height and weight. The normal cardiac index for adults ranges from 2.5 to 4.2 L/minute/m^2; for pregnant women, it ranges from 3.5 to 6.5 L/minute/m^2. There are several other measurements of cardiac function that combine cardiac output values with other values obtained from a PA catheter and an arterial line. (See *Measuring cardiac function*, page 125.)

NURSING CONSIDERATIONS
■ Make sure the patient doesn't move during the procedure because movement can cause an error in measurement.

ANALYZING THERMODILUTION CURVES

The thermodilution curve provides valuable information about cardiac output, injection technique, and equipment problems. When studying the curve, keep in mind that the area under the curve is inversely proportionate to cardiac output: The smaller the area under the curve, the higher the cardiac output; the larger the area under the curve, the lower the cardiac output.

Besides providing a record of cardiac output, the curve may indicate problems related to technique, such as erratic or slow injectate instillations, or other problems, such as respiratory variations or electrical interference. The curves below correspond to those typically seen in clinical practice.

Normal thermodilution curve

With an accurate monitoring system and a patient who has adequate cardiac output, the thermodilution curve begins with a smooth, rapid upstroke and is followed by a smooth, gradual downslope. The curve shown below indicates that the injectate instillation time was within the recommended 4 seconds and that the temperature curve returned to baseline blood temperature.

The height of the curve may vary, depending on whether you use a room-temperature or an iced injectate. Room-temperature injection produces an upstroke of lower amplitude.

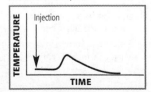

Low cardiac output curve

A thermodilution curve representing low cardiac output shows a rapid, smooth upstroke (from proper injection technique). However, because the heart is ejecting blood less efficiently from the ventricles, the injectate warms slowly and takes longer to be ejected from the ventricle. Consequently, the curve takes longer to return to baseline. This slow return produces a larger area under the curve, corresponding to low cardiac output.

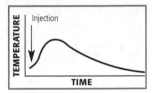

High cardiac output curve

Again, the curve has a rapid, smooth upstroke from proper injection technique. But because the ventricles are ejecting blood too forcefully, the injectate moves through the heart quickly and the curve returns to baseline more rapidly. The smaller area under the curve suggests higher cardiac output.

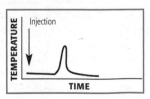

(continued)

ANALYZING THERMODILUTION CURVES *(continued)*

Curve reflecting poor technique

This curve results from an uneven and too slow (taking more than 4 seconds) administration of injectate. The uneven and slower than normal upstroke and the larger area under the curve erroneously indicate low cardiac output. A kinked catheter, unsteady hands during the injection, or improper placement of the injectate lumen in the introducer sheath may also cause this type of curve.

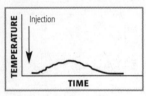

Curve associated with respiratory variations

To obtain a reliable cardiac output measurement, you need a steady baseline pulmonary artery blood temperature. If the patient has rapid or labored respirations or if he's receiving mechanical ventilation, the thermodilution curve may reflect inaccurate cardiac output values. The curve shown below from a patient receiving mechanical ventilation reflects fluctuating pulmonary artery blood temperatures. The thermistor interprets the unsteady temperature as a return to baseline. The result is a curve erroneously showing a high cardiac output (small area under the curve). (*Note:* In some cases, the equipment senses no return to baseline at all and produces a sinelike curve recorded by the computer as 0.00).

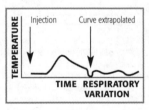

- Perform cardiac output measurements and monitoring at least every 2 to 4 hours, especially if the patient is receiving vasoactive or inotropic agents or if fluids are being added or restricted.
- Discontinue cardiac output measurements when the patient is hemodynamically stable and weaned from his vasoactive and inotropic medications.
- Monitor the patient for signs and symptoms of inadequate perfusion, including restlessness, fatigue, changes in level of consciousness, decreased capillary refill time, diminished peripheral pulses, oliguria, and pale, cool skin.
- Add the fluid volume injected for cardiac output determinations to the patient's total intake.

MEASURING CARDIAC FUNCTION

Listed below are several common measures of cardiac function that are based on information obtained from a pulmonary artery catheter. Most cardiac output (CO) systems will compute these values automatically.

	NORMAL VALUES	FORMULA FOR CALCULATION	CAUSES OF INCREASED VALUES	CAUSES OF DECREASED VALUES
Stroke volume (SV)—Volume of blood pumped by the ventricle in one contraction	60 to 130 ml/beat	SV= CO × 1,000/HR	Sepsis Hypervolemia Inotrope administration	Arrhythmias Hypovolemia Decreased contractility Increased afterload
Stroke volume index (SVI)—Determines if the SV is adequate for patient's body size	30 to 65 ml/beat/ m²	SVI= SV/BSA *or* SVI= CI/HR	Same as SV	Same as SV
Systemic vascular resistance (SVR)—degree of left ventricular resistance, or afterload	800 to 1,400 dynes/ sec/cm⁻⁵	SVR= MAP–CVP/CO × 80	Hypothermia Hypovolemia Vasoconstriction	Vasodilation Vasodilators Shock (anaphylactic, neurogenic, or septic)
Pulmonary vascular resistance (PVR)	20 to 200 dynes/ sec/cm⁻	PVR= MPAP–PAWP/ CO × 80	Hypoxemia Pulmonary embolism Pulmonary hypertension	Pulmonary vasodilating drugs (morphine)

Key:

HR-heart rate
BSA-body surface area
CI-cardiac index

MAP-mean arterial pressure
CVP-central venous pressure
MPAP-mean pulmonary artery pressure

PAWP-pulmonary artery wedge pressure

■ Record the patient's cardiac output, cardiac index, and other hemodynamic values and vital signs at the time of measurement. Note
the patient's position during measurement.

CATHETERIZATION STUDIES

Catheterization studies use a catheter inserted through either an artery
or a vein to go into the heart and examine the coronary arteries, the
heart structure, or determine the location of arrhythmias. Two types of
catheter studies are cardiac catheterization and the electrophysiology
study.

Cardiac catheterization

Cardiac catheterization involves passing a catheter into the right, left,
or both sides of the heart. (See *Differentiating right- and left-side heart
catheterization.*)

This procedure permits measurement of blood pressure and
blood flow in the chambers of the heart. It's used to determine valve
competence and cardiac wall contractility and to detect intracardiac
shunts. The procedure is also used for blood sample collection and
can be used to obtain diagnostic films of the ventricles (contrast ventriculography) and arteries (coronary arteriography or angiography).

Use of thermodilution catheters allows calculation of cardiac output. Such calculations are used to evaluate valvular insufficiency or
stenosis, septal defects, congenital anomalies, myocardial function and
blood supply, and heart wall motion.
Common abnormalities and defects that can be confirmed by cardiac
catheterization include:
■ coronary artery disease
■ myocardial incompetence
■ valvular heart disease
■ septal defects.

NURSING CONSIDERATIONS
When caring for a patient undergoing a cardiac catheterization, describe the procedure and events after it and take steps to prevent postoperative complications.

Before the procedure
■ Explain that this test is used to evaluate the function of the heart
and its vessels. Instruct the patient to restrict food and fluids for at
least 6 hours before the test. Tell him that the procedure takes 1 to

DIFFERENTIATING RIGHT- AND LEFT-SIDE HEART CATHETERIZATION

In catheterization of the left side of the heart, a catheter is inserted into an artery in the antecubital fossa or into the left femoral artery. Left-sided heart catheterization assesses the patency of the coronary arteries, mitral and aortic valve function, and left ventricular function. It aids in the diagnosis of left ventricular enlargement, aortic stenosis and insufficiency aortic root enlargement, mitral insufficiency, aneurysm, and intracardiac shunt.

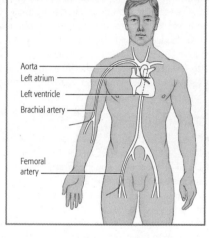

In catheterization of the right side of the heart, the catheter is inserted into an antecubital vein or the femoral vein and advanced through the inferior vena cava or right atrium. Right-sided heart catheterization assesses tricuspid and pulmonic valve function and pulmonary artery pressures.

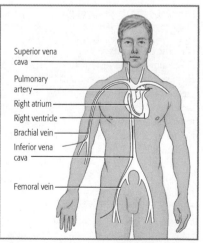

2 hours and that he may receive a mild sedative during the procedure.

- Tell the patient that the catheter is inserted into an artery or vein in the arm or leg. Tell him that he'll experience a transient stinging sensation when a local anesthetic is injected to numb the incision site for catheter insertion.
- Inform the patient that injection of the contrast medium through the catheter may produce a hot, flushing sensation or nausea that quickly passes; instruct him to follow directions to cough or breathe deeply. Explain that he'll be given medication if he experiences chest pain during the procedure. Explain that he may also be given nitroglycerin periodically to dilate coronary vessels and aid visualization. Reassure him that complications, such as myocardial infarction and thromboembolism, are rare.
- Make sure that the patient or a responsible family member has signed a consent form.
- Check for and tell the practitioner about hypersensitivity to shellfish, iodine, or contrast media used in other diagnostic tests.
- Discontinue anticoagulant therapy to reduce the risk of complications from bleeding.
- Review activity restrictions and position requirements that may be necessary for the patient after the procedure, such as lying flat with the limb extended for 4 to 6 hours and using sandbags to apply pressure to the insertion site if a femoral sheath is used.
- Document the presence of peripheral pulses, noting their intensity. Mark the pulses so they may be easily located after the procedure.

After the procedure

- Determine if a hemostatic device, such as a collagen plug or suture closure system, was used to close the vessel puncture site. If either method was used, inspect the site for bleeding or oozing, redness, swelling, or hematoma formation. Maintain the patient on bed rest for 1 to 2 hours.
- Enforce bed rest for 8 hours if no hemostatic device was used. If the femoral route was used for catheter insertion, keep the patient's leg extended for 6 to 8 hours; if the antecubital fossa route was used, keep the arm extended for at least 3 hours.
- Monitor vital signs every 15 minutes for 2 hours, then every 30 minutes for 2 hours, and then every hour for 4 hours. If no hematoma or other problems arise, check every 4 hours. If vital signs are unstable, check every 5 minutes and notify the practitioner.

- Continually assess the insertion site for a hematoma or blood loss, and reinforce the pressure dressing as needed.
- Check the patient's color, skin temperature, and peripheral pulse below the puncture site.
- Administer I.V. fluids as indicated (usually 100 ml/hour) to promote excretion of the contrast medium. Monitor for signs of fluid overload.
- Watch for signs of chest pain, shortness of breath, abnormal heart rate, dizziness, diaphoresis, nausea or vomiting, or extreme fatigue. Notify the practitioner immediately if these complications occur.

Electrophysiology studies

Electrophysiology studies record electrical conduction during slow withdrawal of a bipolar or tripolar electrode catheter from the right ventricle through the bundle of His to the sinoatrial node. The catheter is introduced into the femoral vein, passing through the right atrium and across the septal leaflet of the tricuspid valve.

Normal conduction intervals in adults are as follows: HV interval, 35 to 55 msec; AH interval, 45 to 150 msec; and PA interval, 20 to 40 msec.

NURSING CONSIDERATIONS

When caring for a patient undergoing an electrophysiology study, describe the procedure and events after it and take steps to prevent postoperative complications.

Before the procedure

- Explain that this test is used to evaluate the heart's conduction system. Instruct the patient to restrict food and fluids for at least 6 hours before the test. Tell him that the procedure takes 1 to 3 hours and that he may receive a mild sedative during the procedure.
- Tell the patient that the catheter is inserted into an artery in the leg. Tell him that he'll experience a transient stinging sensation when a local anesthetic is injected to numb the incision site for catheter insertion.
- Have the patient void before the test.
- Make sure that the patient or a responsible family member has signed a consent form.
- Review activity restrictions and position requirements that may be necessary for the patient after the procedure, such as lying flat with the limb extended for 4 to 6 hours and using sandbags to apply pressure to the insertion site.

- Document the presence of peripheral pulses, noting their intensity. Mark the pulses so they may be easily located after the procedure.

After the procedure

- Determine if a hemostatic device, such as a collagen plug or suture closure system, was used to close the vessel puncture site. If either method was used, inspect the site for bleeding or oozing, redness, swelling, or hematoma formation. Maintain the patient on bed rest for 1 to 2 hours.
- Enforce bed rest for 8 hours if no hemostatic device was used. If the femoral route was used for catheter insertion, keep the patient's leg extended for 6 to 8 hours; if the antecubital fossa route was used, keep the arm extended for at least 3 hours.
- Monitor vital signs every 15 minutes for 2 hours, then every 30 minutes for 2 hours, and then every hour for 4 hours. If no hematoma or other problems arise, check every 4 hours. If vital signs are unstable, check every 5 minutes and notify the practitioner.
- Continually assess the insertion site for a hematoma or blood loss, and reinforce the pressure dressing as needed.
- Check the patient's color, skin temperature, and peripheral pulse below the puncture site.
- Obtain a 12-lead electrocardiogram to assess for changes.
- Watch for signs of chest pain, shortness of breath, abnormal heart rate, dizziness, diaphoresis, nausea or vomiting, or extreme fatigue. Notify the practitioner immediately if these complications occur.

IMAGING AND RADIOGRAPHIC TESTS

Imaging and radiographic testing allows for detailed images of the heart and its ability to function. These tests include echocardiography, cardiac magnetic resonance imaging, cardiac positron emission tomography, cardiac blood pool imaging, technetium-99m pyrophosphate scanning, cardiac scoring computed tomography, thallium scanning, Doppler ultrasonography, and venography.

Echocardiography

Echocardiography is used to examine the size, shape, and motion of cardiac structures. In this procedure, a transducer is placed at an acoustic window (an area where bone and lung tissue are absent) on the patient's chest. The transducer directs sound waves toward cardiac structures, which reflect these waves.

The transducer picks up the echoes, converts them to electrical impulses, and relays them to an echocardiography machine for display on a screen and for recording on a strip chart or videotape. The most commonly used echocardiographic techniques are M-mode (motion mode) and two-dimensional.

In M-mode echocardiography, a single, pencil-like ultrasound beam strikes the heart, producing an "ice pick," or vertical, view of cardiac structures. This mode is especially useful for precisely viewing cardiac structures.

In two-dimensional echocardiography, the ultrasound beam rapidly sweeps through an arc, producing a cross-sectional, or fan-shaped, view of cardiac structures; this technique is useful for recording lateral motion and providing the correct spatial relationship between cardiac structures. In many cases, both techniques are performed to complement each other.

Doppler echocardiography may be used to assess speed and direction of blood flow. The sound of blood flow may be heard as the continuous-wave and pulse-wave Doppler sampling of cardiac valves is performed. This technique is used primarily to assess heart sounds and murmurs as they relate to cardiac hemodynamics.

In exercise echocardiography and dobutamine stress echocardiography, a two-dimensional echocardiogram records cardiac wall motion during exercise or while dobutamine is being infused. (See *Teaching about cardiac stress testing,* pages 132 and 133.)

The echocardiogram may detect mitral stenosis, mitral valve prolapse, aortic insufficiency, wall motion abnormalities, and pericardial effusion.

NURSING CONSIDERATIONS

■ Explain the procedure to the patient, and advise him to remain still during the test because movement can distort results. Tell him that conductive gel is applied to the chest and a quarter-sized transducer is placed directly over the gel. Because pressure is exerted to keep the transducer in contact with the skin, warn the patient that he may feel minor discomfort.

■ After the procedure, remove the conductive gel from the skin.

Transesophageal echocardiography

Transesophageal echocardiography combines ultrasound with endoscopy to give a better view of the heart's structures. A small transducer is attached to the end of a gastroscope and inserted into the

TEACHING ABOUT CARDIAC STRESS TESTING

Exercise echocardiography and dobuta-mine stress echocardiography are types of cardiac stress testing that detect changes in heart wall motion through the use of two-dimensional echocardiography during exercise or a dobutamine infusion. Imaging is done before and after either exercise or dobutamine administration. Usually, these tests are performed to:
- identify the cause of chest pain
- detect heart abnormalities, obstructions, or damage
- determine the heart's functional capacity after myocardial infarction or cardiac surgery
- evaluate myocardial perfusion
- measure the heart chambers
- set limits for an exercise program.

Preparing your patient

When preparing your patient for these tests, cover the following points:

- Explain that this test will evaluate how his heart performs under stress and how specific heart structures work under stress.
- Instruct the patient not to eat, smoke, or drink alcohol or caffeinated beverages for at least 4 hours before the test.
- Advise him to ask his practitioner whether he should withhold current medications before the test.
- Tell him to wear a two-piece outfit because he'll be removing all clothing above the waist and will wear a hospital gown.
- Explain that electrodes will be placed on his chest and arms to obtain an initial electrocardiogram (ECG). Mention that the areas where electrodes are placed will be cleaned with alcohol and that the skin will be abraded for optimal electrode contact.
- Tell him that an initial echocardiogram will be performed while he's lying down. Conductive gel, which feels warm, will be placed on his chest. Then a special trans-ducer will be placed at various angles on his chest to visualize different parts of his

esophagus, allowing images to be taken from the posterior aspect of the heart. This causes less tissue penetration and interference from chest wall structures and produces high-quality images of the thoracic aorta, except for the superior ascending aorta, which is shadowed by the trachea.

NURSING CONSIDERATIONS

- Explain to the patient that this test will allow better visualization of heart function and structures.
- Instruct the patient to fast for 6 hours before the test.
- Have the patient remove any dentures or oral prostheses and note any loose teeth.
- Make sure the patient or a responsible family member has signed an informed consent form.

heart. Emphasize that he must remain still to prevent distorting the images.

● Inform the patient that the entire procedure should take 60 to 90 minutes. Explain that the practitioner will compare these echocardiograms to diagnose his heart condition.

Explaining exercise echocardiography

If the patient will have an exercise stress test after the initial echocardiogram, cover these teaching points:

● Tell him that he'll walk on the treadmill at a prescribed rate for a predetermined time to raise his heart rate. After he reaches the prescribed heart rate, he'll lie down and a second echocardiogram will be done.

● Explain that he may feel tired, sweaty, and slightly short of breath during the test. If his symptoms are severe or chest pain develops, the test will be stopped.

● Reassure him that his blood pressure will be monitored during the test. After the test is complete, his ECG and blood pressure will be monitored for 10 minutes.

Describing the dobutamine stress test

If the patient will undergo a dobutamine stress test after the initial echocardiogram, cover these teaching points:

● Explain that an I.V. line will be inserted into his vein for the dobutamine infusion. Tell him that this drug will increase his heart rate without exercise. Tell him to expect initial discomfort when the I.V. line is inserted. Mention that, during the infusion, he may feel palpitations, shortness of breath, and fatigue.

● Inform the patient that a second echocardiogram will be done during the dobutamine infusion. After the drug is infused and his heart rate reaches the desired level, a third echocardiogram will be obtained.

● Reassure the patient that his blood pressure will be monitored during the test.

■ During the procedure, vasovagal responses may occur with gagging, so closely observe the cardiac monitor.

■ After the procedure, don't give the patient food or water until his gag reflex has returned.

Cardiac blood pool imaging

Cardiac blood pool imaging evaluates ventricular performance after the injection of human serum albumin or red blood cells tagged with technetium 99m. A camera records the radioactivity of the isotope while it passes through the left ventricle. A computer is then used to calculate the ejection fraction based on the amount of isotope ejected during each beat; the presence and size of intracardiac shunts can also be determined.

Gated cardiac blood pool imaging uses the camera to record 500 to 1,000 cardiac cycles and determine areas of hypokinesia or akinesia. Multiple-gated acquisition scanning uses sequential images to evaluate wall motion and determine the ejection fraction and other indices of cardiac function.

NURSING CONSIDERATIONS

- Tell the patient that he will receive an I.V. injection of a radioactive tracer, but that the tracer poses no radiation hazard and rarely produces adverse effects.
- Make sure the patient or a responsible family member has signed an informed consent form.

Cardiac magnetic resonance imaging

Also known as *nuclear magnetic resonance,* cardiac magnetic resonance imaging (MRI) yields high-resolution, tomographic, three-dimensional images of body structures. It takes advantage of certain magnetically aligned body nuclei that fall out of alignment after radio frequency transmission. The MRI scanner records the signals the nuclei emit as they realign in a process called precession and then translates the signals into detailed pictures of body structures. The resulting images show tissue characteristics without lung or bone interference.

A cardiac MRI permits visualization of valve leaflets and structures, pericardial abnormalities and processes, ventricular hypertrophy, cardiac neoplasm, infarcted tissue, anatomic malformations, and structural deformities. It can be used to monitor the progression of ischemic heart disease and the effectiveness of treatment.

NURSING CONSIDERATIONS

- Instruct the patient that he'll need to lie still during the test.
- Warn the patient that he'll hear a thumping noise.
- Have the patient remove all jewelry and other metallic objects before testing. A patient with an internal surgical clip, scalp vein needle, pacemaker, gold fillings, heart valve prosthesis, or other metal objects in his body can't undergo an MRI.
- Permit the patient to resume activities as indicated.

Cardiac positron emission tomography

Cardiac positron emission tomography (PET) scanning combines elements of computed tomography scanning and conventional radionuclide imaging.

Radioisotopes are given to the patient by injection, inhalation, or I.V. infusion. One isotope targets blood; one targets glucose. The isotopes emit particles called positrons. The PET scanner detects and reconstructs the positron to form an image.

A PET scan shows coronary blood flow and glucose metabolism. A decrease in blood flow with a corresponding increase in glucose metabolism indicates ischemia; a decrease in blood flow with a decrease in glucose metabolism indicates necrotic or scarred heart tissue.

NURSING CONSIDERATIONS
- Tell the patient that he may be given the isotope by injection, inhalation, or I.V. infusion.
- Stress the importance of remaining still during the test.
- After the test, encourage the patient to increase his fluid intake to help flush the isotope from his bladder.

Cardiac scoring computed tomography

Cardiac scoring computed tomography is a series of tomograms that provide cross-sectional images of the heart. These images are used to reconstruct the horizontal, sagittal, and coronal planes of the heart.

This test helps determine the calcium content in the coronary arteries. Increased calcium content in the coronary arteries indicates an increased risk of myocardial infarction or critical narrowing of the arteries and further testing is indicated.

NURSING CONSIDERATIONS
- Stress the importance of remaining still during the test.
- Tell the patient that he may hear clacking sounds during the test, and reassure him that this is normal.

Technetium-99m pyrophosphate scanning

Technetium-99m (^{99m}Tc) pyrophosphate scanning, also known as *hot spot imaging* or *pyrophosphate scanning,* helps diagnose acute myocardial injury by showing the location and size of newly damaged myocardial tissue. Especially useful for diagnosing transmural infarction, this test works best when performed 12 hours to 6 days after symptom onset. It also helps diagnose right ventricular infarctions; locate true posterior infarctions; assess trauma, ventricular aneurysm, and heart tumors; and detect myocardial damage from a recent electric shock such as defibrillation.

In this test, the patient receives an injection of ^{99m}Tc pyrophosphate, a radioactive material absorbed by injured cells. A scintillation camera scans the heart and displays damaged areas as "hot spots" or bright areas. A spot's size usually corresponds to the injury size.

NURSING CONSIDERATIONS
- Tell the patient that the practitioner will inject ^{99m}Tc pyrophosphate into an arm vein about 3 hours before the start of this

UNDERSTANDING THALLIUM SCANNING

In thallium scanning, areas with poor blood flow and ischemic cells fail to take up the isotope (thallium-201 or Cardiolite) and thus appear as cold spots on a scan. Thallium imaging should show normal distribution of the isotope throughout the left ventricle with no defects (cold spots).

What resting reveals

To distinguish normal from infarcted myocardial tissue, the practitioner may order an exercise thallium scan followed by a resting perfusion scan. A resting perfusion scan helps differentiate between an ischemic area and an infarcted or scarred area of the myocardium. Ischemic myocardium appears as a reversible defect (the cold spot disappears). Infarcted myocardium shows up as a nonreversible defect (the cold spot remains).

45-minute test. Reassure him that the injection causes only transient discomfort and that it involves only negligible radiation exposure.

- Instruct the patient to remain still during the test.
- Permit the patient to resume activities, as indicated.

Thallium scanning

Also known as *cold spot imaging,* thallium scanning evaluates myocardial blood flow and myocardial cell status. This test helps determine areas of ischemic myocardium and infarcted tissue. It can also help evaluate coronary artery and ventricular function as well as pericardial effusion. Thallium imaging can also detect a myocardial infarction in its first few hours. (See *Understanding thallium scanning.*)

The test uses thallium-201, a radioactive isotope that emits gamma rays and closely resembles potassium. When injected I.V., the isotope enters healthy myocardial tissue rapidly but enters areas with poor blood flow and damaged cells slowly. A camera counts the gamma rays and displays an image. Areas with heavy isotope uptake appear light, whereas areas with poor uptake, known as "cold spots," look dark. Cold spots represent areas of reduced myocardial perfusion.

NURSING CONSIDERATIONS

- Tell the patient to avoid heavy meals, cigarette smoking, and strenuous activity for 24 hours before the test.

■ If your patient is scheduled for an exercise thallium scan, advise him to wear comfortable clothes or pajamas and snug-fitting shoes or slippers.

■ After the procedure, permit the patient to resume activities, as indicated.

Doppler ultrasonography

Doppler ultrasonography evaluates blood flow in the major blood vessels of the arms and legs and in the extracranial cerebrovascular system. A handheld transducer directs high-frequency sound waves to the artery or vein being tested.

The sound waves strike moving red blood cells and are reflected back to the transducer at frequencies that correspond to blood flow velocity through the vessel. The transducer then amplifies the sound waves to permit direct listening and graphic recording of blood flow. Measurement of systolic pressure helps detects the presence, location, and extent of peripheral arterial occlusive disease.

Pulse volume recorder testing may be performed along with Doppler ultrasonography to yield a quantitative recording of changes in blood volume or flow in an extremity or organ. (See *Measuring the ankle-brachial index,* pages 138 and 139.)

Normally, venous blood flow fluctuates with respiration, so observing changes in sound wave frequency during respiration helps detect venous occlusive disease. Compression maneuvers can also help detect occlusion of the veins as well as occlusion or stenosis of carotid arteries. Abnormal images and Doppler signals may indicate plaque, stenosis, occlusion, dissection, aneurysm, carotid body tumor, and arteritis.

NURSING CONSIDERATIONS

■ Explain the test to the patient, and tell him that it takes about 20 minutes.

■ Check with the vascular laboratory to determine whether special equipment will be used and whether special instructions are necessary.

■ Water-soluble conductive gel is applied to the tip of the transducer to provide coupling between the skin and the transducer.

Venography of the leg

Also known as *ascending contrast phlebography,* a venography is a radiographic examination of veins in the lower extremity that's commonly used to assess the condition of the deep leg veins after injection of a contrast medium.

MEASURING THE ANKLE-BRACHIAL INDEX

A Doppler ultrasound device can also be used to measure ankle-brachial index (ABI) to help identify peripheral vascular disease. To perform this test, follow these steps.

- Explain the procedure to the patient.
- Gather your materials.
- Wash your hands.
- Apply warm conductivity gel to the patient's arm where the brachial pulse has been palpated and then obtain the systolic reading.

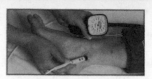

- Locate the dorsalis pedis pulse and repeat the procedure.

- Use the chart below to calculate the ABI. Document your findings.

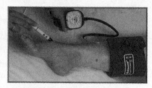

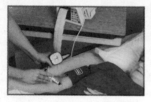

- Locate the posterior tibial pulse and repeat the procedure, recording your reading.

Calculating ABI

To calculate ABI, divide the higher systolic pressure obtained for each leg (dorsalis pedis or posterior tibial) by the higher brachial systolic pressure.

SAMPLE SYSTOLIC READINGS (MM HG)	LEFT	RIGHT
Posterior tibial	128	96
Dorsalis pedis	130	90
Brachial	132	130
Calculations	130 ÷ 132 = 0.98	96 ÷ 132 = 0.73

MEASURING THE ANKLE-BRACHIAL INDEX *(continued)*

What the results mean

- Greater than 1.3: Unreliable and in-conclusive; possibly false-high readings produced by calcified vessels (such as occurs in diabetes)
- 1.01 to 1.3: Correlates with patient history (especially in diabetes)

- 0.97 to 1: Normal
- 0.8 to 0.96: Mild ischemia
- 0.4 to 0.79: Moderate to severe ischemia
- 0.39 or less: Severe ischemia; danger of limb loss

This procedure isn't used for routine screening because it exposes the patient to relatively high doses of radiation and can cause such complications as phlebitis, local tissue damage and, occasionally, deep vein thrombosis (DVT). It's used in patients whose duplex ultrasound findings are unclear.

NURSING CONSIDERATIONS

- Make sure the patient has signed an appropriate consent form.
- Note and report allergies.
- Check the patient's history for and report hypersensitivity to iodine, iodine-containing foods, or contrast media.
- Reassure the patient that contrast media complications are rare, but tell him to report nausea, severe burning or itching, constriction in the throat, or dyspnea at once.
- Discontinue anticoagulation therapy, as indicated.
- Administer sedation indicated.
- Instruct the patient to restrict food and to drink only clear liquids for 4 hours before the test.
- Warn the patient that he might experience a burning sensation in the leg when the contrast medium is injected as well as some discomfort during the procedure.
- If DVT is documented, initiate therapy (heparin infusion, bed rest, leg elevation or support) as indicated.

Treatments

Many treatments are available for patients with cardiovascular disease. The dramatic ones, such as heart transplantation and artificial heart insertion, have received a lot of publicity. However, some more commonly used treatment measures include:

- drug therapy
- surgery
- balloon catheter treatments
- defibrillation
- synchronized cardioversion
- pacemaker insertion.

DRUG THERAPY

Types of drugs used to improve cardiovascular function include:

- cardiac glycosides and phosphodiesterase (PDE) inhibitors
- antiarrhythmics
- antianginals
- antihypertensives
- diuretics
- adrenergics
- beta-adrenergic receptor blockers
- antilipemics.

Cardiac glycosides and PDE inhibitors

Cardiac glycosides and PDE inhibitors increase the force of the heart's contractions. Increasing the force of contractions is known as a *positive inotropic effect,* so these drugs are also called *inotropic drugs* (affecting the force or energy of muscular contractions). (See *Understanding cardiac glycosides and PDE inhibitors.*)

UNDERSTANDING CARDIAC GLYCOSIDES AND PDE INHIBITORS

Cardiac glycosides and phosphodiesterase (PDE) inhibitors have a positive inotropic effect on the heart, meaning they increase the force of contraction. Use this table to learn about the indications, adverse reactions, and nursing considerations associated with these drugs.

DRUGS	INDICATIONS	ADVERSE REACTIONS	NURSING CONSIDERATIONS
CARDIAC GLYCOSIDE			
Digoxin (Lanoxin)	Heart failure, supraventricular arrhythmias	● Digoxin toxicity (nausea, abdominal pain, headache, irritability, depression, insomnia, vision disturbances, arrhythmias) ● Arrhythmias ● Anorexia	● If immediate effects are required (as with a supraventricular arrhythmia), a loading dose of digoxin is required. ● Check apical pulse for 1 minute before administration; withhold drug and report pulse less than 60 beats/minute. ● Therapeutic levels are 0.5 to 2 ng/ml.
PDE INHIBITORS			
Inamrinone, milrinone (Primacor)	Heart failure refractory to digoxin, diuretics, and vasodilators	● Arrhythmias ● Nausea ● Vomiting ● Headache ● Fever ● Chest pain ● Hypokalemia ● Thrombocytopenia	● These drugs are contraindicated in patients in the acute phase of myocardial infarction (MI) and after an MI. ● Serum potassium levels should be within normal limits before and during therapy.

Cardiac glycosides, such as digoxin (Lanoxin), also slow the heart rate (called a *negative chronotropic effect*) and slow electrical impulse conduction through the atrioventricular (AV) node (called a *negative dromotropic effect*).

PDE inhibitors, such as inamrinone and milrinone (Primacor), are typically used for short-term management of heart failure or long-term management in patients awaiting heart transplant surgery. PDE inhibitors improve cardiac output by strengthening contractions. These drugs are thought to help move calcium into the cardiac cell or to increase calcium storage in the sarcoplasmic reticulum. By directly relaxing vascular smooth muscle, they also decrease peripheral vascular resistance (afterload) and the amount of blood returning to the heart (preload).

Antiarrhythmics

Antiarrhythmics are used to treat arrhythmias, which are disturbances of the normal heart rhythm. (See *Understanding antiarrhythmics.*)

Unfortunately, many antiarrhythmics can worsen or cause arrhythmias, too. In any case, the benefits of antiarrhythmic therapy need to be weighed against its risks.

Antiarrhythmics are categorized into four major classes: I (which includes IA, IB, and IC), II, III, and IV. The mechanisms of action of antiarrhythmics vary widely, and a few drugs exhibit properties common to more than one class. One drug, adenosine (Adenocard), doesn't fall into any of these classes.

CLASS I ANTIARRHYTHMICS

Class I antiarrhythmics are sodium channel blockers. This is the largest group of antiarrhythmic drugs. Class I drugs are commonly subdivided into classes IA, IB, and IC. With the development of many newer drugs, the use of this class of antiarrhythmics is decreasing.

Class IA antiarrhythmics

Class IA antiarrhythmics control arrhythmias by altering the myocardial cell membrane and interfering with autonomic nervous system control of pacemaker cells. Class IA antiarrhythmics include:
- disopyramide (Norpace)
- procainamide (Procanbid)
- quinidine sulfate (Quinidex)
- quinidine gluconate (Quinaglute).

Class IA antiarrhythmics also block parasympathetic stimulation of the sinoatrial (SA) and AV nodes. Because stimulation of the parasympathetic nervous system causes the heart rate to slow down, drugs that block the parasympathetic nervous system increase the AV node's conduction rate.

This increase in the conduction rate can produce dangerous increases in the ventricular heart rate if rapid atrial activity is present, as in a patient with atrial fibrillation. In turn, the increased ventricular heart rate can offset the ability of the antiarrhythmics to convert atrial arrhythmias to a regular rhythm.

UNDERSTANDING ANTIARRHYTHMICS

Antiarrhythmics are used to restore normal heart rhythm in patients with arrhythmias. Check this table for information about the indications, adverse reactions, and nursing considerations associated with these drugs.

DRUGS	INDICATIONS	ADVERSE REACTIONS	NURSING CONSIDERATIONS
CLASS IA ANTIARRHYTHMICS			
Disopyramide (Norpace), procainamide (Procanbid), quinidine sulfate (Quinidex), quinidine gluconate (Quinaglute)	● Ventricular tachycardia ● Atrial fibrillation ● Atrial flutter ● Paroxysmal atrial tachycardia	● Diarrhea ● Nausea ● Vomiting ● Arrhythmias ● Electrocardiogram (ECG) changes ● Hepatotoxicity ● Respiratory arrest	● Check apical pulse rate before therapy. If you note extremes in pulse rate, hold the dose and notify the practitioner. ● Use cautiously in patients with asthma.
CLASS IB ANTIARRHYTHMICS			
Lidocaine (Xylocaine), mexiletine (Mexitil)	● Ventricular tachycardia, ventricular fibrillation	● Drowsiness ● Hypotension ● Bradycardia ● Arrhythmias ● Widened QRS complex	● IB antiarrhythmics may potentiate the effects of other antiarrhythmics. ● Administer I.V. infusions using an infusion pump.
CLASS IC ANTIARRHYTHMICS			
Flecainide (Tambocor), moricizine (Ethmozine), propafenone (Rythmol)	● Ventricular tachycardia, ventricular fibrillation, supraventricular arrhythmias	● New arrhythmias ● Heart failure ● Cardiac death	● Correct electrolyte imbalances before giving. ● Monitor the patient's ECG before and after dosage adjustments.

(continued)

UNDERSTANDING ANTIARRHYTHMICS *(continued)*

DRUGS	INDICATIONS	ADVERSE REACTIONS	NURSING CONSIDERATIONS
CLASS II ANTIARRHYTHMICS			
Acebutolol (Sectral), esmolol (Brevibloc), propranolol (Inderal)	● Atrial flutter, atrial fibrillation, paroxysmal atrial tachycardia ● Ventricular arrhythmias	● Arrhythmias ● Bradycardia ● Heart failure ● Hypotension ● Nausea and vomiting ● Bronchospasm	● Monitor apical heart rate and blood pressure. ● Abruptly stopping these drugs can exacerbate angina and precipitate myocardial infarction.
CLASS III ANTIARRHYTHMICS			
Amiodarone (Cordarone), ibutilide fumarate (Corvert)	● Life-threatening arrhythmias resistant to other antiarrhythmics	● Aggravation of arrhythmias ● Hypotension ● Anorexia ● Severe pulmonary toxicity (amiodarone) ● Hepatic dysfunction	● Amiodarone increases the risk of digoxin toxicity in patients also taking digoxin. ● Monitor blood pressure and heart rate and rhythm for changes. ● Monitor for signs of pulmonary toxicity (dyspnea, nonproductive cough, and pleuritic chest pain) in patient taking amiodarone.
CLASS IV ANTIARRHYTHMICS			
Diltiazem (Cardizem), verapamil (Calan)	● Supraventricular arrhythmias	● Peripheral edema ● Hypotension ● Bradycardia ● Atrioventricular block ● Flushing (with diltiazem) ● Heart failure ● Pulmonary edema	● Monitor heart rate and rhythm and blood pressure carefully when initiating therapy or increasing dose. ● Calcium supplements may reduce effectiveness.

UNDERSTANDING ANTIARRHYTHMICS *(continued)*

DRUGS	INDICATIONS	ADVERSE REACTIONS	NURSING CONSIDERATIONS
MISCELLANEOUS			
Adenosine (Adenocard)	• Paroxysmal supraventricular tachycardia	• Facial flushing • Shortness of breath • Dyspnea • Chest discomfort	• Adenosine must be given over 1 to 2 seconds, followed by a 20 ml flush of normal saline solution. • Record rhythm strip during administration.

Class IB antiarrhythmics

Lidocaine (Xylocaine), a class IB antiarrhythmic, is one of the antiarrhythmics commonly used in treating patients with acute ventricular arrhythmias. Other IB antiarrhythmics include mexiletine (Mexitil).

Class IB drugs work by blocking the rapid influx of sodium ions during the depolarization phase of the heart's depolarization-repolarization cycle, resulting in a decreased refractory period, which reduces the risk of arrhythmia.

Because class IB antiarrhythmics especially affect the Purkinje fibers (fibers in the heart's conducting system) and myocardial cells in the ventricles, they're used only in treating patients with ventricular arrhythmias.

Class IC antiarrhythmics

Class IC antiarrhythmics are used to treat patients with certain severe, refractory (resistant) ventricular arrhythmias. Class IC antiarrhythmics include flecainide (Tambocor), moricizine (Ethmozine), and propafenone (Rythmol).

Class IC antiarrhythmics primarily slow conduction along the heart's conduction system. Moricizine decreases the fast inward current of sodium ions of the action potential. This depresses the depolarization rate and effective refractory period.

CLASS II ANTIARRHYTHMICS

Class II antiarrhythmics include the beta-adrenergic antagonists, also known as *beta-adrenergic receptor blockers*. Beta-adrenergic receptor blockers used as antiarrhythmics include:

- acebutolol (Sectral)
- esmolol (Brevibloc)
- propranolol (Inderal).

Class II antiarrhythmics block beta-adrenergic receptor sites in the heart's conduction system. As a result, the SA node's ability to fire spontaneously (automaticity) is slowed. The ability of the AV node and other cells to receive and conduct an electrical impulse to nearby cells (conductivity) is also reduced.

Class II antiarrhythmics also reduce the strength of the heart's contractions. When the heart beats less forcefully, it doesn't require as much oxygen to do its work.

CLASS III ANTIARRHYTHMICS

Class III antiarrhythmics are used to treat patients with ventricular arrhythmias. Amiodarone (Cordarone) is the most widely used class III antiarrhythmic.

Although the exact mechanism of action isn't known, class III antiarrhythmics are thought to suppress arrhythmias by converting a unidirectional block to a bidirectional block. They have little or no effect on depolarization.

CLASS IV ANTIARRHYTHMICS

The class IV antiarrhythmics include the calcium channel blockers. These drugs block the movement of calcium during phase 2 of the action potential and slow conduction and the refractory period of calcium-dependent tissues, including the AV node. The calcium channel blockers used to treat patients with arrhythmias are verapamil (Calan) and diltiazem (Cardizem).

ADENOSINE

Adenosine is an injectable antiarrhythmic drug indicated for acute treatment for paroxysmal supraventricular tachycardia. Adenosine depresses the pacemaker activity of the SA node, reducing the heart rate and the AV node's ability to conduct impulses for the atria to the ventricles.

Antianginals

When the heart's oxygen demand exceeds the amount of oxygen being supplied, areas of heart muscle become ischemic. When the heart muscle is ischemic, a person experiences chest pain. This condition is known as *angina* or *angina pectoris*.

Although angina's cardinal symptom is chest pain, the drugs used to treat angina aren't typically analgesics. Instead, antianginal drugs

HOW ANTIANGINALS WORK

When the coronary arteries can't supply enough oxygen to the myocardium, angina occurs. This forces the heart to work harder, increasing heart rate, preload, afterload, and the force of myocardial contractility. Antianginals relieve angina by decreasing one or more of these four factors.

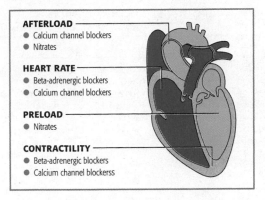

AFTERLOAD
- Calcium channel blockers
- Nitrates

HEART RATE
- Beta-adrenergic blockers
- Calcium channel blockers

PRELOAD
- Nitrates

CONTRACTILITY
- Beta-adrenergic blockers
- Calcium channel blockerss

correct angina by reducing myocardial oxygen demand (the amount of oxygen the heart needs to do its work, increasing the supply of oxygen to the heart, or both. (See *How antianginals work.*)

The three classes of commonly used antianginals include:
- nitrates (for acute angina)
- beta-adrenergic receptor blockers (for long-term prevention of angina)
- calcium channel blockers (used when other drugs fail to prevent angina). (See *Understanding antianginals,* pages 148 and 149.)

NITRATES
Nitrates are the drug of choice for relieving acute angina. Nitrates commonly prescribed to correct angina include:
- isosorbide dinitrate (Isordil)
- isosorbide mononitrate (Imdur)
- nitroglycerin (Nitro-Bid).

Nitrates cause the smooth muscle of the veins and, to a lesser extent, the arteries to relax and dilate. This is what happens:
- When the veins dilate, less blood returns to the heart.

UNDERSTANDING ANTIANGINALS

Antianginal drugs are effective in treating patients with angina because they reduce myocardial oxygen demand, increase the supply of oxygen to the heart, or both. Use this table to learn about the indications, adverse reactions, and nursing considerations associated with these drugs.

DRUGS	INDICATIONS	ADVERSE REACTIONS	NURSING CONSIDERATIONS
NITRATES			
Isosorbide dinitrate (Isordil), isosorbide mononitrate (Imdur), nitroglycerin (Nitro-Bid)	● Relief and prevention of angina	● Headache ● Hypotension ● Dizziness ● Increased heart rate	● Only sublingual and translingual forms should be used to treat an acute angina attack. ● Monitor the patient's blood pressure before and after administration. ● Avoid giving nitrates to patients taking erectile dysfunction drugs because of the risk of severe hypotension.
BETA-ADRENERGIC RECEPTOR BLOCKERS			
Atenolol (Tenormin), Carvedilol (Coreg), metoprolol (Lopressor), propranolol (Inderal)	● Long-term prevention of angina ● First-line therapy for hypertension ● Stable heart failure due to decreased left ventricle ejection fraction	● Bradycardia ● Fainting ● Fluid retention ● Heart failure ● Arrhythmias ● Nausea ● Diarrhea ● Atrioventricular blocks ● Bronchospasm ● Hypoglycemia	● Monitor apical pulse rate before giving. Monitor blood pressure, electrocardiogram, and heart rate and rhythm frequently. ● Signs of hypoglycemic shock may be masked; watch diabetic patients for sweating, fatigue, and hunger. ● Monitor patients with a history of respiratory problems for breathing difficulty if using a nonselective beta-adrenergic receptor blocker.

UNDERSTANDING ANTIANGINALS *(continued)*

DRUGS	INDICATIONS	ADVERSE REACTIONS	NURSING CONSIDERATIONS
CALCIUM CHANNEL BLOCKERS			
Amlodipine (Norvasc), diltiazem (Cardizem), nifedipine (Adalat), verapamil (Calan)	● Long-term prevention of angina (especially Prinzmetal's angina) ● Hypertension	● Orthostatic hypotension ● Heart failure ● Hypotension ● Arrhythmias ● Dizziness ● Headache ● Persistent peripheral edema ● Pulmonary edema	● Monitor cardiac rate and rhythm and blood pressure carefully when initiating therapy or increasing the dose. ● Calcium supplementation may decrease the effects of calcium channel blockers.

■ This, in turn, reduces the amount of blood in the ventricles at the end of diastole, when the ventricles are full. (This blood volume in the ventricles just before contraction is called *preload*).

■ By reducing preload, nitrates reduce ventricular size and ventricular wall tension so the left ventricle doesn't have to stretch as much to pump blood. This, in turn, reduces the heart's oxygen requirements.

■ As the coronary arteries dilate, more blood is delivered to the myocardium, improving oxygenation of the ischemic tissue.

The arterioles provide the most resistance to the blood pumped by the left ventricle (called *peripheral vascular resistance*). Nitrates decrease afterload by dilating the arterioles, reducing resistance, easing the heart's workload, and easing oxygen demand.

BETA-ADRENERGIC RECEPTOR BLOCKERS

Beta-adrenergic receptor blockers are used for long-term prevention of angina, and they're one of the main types of drugs used to treat hypertension. Beta-adrenergic receptor blockers include:

■ atenolol (Tenormin)
■ carvedilol (Coreg)
■ metoprolol tartrate (Lopressor)
■ propranolol (Inderal)

Beta-adrenergic receptor blockers decrease blood pressure and block beta-adrenergic receptor sites in the heart muscle and conduction system. Decreasing the heart rate and reducing the force of the heart's contractions result in a lower demand for oxygen.

CALCIUM CHANNEL BLOCKERS

Calcium channel blockers are commonly used to prevent angina that doesn't respond to drugs in either of the other antianginal classes. Some calcium channel blockers are also used as antiarrhythmics.

Calcium channel blockers include:

- amlodipine (Norvasc)
- diltiazem (Cardizem)
- nifedipine (Adalat)
- verapamil (Calan).

Calcium channel blockers prevent the passage of calcium ions across the myocardial cell membrane and vascular smooth-muscle cells. This causes dilation of the coronary and peripheral arteries, which decreases the force of the heart's contraction and reduces the heart's workload.

By preventing arterioles from constriction, calcium channel blockers also reduce afterload. In addition, decreasing afterload decreases the heart's oxygen demands.

Calcium channel blockers also reduce the heart rate by slowing conduction through the SA and AV nodes. A slower heart rate reduces the heart's need for oxygen.

Antihypertensives

Antihypertensives, which reduce blood pressure, are used in patients with hypertension, a disorder characterized by high systolic blood pressure, diastolic blood pressure, or both.

Treatment for hypertension begins with beta-adrenergic receptor blockers and diuretics. (See *Treating hypertension*.) If those drugs aren't effective, treatment continues with sympatholytic drugs (other than beta-adrenergic receptor blockers), vasodilators, angiotensin-converting enzyme (ACE) inhibitors, angiotensin receptor blockers (ARBs), or a combination of drugs. (See *Understanding antihypertensives,* pages 152 and 153.)

Sympatholytics

The sympatholytics include several types of drugs but work by inhibiting or blocking the sympathetic nervous system, which causes dilation of the peripheral blood vessels or decreases cardiac output, thereby reducing blood pressure.

(Text continues on page 154.)

TREATING HYPERTENSION

Below is a flowchart for treating hypertension based on the recommendations of the Joint National Committee on the Detection, Evaluation, and Treatment of High Blood Pressure.

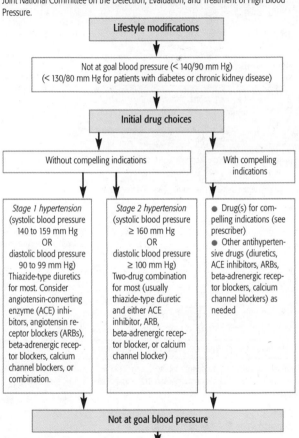

Lifestyle modifications

↓

Not at goal blood pressure (< 140/90 mm Hg)
(< 130/80 mm Hg for patients with diabetes or chronic kidney disease)

↓

Initial drug choices

Without compelling indications

With compelling indications

Stage 1 hypertension
(systolic blood pressure 140 to 159 mm Hg
OR
diastolic blood pressure 90 to 99 mm Hg)
Thiazide-type diuretics for most. Consider angiotensin-converting enzyme (ACE) inhibitors, angiotensin receptor blockers (ARBs), beta-adrenergic receptor blockers, calcium channel blockers, or combination.

Stage 2 hypertension
(systolic blood pressure ≥ 160 mm Hg
OR
diastolic blood pressure ≥ 100 mm Hg)
Two-drug combination for most (usually thiazide-type diuretic and either ACE inhibitor, ARB, beta-adrenergic receptor blocker, or calcium channel blocker)

● Drug(s) for compelling indications (see prescriber)
● Other antihypertensive drugs (diuretics, ACE inhibitors, ARBs, beta-adrenergic receptor blockers, calcium channel blockers) as needed

Not at goal blood pressure

↓

● Optimize dosages or add additional drugs until goal blood pressure is achieved.
● Consider consultation with hypertension specialist.

UNDERSTANDING ANTIHYPERTENSIVES

Antihypertensives are prescribed to reduce blood pressure in patients with hypertension.
Use this table to learn about the indications, adverse reactions, and nursing considerations
associated with these drugs.

DRUGS	INDICATIONS
SYMPATHOLYTIC DRUGS	
Central-acting sympathetic nervous system inhibitors (such as clonidine [Catapres], guanabenz [Wytensin], guanfacine [Tenex], and methyldopa)	● Hypertension
Alpha blockers (such as doxazosin [Cardura], phentolamine [Regitine], prazosin [Minipress], and terazosin [Hytrin])	
Mixed alpha- and beta-adrenergic receptor blockers (such as labetalol [Normodyne])	
Norepinephrine depletors (such as guanadrel [Hylorel])	
VASODILATORS	
Diazoxide (Hyperstat I.V.), hydralazine (Apresoline) , minoxidil, nitroprusside (Nitropress)	● Used in combination with other drugs to treat moderate to severe hypertension ● Hypertensive crisis
ANGIOTENSIN-CONVERTING ENZYME (ACE) INHIBITORS	
Benazepril (Lotensin), captopril (Capoten), enalapril (Vasotec), lisinopril (Prinivil), quinapril (Accupril), ramipril (Altace)	● Hypertension ● Heart failure
ANGIOTENSIN II RECEPTOR BLOCKERS	
Candesartan (Atacand), irbesartan (Avapro), losartan (Cozaar), olmesartan (Benicar), valsartan (Diovan)	● Hypertension ● Heart failure resistant to ACE inhibitors

ADVERSE REACTIONS	NURSING CONSIDERATIONS
● Hypotension (alpha blockers) ● Depression ● Drowsiness ● Edema ● Vertigo (central-acting drugs) ● Bradycardia ● Hepatic necrosis ● Arrhythmias	● Monitor blood pressure and pulse before and after administration.
● Tachycardia ● Palpitations ● Angina ● Fatigue ● Headache ● Severe pericardial effusion ● Hepatotoxicity ● Nausea ● Stevens-Johnson syndrome	● Monitor blood pressure and pulse before and after administration. ● Monitor patient receiving nitroprusside for signs of cyanide toxicity.
● Angioedema ● Persistent cough ● Rash ● Renal insufficiency	● Monitor blood pressure and pulse before and after administration.
● Fatigue ● Abdominal pain ● Rash ● Hypotension	● Monitor blood pressure and pulse before and after administration.

The sympatholytic drugs are classified by their site or mechanisms of action and include:

- central-acting sympathetic nervous system inhibitors, such as clonidine (Catapres), guanabenz (Wytensin), guanfacine (Tenex), and methyldopa (Aldomet)
- alpha blockers, such as doxazosin (Cardura), phentolamine (Regitine), prazosin (Minipress), and terazosin (Hytrin)
- mixed alpha- and beta-adrenergic receptor blockers such as labetalol (Normodyne)
- norepinephrine depletors such as guanadrel (Hylorel).

Vasodilators

The two types of vasodilators include calcium channel blockers and direct vasodilators. Theses drugs decrease systolic and diastolic blood pressure.

Calcium channel blockers produce arteriolar relaxation by preventing the entry of calcium into the cells. This prevents the contraction of vascular smooth muscle.

Direct vasodilators act on arteries, veins, or both. They work by relaxing peripheral vascular smooth muscles, causing the blood vessels to dilate. This decreases blood pressure by increasing the diameter of the blood vessels, reducing total peripheral resistance.

The direct vasodilators include:

- hydralazine (Apresoline)
- minoxidil (Loniten)
- diazoxide (Hyperstat I.V.)
- nitroprusside (Nipride).

Hydralazine and minoxidil are usually used to treat patients with resistant and refractory hypertension. Diazoxide and nitroprusside are reserved for use in hypertensive crisis.

ACE inhibitors

ACE inhibitors reduce blood pressure by interrupting the renin-angiotensin-aldosterone system (RAAS). (See *Antihypertensives and the RAAS.*)

Commonly prescribed ACE inhibitors include:

- benazepril (Lotensin)
- captopril (Capoten)
- enalapril (Vasotec)
- lisinopril (Prinivil)
- quinapril (Accupril)
- ramipril (Altace).

Here's how the RAAS works:

ANTIHYPERTENSIVES AND THE RAAS

The renin-angiotensin-aldosterone system (RAAS) regulates the body's sodium and water levels and blood pressure.

1. Juxtaglomerular cells near the glomeruli in each kidney secrete the enzyme renin into the blood.

2. Renin circulates throughout the body and converts angiotensinogen, made in the liver, to angiotensin I.

3. In the lungs, angiotensin I is converted by hydrolysis to angiotensin II.

4. Angiotensin II acts on the adrenal cortex to stimulate production of the hormone aldosterone. Aldosterone acts on the juxtaglomerular cells to increase sodium and water retention and to stimulate or depress further renin secretion, completing the feedback system that automatically readjusts homeostasis.

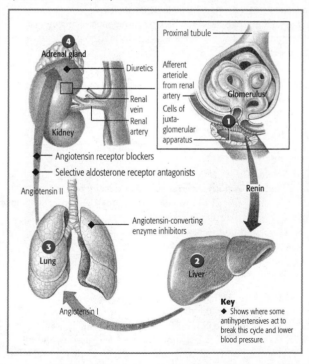

Key
◆ Shows where some antihypertensives act to break this cycle and lower blood pressure.

- Normally, the kidneys maintain blood pressure by releasing the hormone renin.
- Renin acts on the plasma protein angiotensinogen to form angiotensin I.
- Angiotensin I is then converted to angiotensin II.
- Angiotensin II, a potent vasoconstrictor, increases peripheral resistance and promotes the excretion of aldosterone.
- Aldosterone, in turn, promotes the retention of sodium and water, increasing the volume of blood the heart needs to pump.

ACE inhibitors work by preventing the conversion of angiotensin I to angiotensin II. As angiotensin II is reduced, arterioles dilate, reducing peripheral vascular resistance.

By reducing aldosterone secretion, ACE inhibitors promote the excretion of sodium and water, reducing the amount of blood the heart needs to pump, resulting in a lowered blood pressure.

ANGIOTENSIN II RECEPTOR BLOCKERS

Unlike ACE inhibitors, which prevent production of angiotensin, ARBs inhibit the action of angiotensin II by attaching to tissue-binding receptor sites.

Commonly prescribed ARBs include:
- candesartan (Atacand)
- irbesartan (Avapro)
- losartan (Cozaar)
- olmesartan (Benicar)
- valsartan (Diovan).

Diuretics

Diuretics are used to promote the excretion of water and electrolytes by the kidneys. By doing so, diuretics play a major role in treating hypertension and other cardiovascular conditions. (See *Understanding diuretics*.)

The major diuretics used as cardiovascular drugs include:
- thiazide and thiazide-like diuretics
- loop diuretics
- potassium-sparing diuretics.

THIAZIDE AND THIAZIDE-LIKE DIURETICS

Thiazide and thiazide-like diuretics are sulfonamide derivatives. Thiazide diuretics include bendroflumethiazide (Naturetin), hydrochlorothiazide (HydroDIURIL), hydroflumethiazide (Saluron), and methyclothiazide (Enduron). Thiazide-like diuretics include chlorthalidone (Hygroton) and indapamide (Lozol).

UNDERSTANDING DIURETICS

Diuretics are used to treat patients with various cardiovascular conditions. They work by promoting the excretion of water and electrolytes by the kidneys. Use this table to learn about the indications, adverse reactions, and nursing considerations associated with these drugs.

DRUGS	INDICATIONS	ADVERSE REACTIONS	NURSING CONSIDERATIONS
THIAZIDE AND THIAZIDE-LIKE DIURETICS			
Bendroflume-thiazide (Naturetin), chlorthali-done (Hygroton), hydrochloro-thiazide (HydroDIURIL), hydroflume-thiazide (Saluron), indapamide (Lozol), methyclothiazide (Enduron)	● Hypertension ● Edema	● Hypokalemia ● Orthostatic hypotension ● Hyponatremia ● Dizziness ● Nausea	● Monitor potassium level. ● Monitor intake and output. ● Monitor glucose level in diabetic patients. Thiazide diuretics can cause hyperglycemia.
LOOP DIURETICS			
Bumetanide (Bumex), ethacrynic acid (Edecrin), furosemide (Lasix)	● Hypertension ● Heart failure ● Edema	● Dehydration ● Orthostatic hypotension ● Hyperuricemia ● Hypokalemia ● Hyponatremia ● Dizziness ● Muscle cramps ● Rash	● Monitor for signs of excess diuresis (hypotension, tachycardia, poor skin turgor, and excessive thirst). ● Monitor blood pressure, heart rate, and intake and output. ● Monitor electrolyte levels.

(continued)

UNDERSTANDING DIURETICS *(continued)*

DRUGS	INDICATIONS	ADVERSE REACTIONS	NURSING CONSIDERATIONS
POTASSIUM-SPARING DIURETICS			
Amiloride (Midamor), spironolactone (Aldactone), triamterene (Dyrenium)	● Edema ● Diuretic-induced hypokalemia in patients with heart failure ● Cirrhosis ● Nephrotic syndrome ● Hypertension	● Hyperkalemia ● Headache ● Nausea ● Rash	● Monitor electrocardiogram for arrhythmias. ● Monitor potassium levels. ● Monitor intake and output.

Thiazide and thiazide-like diuretics work by preventing sodium from being reabsorbed in the kidneys. As sodium is excreted, it pulls water along with it. Thiazide and thiazide-like diuretics also increase the excretion of chloride, potassium, and bicarbonate, which can result in electrolyte imbalances.

Initially, these drugs decrease circulating blood volume, leading to a reduced cardiac output. However, if the therapy is maintained, cardiac output stabilizes, but plasma fluid volume decreases.

LOOP DIURETICS

Loop (high-ceiling) diuretics are highly potent drugs. They include:

- bumetanide (Bumex)
- ethacrynic acid (Edecrin)
- furosemide (Lasix).

The loop diuretics are the most potent diuretics available, producing the greatest volume of diuresis (urine production). They also have a high potential for causing severe adverse reactions.

Bumetanide is the shortest-acting diuretic. It's even 40 times more potent than another loop diuretic, furosemide.

Loop diuretics receive their name because they act primarily on the thick ascending loop of Henle (the part of the nephron responsible for concentrating urine) to increase the secretion of sodium, chloride, and water. These drugs may also inhibit sodium, chloride, and water reabsorption.

POTASSIUM-SPARING DIURETICS

Potassium-sparing diuretics have weaker diuretic and antihypertensive effects than other diuretics, but they have the advantage of conserving potassium.

The potassium-sparing diuretics include:

- amiloride (Midamor)
- spironolactone (Aldactone)
- triamterene (Dyrenium).

The direct action of the potassium-sparing diuretics on the distal tubule of the kidney produces:

- increased urinary excretion of sodium and water
- increased excretion of chloride and calcium ion
- decreased excretion of potassium and hydrogen ion.

These effects lead to reduced blood pressure and increased serum potassium levels.

Spironolactone, one of the main potassium-sparing diuretics, is structurally similar to aldosterone and acts as an aldosterone antagonist.

Aldosterone promotes the retention of sodium and water and loss of potassium; spironolactone counteracts these effects by competing with aldosterone for receptor sites. As a result, sodium, chloride, and water are excreted, and potassium is retained.

Anticoagulants

Anticoagulants are used to reduce the blood's ability to clot. (See *Understanding anticoagulants,* pages 160 and 161.) Major categories of anticoagulants include:

- heparin
- factor Xa inhibitors
- oral anticoagulants
- antiplatelet drugs.

HEPARIN

Heparin, prepared commercially from animal tissue, is used to prevent clot formation. Low-molecular-weight heparin, such as dalteparin (Fragmin) and enoxaparin (Lovenox), prevents deep vein thrombosis (a blood clot in the deep veins, usually of the legs) in surgical patients.

Because it doesn't affect the synthesis of clotting factors, heparin can't dissolve already formed clots. It does prevent the formation of new thrombi, though. Here's how it works:

- Heparin inhibits the formation of thrombin and fibrin by activating antithrombin III.

UNDERSTANDING ANTICOAGULANTS

Anticoagulants reduce the blood's ability to clot and are included in the treatment plans for many patients with cardiovascular disorders. Use this table to learn about the indications, adverse reactions, and nursing considerations associated with these drugs.

DRUGS	INDICATIONS	ADVERSE REACTIONS	NURSING CONSIDERATIONS
HEPARINS			
Heparin and low-molecular-weight heparins, such as dalteparin (Fragmin) and enoxaparin (Lovenox)	● Deep vein thrombosis (prevention and treatment) ● Embolism prophylaxis ● Disseminated intravascular coagulation (heparin) ● Prevention of complications after myocardial infarction (MI)	● Bleeding ● Hemorrhage ● Thrombocytopenia	● Monitor thromboplastin time; the therapeutic range is 1½ to 2½ times the control. ● Monitor the patient for signs of bleeding. ● Concomitant administration with nonsteroidal anti-inflammatory drugs, iron dextran, or an antiplatelet drug increases the risk of bleeding. ● Protamine sulfate reverses the effects of heparin.
FACTOR XA INHIBITORS			
Fondaparinux (Arixtra)	● Deep vein thrombosis (prevention and treatment) ● acute pulmonary embolism	● Hemorrhage ● Thrombocytopenia ● Nausea ● Fever	● Not interchangeable with heparin or low-dose heparins. ● Monitor the patient for signs of bleeding. ● Monitor complete blood count and platelet count. ● Monitor anti-Xa levels. Goal for prophylaxis is 0.2 to 0.4 anti-Xa units/ml; goal for therapy is 0.5 anti-Xa units/ml.

UNDERSTANDING ANTICOAGULANTS *(continued)*

DRUGS	INDICATIONS	ADVERSE REACTIONS	NURSING CONSIDERATIONS
ORAL ANTICOAGULANTS			
Warfarin (Coumadin)	● Deep vein thrombosis pro- phylaxis ● Prevention of complications of prosthetic heart valves or diseased mitral valves ● Atrial arrhyth- mias	● Bleeding (may be severe) ● Hepatitis ● Diarrhea	● Monitor prothrombin time and International Normalized Ratio. ● Monitor the patient for signs of bleeding. ● The effects of oral anti- coagulants can be re- versed with phytonadione (vitamin K).
ANTIPLATELET DRUGS			
Aspirin (Ecotrin), dipyri- damole (Persantine), ticlopidine (Ticlid), clopidogrel (Plavix)	● Decreases the risk of death post- MI ● Prevention of complications of prosthetic heart valves ● Reduction of risk of MI after pre- vious MI or in pa- tients with unstable angina ● Prevention of reocclusion in coro- nary revasculariza- tion procedures	● GI distress ● Bleeding ● Thrombocy- topenia ● Angioedema	● Monitor the patient for signs of bleeding. ● Aspirin and ticlopidine should be taken with meals to prevent GI irrita- tion. ● Dipyridamole should be taken with a full glass of fluid at least 1 hour before meals.

- Antithrombin III then inactivates factors IXa, Xa, XIa, and XIIa in the intrinsic and common pathways. The end result is prevention of a stable fibrin clot.
- In low doses, heparin increases the activity of antithrombin III against factor Xa and thrombin and inhibits clot formation. Much larger doses are necessary to inhibit fibrin formation after a clot has formed. This relationship between dose and effect is the rationale for using low-dose heparin to prevent clotting.

- Whole blood clotting time, thrombin time, and partial thrombo-plastin time are prolonged during heparin therapy. However, these times may be only slightly prolonged with low or ultra-low preventive doses.

  Heparin can be used to prevent clotting when a patient's blood must circulate outside the body through a machine, such as a cardiopulmonary bypass machine or hemodialysis machine.

FACTOR XA INHIBITORS

Factor Xa inhibitors are a new class of anticoagulants. At this time, the only drug in this class is fondaparinux (Arixtra). Fondaparinux works by inhibiting only factor Xa. Factor Xa is the common point in the intrinsic and extrinsic clotting pathways. Inhibition of factor Xa prevents the formation of thrombin and the formation of a stable fibrin clot.

ORAL ANTICOAGULANTS

Oral anticoagulants alter the liver's ability to synthesize vitamin K-dependent clotting factors, including prothrombin and factors VII, IX, and X. Clotting factors already in the bloodstream continue to coagulate blood until they become depleted, so anticoagulation doesn't begin immediately. The major oral anticoagulant used in the United States is warfarin (Coumadin).

ANTIPLATELET DRUGS

Examples of antiplatelet drugs are:

- aspirin (Ecotrin)
- dipyridamole (Persantine)
- ticlopidine (Ticlid)
- clopidogrel (Plavix).

  Antiplatelet drugs are used to prevent arterial thromboembolism, especially in patients at risk for myocardial infarction (MI), stroke, and arteriosclerosis (hardening of the arteries). They interfere with platelet activity in different drug-specific and dose-related ways.

  Low dosages of aspirin (81 mg/day) appear to inhibit clot formation by blocking the synthesis of prostaglandins, which in turn prevents formation of the platelet-aggregating substance thromboxane A_2. Dipyridamole and clopidogrel may inhibit platelet aggregation.

  Ticlopidine inhibits the binding of fibrinogen to platelets during the first stage of the clotting cascade.

HOW THROMBOLYTICS DISSOLVE CLOTS

When a thrombus forms in an artery, it obstructs the blood supply, causing ischemia and necrosis. Thrombolytics can dissolve thrombi in the coronary and pulmonary arteries, restoring the blood supply to the area beyond the blockage.

Obstructed artery

A thrombus blocks blood flow through the artery, causing distal ischemia.

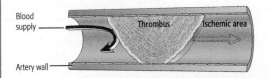

Blood supply | Thrombus | Ischemic area

Artery wall

Inside the thrombus

The thrombolytic enters the thrombus and binds to the fibrin-plasminogen complex, converting inactive plasminogen into active plasmin. Active plasmin digests fibrin, dissolving the thrombus. As the thrombus dissolves, blood flow resumes.

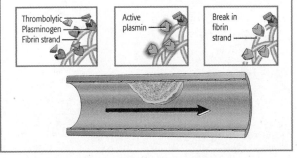

Thrombolytic
Plasminogen
Fibrin strand

Active plasmin

Break in fibrin strand

Thrombolytics

Thrombolytics dissolve preexisting clots or thrombi, and they're commonly used in acute or emergency situations. They work by converting plasminogen to plasmin, which lyses (dissolves) thrombi, fibrinogen, and other plasma proteins. (See *How thrombolytics dissolve clots*. Also see *Understanding thrombolytics,* page 164.)

UNDERSTANDING THROMBOLYTICS

Sometimes called *clot busters*, thrombolytics are prescribed to dissolve a preexisting clot or thrombus. These drugs are typically used in acute or emergency situations. Use this table to learn about the indications, adverse reactions, and nursing considerations associated with these drugs.

DRUGS	INDICATIONS	ADVERSE REACTIONS	NURSING CONSIDERATIONS
THROMBOLYTICS			
Alteplase (Activase), reteplase (Retavase), streptokinase (Streptase)	● Acute myocardial infarction ● Acute ischemic stroke ● Pulmonary embolus ● Catheter occlusion ● Arterial thrombosis	● Bleeding ● Allergic reaction	● Monitor partial thromboplastin time, prothrombin time, International Normalized Ratio, hemoglobin levels, and hematocrit before, during, and after administration. ● Monitor vital signs frequently during and immediately after administration. Don't use an automatic blood pressure cuff to monitor blood pressure. ● Monitor puncture sites for bleeding. Don't use a tourniquet when obtaining blood samples. ● Monitor for signs of bleeding.

Some commonly used thrombolytics include:
- alteplase (Activase)
- reteplase (Retavase)
- streptokinase (Streptase).

Adrenergics

Adrenergics are also called *sympathomimetics* because they produce effects similar to those produced by the sympathetic nervous system.

Adrenergics are classified based on their chemical structure: catecholamines (both naturally occurring and synthetic) and noncatecholamines (See *Understanding adrenergics*, pages 166 to 169.)

Therapeutic use of adrenergics depends on which receptors they stimulate and to what degree. Adrenergics can affect:

- alpha-adrenergic receptors
- beta-adrenergic receptors
- dopamine receptors.

Most of the adrenergic drugs produce their effects by stimulating alpha- and beta-adrenergic receptors. These drugs mimic the action of norepinephrine or epinephrine.

Dopaminergic drugs act primarily on receptors in the sympathetic nervous system that are stimulated by dopamine.

CATECHOLAMINES

Because of their common basic chemical structure, catecholamines share certain properties. They stimulate the nervous system, constrict peripheral blood vessels, increase heart rate, and dilate the bronchi. They can be manufactured in the body or in a laboratory. Common catecholamines include:

- dobutamine (Dobutrex)
- dopamine (Intropin)
- epinephrine (Adrenalin)
- norepinephrine (Levophed)

Catecholamines are primarily direct-acting. When catecholamines combine with alpha or beta receptors, they cause either an excitatory or inhibitory effect. Typically, activation of alpha receptors generates an excitatory response except for intestinal relaxation. Activation of the beta receptors mostly produces an inhibitory response except in the cells of the heart, where norepinephrine produces excitatory effects. (See *Learning about adrenergic receptor uses and effects,* page 170.)

The effects of catecholamines depend on the dosage and the route of administration. Catecholamines are potent inotropes, meaning they make the heart contract more forcefully. As a result, the ventricles empty more completely with each heartbeat, increasing the heart's workload and the amount of oxygen it needs to do this harder work.

Catecholamines also produce a positive chronotropic effect, which means they cause the heart to beat faster. That's because the pacemaker cells in the heart's SA node depolarize at a faster rate. As catecholamines cause blood vessels to constrict and blood pressure to increase, the heart rate decreases as the body tries to prevent an excessive increase in blood pressure.

Catecholamines can cause the Purkinje fibers to fire spontaneously, possibly producing abnormal heart rhythms, such as premature

(Text continues on page 168.)

UNDERSTANDING ADRENERGICS

Adrenergic drugs produce effects similar to those produced by the sympathetic nervous system. Adrenergic drugs can affect alpha-adrenergic receptors, beta-adrenergic receptors, or dopamine receptors. However, most of the drugs stimulate the alpha and beta receptors, mimicking the effects of norepinephrine and epinephrine. Dopaminergic drugs act on receptors typically stimulated by dopamine.

Use this table to learn about the indications, adverse reactions, and nursing considerations associated with these drugs.

DRUGS	INDICATIONS	ADVERSE REACTIONS
CATECHOLAMINES		
Dobutamine (Dobutrex)	● Increase cardiac output in short-term treatment of cardiac decompensation from depressed contractility	Headache, tingling sensation, bronchospasm, palpitations, tachycardia, cardiac arrhythmias (premature ventricular contractions), hypotension, hypertension and hypertensive crisis, angina, nausea, vomiting, tissue necrosis and sloughing (if catecholamine given I.V. leaks into surrounding tissue)
Dopamine (Intropin)	● Treat shock and correct hemodynamic imbalances ● Increase cardiac output ● Hypotension	Headache, bradycardia, palpitations, tachycardia, conduction disturbance, cardiac arrhythmias (ventricular), hypotension, hypertension and hypertensive crisis, azotemia, angina, nausea, vomiting, gangrene of extremities in high dose, tissue necrosis and sloughing (if catecholamine given I.V. leaks into surrounding tissue), bronchospasm
Epinephrine (Adrenalin)	● Bronchospasm ● Hypersensitivity reactions ● Anaphylaxis ● Restoration of cardiac rhythm in cardiac arrest	Restlessness, anxiety, dizziness, headache, tachycardia, palpitations, cardiac arrhythmias (ventricular fibrillation), hypertension, stroke, cerebral hemorrhage, angina, increased blood glucose levels, tissue necrosis and sloughing (if catecholamine given I.V. leaks into surrounding tissue)

NURSING
CONSIDERATIONS

- Correct hypovolemia before administering drug.
- Incompatible with alkaline solution (sodium bicarbonate); don't mix or give through same line; don't mix with other drugs.
- Administer continuous drip on infusion pump.
- Give drug into a large vein to prevent irritation or extravasation at site.
- Monitor cardiac rate and rhythm and blood pressure carefully when initiating therapy or increasing the dose.

- Correct hypovolemia before giving drug.
- Administer continuous drip on infusion pump.
- Give drug into a large vein to prevent extravasation; if extravasation occurs, stop infusion and treat site with phentolamine (Regitine) infiltrate to prevent tissue necrosis.
- Monitor cardiac rate and rhythm and blood pressure carefully when initiating therapy or increasing the dose.
- Monitor urine output during treatment, especially at high doses.

- Correct hypovolemia before giving drug.
- Administer continuous drip on infusion pump.
- Give drug into a large vein to prevent irritation or extravasation at site.
- Monitor cardiac rate and rhythm and blood pressure carefully when starting therapy or increasing the dose.

(continued)

UNDERSTANDING ADRENERGICS *(continued)*		
DRUGS	**INDICATIONS**	**ADVERSE REACTIONS**
CATECHOLAMINES		
Norepineph-rine (Levophed)	● Maintain blood pressure in acute hypotensive states	Anxiety, dizziness, headache, bradycardia, cardiac arrhythmias, hypotension, hypertension, tissue necrosis and sloughing (if catecholamine given I.V. leaks into surrounding tissue), fever, metabolic acidosis, increased blood glucose levels, dyspnea
NONCATECHOLAMINES		
Ephedrine	● Maintain blood pressure in acute hypotensive states, especially with spinal anesthesia ● Treatment of orthostatic hypotension and bronchospasm	Anxiety, dizziness, headache, palpitations, hypotension, hypertension, nausea, vomiting
Phenylephrine (Neo-Synephrine)	● Maintain blood pressure in hypotensive states, especially hypotensive emergencies with spinal anesthesia	Restlessness, anxiety, dizziness, headache, palpitations, cardiac arrhythmias, hypertension, tissue necrosis and sloughing (if catecholamine given I.V. leaks into surrounding tissue)

ventricular contractions and fibrillation. Epinephrine is likelier than norepinephrine to produce this spontaneous firing,

NONCATECHOLAMINES

Noncatecholamine adrenergic drugs have various therapeutic uses because of the many effects these drugs can have on the body such as the local or systemic constriction of blood vessels by phenylephrine (Neo-Synephrine).

Direct-acting noncatecholamines that stimulate alpha activity include methoxamine (Vasoxyl) and phenylephrine.

Those that selectively exert $beta_2$ activity include:
■ albuterol (Proventil)

**NURSING
CONSIDERATIONS**

- Correct hypovolemia before giving drug.
- Administer continuous drip on infusion pump.
- Give drug into a large vein to prevent extravasation; if extravasation occurs, stop infusion, and treat site with phentolamine infiltrate to prevent tissue necrosis.
- Monitor cardiac rate and rhythm and blood pressure carefully when starting therapy or increasing the dose.

- Correct hypovolemia before giving drug.
- Give drug into a large vein to prevent irritation or extravasation at site.
- Monitor cardiac rate and rhythm and blood pressure carefully when initiating therapy or increasing the dose.

- Correct hypovolemia before giving drug.
- Administer continuous drip on infusion pump.
- Give drug into a large vein to prevent extravasation; if extravasation occurs, stop infusion, and treat site with phentolamine infiltrate to prevent tissue necrosis.
- Monitor cardiac rate and rhythm and blood pressure carefully when starting therapy or increasing the dose.

■ isoetharine (Bronkosol)
■ metaproterenol (Alupent)

Dual-acting noncatecholamines combine both actions and include ephedrine.

Adrenergic blockers

Adrenergic blockers, also called *sympatholytics*, are used to disrupt sympathetic nervous system function. (See *Understanding adrenergic blockers*, page 171.)

These drugs work by blocking impulse transmission (and thus sympathetic nervous system stimulation) at adrenergic neurons or

LEARNING ABOUT ADRENERGIC RECEPTOR USES AND EFFECTS

RECEPTOR ACTIVATED	THERAPEUTIC USES	ADVERSE EFFECTS
Alpha$_1$	● Control topical superficial bleeding ● Treat nasal decongestion ● Elevate blood pressure ● Delay absorption of local anesthetics ● Decrease intraocular pressure	● Hypertension ● Necrosis with extravasation ● Bradycardia
Alpha$_2$	● Treat glaucoma	● Burning sensation ● Ptosis ● Redness and swelling of eyelid
Beta$_1$	● Treat heart failure, cardiac arrest, and shock	● Tachycardia ● Arrhythmias ● Angina
Beta$_2$	● Produce bronchodilation ● Delay preterm labor	● Hyperglycemia ● Tremors
Dopamine	● Increase renal blood flow ● Increase cardiac output ● Elevate blood pressure	● Ectopy ● Nausea and vomiting ● Tachycardia ● Palpitations

adrenergic receptor sites. The action of the drugs at these sites can be exerted by:

■ interrupting the action of sympathomimetics (adrenergics)
■ reducing available norepinephrine
■ preventing the action of cholinergics.

Adrenergic-blocking drugs are classified according to their site of action as alpha-adrenergic receptor blockers or beta-adrenergic receptor blockers.

UNDERSTANDING ADRENERGIC BLOCKERS

Adrenergic blockers block impulse transmission at adrenergic receptor sites by interrupting the action of adrenergic drugs, reducing the amount of norepinephrine available, and blocking the action of cholinergics.

Use this table to learn the indications, adverse reactions, and nursing considerations needed to safely administer these drugs.

DRUGS	INDICATIONS	ADVERSE REACTIONS	NURSING CONSIDERATIONS
ALPHA-ADRENERGIC RECEPTOR BLOCKERS			
Phentolamine (Regitine), prazosin (Minipress)	● Hypertension ● Pheochromocytoma	Orthostatic hypotension, bradycardia, tachycardia, edema, difficulty breathing, flushing, weakness, palpitations, shock	● Monitor vital signs and heart rhythm before, during, and after administration. ● Instruct the patient to rise slowly to a standing position to avoid orthostatic hypotension.
BETA-ADRENERGIC RECEPTOR BLOCKERS			
Nonselective Carvedilol (Coreg), labetalol (Normodyne), propranolol (Inderal), sotalol (Betapace), timolol (Blocadren) **Selective** Acebutolol (Sectral), atenolol (Tenormin), esmolol (Brevibloc), metoprolol (Lopressor)	● Prevention of complications after myocardial infarction, angina, hypertension, supraventricular arrhythmias, anxiety, essential tremor, cardiovascular symptoms associated with thyrotoxicosis, migraine headaches, pheochromocytoma	Hypotension, bradycardia, peripheral vascular insufficiency, bronchospasm (nonselective), sore throat, atrioventricular block, thrombocytopenia, hypoglycemia	● Monitor vital signs and heart rhythm frequently. ● Beta-adrenergic receptor blockers can alter the requirements for insulin and oral antidiabetics.

ALPHA-ADRENERGIC RECEPTOR BLOCKERS

Alpha-adrenergic receptor blockers work by interrupting the actions of sympathomimetic drugs at alpha-adrenergic receptors. This results in:

- relaxation of the smooth muscle in the blood vessels
- increased dilation of blood vessels
- decreased blood pressure.

Drugs in this class include phentolamine and prazosin.

Ergotamine (Ergomar) is a mixed alpha agonist and antagonist. At high dose, it acts as an alpha-adrenergic receptor blocker.

Alpha-adrenergic receptor blockers work in one of two ways:

- They interfere with or block the synthesis, storage, release, and re-uptake of norepinephrine by neurons.
- They antagonize epinephrine, norepinephrine, or adrenergic (sympathomimetic) drugs at alpha-receptor sites.

Alpha-receptor sites are either $alpha_1$ or $alpha_2$ receptors. Alpha-adrenergic receptor blockers include drugs that block stimulation of $alpha_1$ receptors and that may block $alpha_2$ stimulation.

Alpha-adrenergic receptor blockers occupy alpha-receptor sites on the smooth muscle of blood vessels.

This prevents catecholamines from occupying and stimulating the receptor sites. As a result, blood vessels dilate, increasing local blood flow to the skin and other organs. The decreased peripheral vascular resistance helps to decrease blood pressure.

BETA-ADRENERGIC RECEPTOR BLOCKERS

Beta-adrenergic receptor blockers, the most widely used adrenergic blockers, prevent stimulation of the sympathetic nervous system by inhibiting the action of catecholamines and other sympathomimetic drugs at beta-adrenergic receptors.

Beta-adrenergic drugs are selective or nonselective. Nonselective beta-adrenergic drugs affect:

- $beta_1$-receptor sites (located mainly in the heart)
- $beta_2$-receptor sites (located in the bronchi, blood vessels, and the uterus).

Nonselective beta-adrenergic drugs include carvedilol, labetalol, propranolol, sotalol (Betapace), and timolol (Blocadren).

Selective beta-adrenergic receptor blockers primarily affect the $beta_1$-adrenergic sites. They include acebutolol, atenolol, esmolol and metoprolol.

Some beta-adrenergic receptor blockers such as acebutolol have intrinsic sympathetic activity. This means that instead of attaching to beta receptors and blocking them, these beta-adrenergic receptor blockers attach to beta receptors and stimulate them. These drugs are sometimes classified as partial agonists.

Beta-adrenergic receptor blockers have widespread effects in the body because they produce their blocking action not only at the adrenergic nerve endings but also in the adrenal medulla. Effects on the heart include:

- increased peripheral vascular resistance
- decreased blood pressure
- decreased force of contractions of the heart
- decreased oxygen consumption of the heart
- slowed conduction of impulses between the atria and ventricles
- decreased cardiac output.

Some of the effects of beta-adrenergic receptor blockers depend on whether the drug is classified as selective or nonselective. Selective beta-adrenergic receptor blockers, which preferentially block beta$_1$-receptor sites, reduce stimulation of the heart. They're commonly called *cardioselective beta-adrenergic receptor blockers.*

Nonselective beta-adrenergic receptor blockers, which block both beta$_1$- and beta$_2$-receptor sites, reduce stimulation of the heart and cause the bronchioles of the lungs to constrict. This can cause bronchospasm in patients with chronic obstructive lung disorders.

Antilipemics

Antilipemics are used to lower abnormally high blood levels of lipids, such as cholesterol, triglycerides, and phospholipids.

Examples of antilipemic drug classes include:

- bile-sequestering drugs
- fibric acid derivatives
- HMG-CoA reductase inhibitors
- cholesterol absorption inhibitors. (See *Understanding antilipemics*, pages 174 and 175.)

These drugs are used in combination with lifestyle changes, such as proper diet, weight loss, and exercise.

BILE-SEQUESTERING DRUGS

Bile-sequestering drugs help lower blood levels of low-density lipoproteins (LDLs). They combine with bile acids in the intestines to form an insoluble compound that's then excreted in the feces. The decreasing level of bile acid in the gallbladder triggers the liver to synthesize more bile acids from their precursor, cholesterol. As cholesterol leaves the bloodstream and other storage areas to replace the lost bile acids, blood cholesterol levels decrease.

UNDERSTANDING ANTILIPEMICS

Antilipemics are used to lower high blood levels of lipids by combining with bile acids, reducing cholesterol formation, inhibiting enzymes, and inhibiting cholesterol absorption.

Use this table to learn the indications, adverse reactions, and nursing considerations needed to safely give these drugs.

DRUGS	INDICATIONS	ADVERSE REACTIONS	NURSING CONSIDERATIONS
BILE-SEQUESTERING DRUGS			
cholestyramine (Questran), colesevelam (Welchol), colestipol (Colestid)	• Elevated cholesterol level	• Constipation • Increased bleeding tendencies • Muscle and joint pain • Nausea, heartburn • Headache	• Instruct patient that he'll need to return for periodic blood tests. • Give before meals. • Don't give the powder form dry; mix with fluid. • Give other drugs 1 hour before or 4 to 6 hours after these drugs.
FIBRIC ACID DERIVATIVES			
fenofibrate (Tricor), gemfibrozil (Lopid)	• Hypercholesterolemia • Hypertriglyceridemia	• Rash, nausea, vomiting, diarrhea • Myalgia, flu-like syndrome • Impotence • Dizziness, blurred vision • Abdominal pain, epigastric pain	• Instruct the patient that he'll need to return for periodic blood tests. • Educate the patient on dietary and lifestyle changes to help lower cholesterol and triglyceride levels. • Give with meals.

Examples of bile-sequestering drugs include:

- cholestyramine (Questran)
- colesevelam (Welchol)
- colestipol hydrochloride (Colestid).

Bile-sequestering drugs are the drugs of choice for treating a patient who can't reduce his LDL levels through dietary changes because of familial hypercholesterolemia.

UNDERSTANDING ANTILIPEMICS *(continued)*

DRUGS	INDICATIONS	ADVERSE REACTIONS	NURSING CONSIDERATIONS
HMG-CoA REDUCTASE INHIBITORS			
atorvastatin (Lipitor), fluvastatin (Lescol), lovastatin (Mevacor), pravastatin (Pravachol), simvastatin (Zocor), rosuvastatin (Crestor)	● Elevated cholesterol, triglyceride, and low-density lipoprotein (LDL) levels ● Prevention of cardiovascular disease in adults without clinically evident coronary disease but with multiple risk factors	● Rhabdomyolysis with acute renal failure ● Headache ● Flatulence, abdominal pain, constipation, nausea	● Instruct the patient that he'll need to return for periodic blood tests. ● Monitor periodic liver function tests. ● Give the drug at the same time each day; it doesn't need to be given with food. ● Educate the patient on dietary and lifestyle changes to help lower cholesterol and triglyceride levels.
CHOLESTEROL ABSORPTION INHIBITORS			
ezetimibe (Zetia)	● Elevated cholesterol, triglyceride, and LDL levels ● Given as adjunctive treatment with simvastatin	● Cough ● Myalgia, arthralgia ● Headache, dizziness	● Instruct the patient that he'll need to return for periodic blood tests. ● Educate the patient on dietary and lifestyle changes to help lower cholesterol and triglyceride levels. ● If giving with an HMG-CoA reductase inhibitor, give both drugs together.

FIBRIC ACID DERIVATIVES

Fibric acid derivatives reduce high triglyceride levels and, to a lesser extent, high LDL levels. It isn't known exactly how these drugs work, although it's thought that they:

- reduce cholesterol production early in its formation
- mobilize cholesterol from the tissues
- increase cholesterol excretion
- decrease synthesis and secretion of lipoproteins

■ decrease synthesis of triglycerides.

Fenofibrate (Tricor) and gemfibrozil (Lopid) are two commonly used fibric acid derivatives.

Fibric acid drugs are primarily used to reduce triglyceride levels and also reduce blood cholesterol levels. Gemfibrozil also increases the high-density lipoprotein (HDL) levels in the blood and increases the serum's capacity to dissolve additional cholesterol.

HMG-CoA REDUCTASE INHIBITORS

HMG-CoA reductase inhibitors (also known as the *statins*) lower lipid levels by interfering with cholesterol synthesis. They inhibit the enzyme that's responsible for converting HMG-CoA to mevalonate, an early rate-limiting step in the biosynthesis of cholesterol.

Commonly prescribed HMG-CoA reductase inhibitors include:

■ atorvastatin (Lipitor)
■ fluvastatin (Lescol)
■ lovastatin (Mevacor)
■ pravastatin (Pravachol)
■ simvastatin (Zocor)
■ rosuvastatin (Crestor)

Statin drugs are used primarily to reduce LDLs and also reduce total blood cholesterol levels. They also produce a mild increase in HDLs. Because of their effect on LDL and total cholesterol, these drugs are used to not only treat hypercholesterolemia, but also for primary and secondary prevention of cardiovascular events.

CHOLESTEROL ABSORPTION INHIBITORS

As their name implies, cholesterol absorption inhibitors inhibit the absorption of cholesterol and related phytosterols from the intestine. At this time, ezetimibe (Zetia) is the only drug in the class.

Ezetimibe reduces blood cholesterol levels by inhibiting the absorption of cholesterol by the small intestine. This leads to a decrease in delivery of intestinal cholesterol to the liver, causing a reduction in hepatic cholesterol stores and an increase in clearance from the blood.

Ezetimibe may be used alone or with statins to help lower cholesterol. One drug currently on the market combines a statin (simvastatin) and ezetimibe to help decrease total cholesterol and LDLs, and increase HDL cholesterol.

SURGERY

Despite the drama of successful single- and multiple-organ transplants, treatment with improved immunosuppressants, and advances in ventricular assist devices (VADs), far more patients undergo conventional surgeries such as coronary artery bypass graft (CABG). Surgeries for the treatment of disorders of the cardiovascular system include:

- CABG
- minimally invasive direct coronary artery bypass (MIDCAB)
- heart transplantation
- vascular repair
- valve surgery
- VAD insertion.

Coronary artery bypass graft

A CABG circumvents an occluded coronary artery with an autogenous graft (usually a segment of the saphenous vein or internal mammary artery), thereby restoring blood flow to the myocardium.

The most common procedure, aortocoronary bypass, involves suturing one end of the autogenous graft to the ascending aorta and the other end to a coronary artery distal to the occlusion. (See *Bypassing coronary occlusions,* page 178.)

Other surgical techniques, such as the mini-CABG and direct coronary artery bypass, can reduce the risk of cerebral complications and accelerate recovery for patients requiring grafts of only one or two arteries.

More than 450,000 Americans (most of them men) undergo CABG surgery each year, making it one of the most common cardiac surgeries. Prime candidates include patients with severe angina from atherosclerosis and others with coronary artery disease (CAD) who have a high risk of MI. A successful CABG can relieve anginal pain, improve cardiac function and, possibly, enhance the patient's quality of life.

Although the surgery relieves pain in about 90% of patients, its long-term effectiveness is unclear. Such problems as graft closure and development of atherosclerosis in other coronary arteries may make repeat surgery necessary. In addition, because a CABG doesn't resolve the underlying disease associated with arterial blockage, a CABG may not reduce the risk of MI recurrence. Patients most likely to benefit from a CABG include those with left main CAD, severe proximal left anterior descending CAD, three-vessel CAD with proximal stenoses or

BYPASSING CORONARY OCCLUSIONS

After the patient receives general anesthesia, surgery begins with graft harvesting. The surgeon makes a series of incisions in the patient's thigh or calf and removes a saphenous vein segment for grafting. Most surgeons prefer to use a segment of the internal mammarian artery.

Exposing the heart

Once the autografts are obtained, the surgeon performs a medial sternotomy to expose the heart and then initiates cardiopulmonary bypass.

To reduce myocardial oxygen demands during surgery and to protect the heart, the surgeon induces cardiac hypothermia and standstill by injecting a cold, cardioplegic solution (potassium-enriched saline solution) into the aortic root.

Securing the graft

After the patient is prepared, the surgeon sutures one end of the venous graft to the ascending aorta and the other end to a patent coronary artery that's distal to the occlusion. The graft is sutured in a reversed position to promote proper blood flow. The surgeon repeats this procedure for each occlusion to be bypassed.

In the example depicted below, saphenous vein segments bypass occlusions in three sections of the coronary artery.

Finishing the surgery

When the grafts are in place, the surgeon flushes the cardioplegic solution from the heart and discontinues cardiopulmonary bypass. He then implants epicardial pacing electrodes, inserts a chest tube, closes the incision, and applies a sterile dressing.

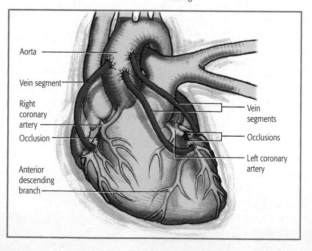

Aorta

Vein segment

Right coronary artery

Occlusion

Anterior descending branch

Vein segments

Occlusions

Left coronary artery

left ventricular dysfunction, and those with three-vessel CAD with normal left ventricular function at rest, but with inducible ischemia and poor exercise capacity.

During the procedure, the patient may be placed on cardiopulmonary bypass so the surgeon can work on a nonbeating heart. This is called an *on-pump CABG*. If cardiopulmonary bypass isn't used, the surgeon works on a beating heart, and this is known as an *off-pump CABG*. An off-pump CABG has several advantages over an on-pump CABG including decreased risk of complications and shorter hospital stay and recovery time.

PREPARING THE PATIENT
- Reinforce the physician's explanation of the surgery.
- Explain the complex equipment and procedures used on the intensive care unit (ICU) or postanesthesia care unit (PACU).
- Explain that the patient awakens from surgery with an endotracheal (ET) tube in place, and he'll be connected to a mechanical ventilator. He'll also be connected to a cardiac monitor and may have in place a nasogastric (NG) tube, a chest tube, an indwelling urinary catheter, arterial lines, epicardial pacing wires and, possibly, a pulmonary artery (PA) catheter. Tell him that discomfort is minimal and that the equipment is removed as soon as possible.
- Review incentive spirometry techniques and range-of-motion (ROM) exercises with the patient.
- Make sure that the patient or a responsible family member has signed a consent form.
- Before surgery, prepare the patient's skin.
- Immediately before surgery, begin cardiac monitoring, and then assist with PA catheterization and insertion of arterial lines. Some facilities insert PA catheters and arterial lines in the operating room before surgery.

MONITORING AND AFTERCARE
- After a CABG, look for signs of hemodynamic compromise, such as severe hypotension, decreased cardiac output, and shock.
- Keep emergency resuscitative equipment immediately available.
- Begin warming procedures according to your facility's policy.
- Check and record vital signs and hemodynamic parameters every 5 to 15 minutes until the patient's condition stabilizes.
- To ensure adequate myocardial perfusion, keep arterial pressure within the limits set by the physician. Usually, mean arterial pressure (MAP) less than 70 mm Hg results in inadequate tissue perfusion; pressure greater than 110 mm Hg can cause hemorrhage and

graft rupture. Monitor pulmonary artery pressure (PAP), central venous pressure (CVP), left atrial pressure, and cardiac output.

- Be alert for changes in hemodynamics that indicate either hypervolemia or hypovolemia, especially an increase or decrease in CVP and PAP.
- Give drugs as indicated and adjust according to the patient's response. Vasopressors may be used to help increase perfusion of the coronary arteries. Nitroglycerin may be administered to help minimize spasm of the newly grafted artery.
- Monitor the patient's hemoglobin levels and hematocrit and be prepared to transfuse blood or blood products as necessary.
- Monitor electrocardiograms (ECGs) continuously for disturbances in heart rate and rhythm. If you detect serious abnormalities, notify the physician and be prepared to assist with epicardial pacing or, if necessary, cardioversion or defibrillation.
- Frequently evaluate the patient's peripheral pulses, capillary refill time, and skin temperature and color and auscultate for heart sounds; report abnormalities.
- Evaluate tissue oxygenation by assessing breath sounds, chest excursion, and symmetry of chest expansion. Check arterial blood gas (ABG) results every 2 to 4 hours, and adjust ventilator settings to keep ABG values within ordered limits.
- Maintain chest tube drainage at the ordered negative pressure (usually –10 to –40 cm), and assess regularly for hemorrhage, excessive drainage (greater than 200 ml/hour), and sudden decrease or cessation of drainage.
- Monitor the patient's intake and output, and assess for electrolyte imbalance, especially hypokalemia and hypomagnesemia. Assess urine output at least hourly during the immediate postoperative period and then less frequently as the patient's condition stabilizes.
- As the patient's incisional pain increases, give an analgesic or other drugs as indicated.
- After weaning the patient from the ventilator and removing the ET tube, provide chest physiotherapy. Start with incentive spirometry, and encourage the patient to cough, turn frequently, and deep-breathe. Assist with ROM exercises to enhance peripheral circulation and prevent thrombus formation.
- Explain that postpericardiotomy syndrome commonly develops after open-heart surgery. Instruct the patient about signs and symptoms, such as fever, muscle and joint pain, weakness, and chest discomfort.

USING CARDIAC REHAB

Cardiac rehab is an exercise program designed to monitor and improve cardiovascular status and help the patient learn how to manage heart disease.

Elements of cardiac rehab include:
- individualized exercise program
- diet, nutrition, and weight control
- stress management
- reduction of risk factors
- lipid and cholesterol control.

Sessions are held weekly, based on patient need and tolerance. Heart rate, blood pressure, and symptoms are continuously monitored during the session. Education is provided based on the patient's individual needs.

- Prepare the patient for the possibility of postoperative depression, which may not develop until weeks after discharge. Reassure him that this depression is normal and should pass quickly.
- Maintain nothing-by-mouth status until bowel sounds return. Then begin the patient on clear liquids, and advance his diet as tolerated. Tell the patient to expect sodium and cholesterol restrictions, and explain that this diet can help reduce the risk of recurrent arterial occlusion.
- Monitor the patient's sternal incision and graft harvest sites for signs of infection, including redness, warmth, and drainage. Monitor the patient's temperature, and notify the physician if the patient has a fever over 101° F (38.3° C).
- Monitor for postoperative complications, such as stroke, pulmonary embolism, pneumonia, impaired renal perfusion, hypertension, MI, and infection.
- Gradually allow the patient to increase activities as indicated. (See *Using cardiac rehab.*)
- Provide support to the patient and his family to help them cope with recovery and lifestyle changes. (See *Teaching the patient after a CABG,* page 182.)

Minimally invasive direct coronary artery bypass

Until recently, cardiac surgery required stopping the heart and using cardiopulmonary bypass to oxygenate and circulate blood. Now, a MIDCAB can be performed on a pumping heart through a small thoracotomy incision. The patient may receive only right lung ventilation along with drugs, such as beta-adrenergic receptor blockers, to slow the heart rate and reduce heart movement during surgery.

TEACHING THE PATIENT AFTER A CABG

Before discharge from the hospital, instruct the patient to:

● watch for and immediately notify the practitioner of any signs of infection (redness, swelling, or drainage from the leg or chest incisions; fever; or sore throat) or possible arterial reocclusion (angina, dizziness, dyspnea, rapid or irregular pulse, or prolonged recovery time from exercise)

● call the practitioner in the case of weight gain greater than 3 lb (1.4 kg) in 1 week

● follow his prescribed diet, especially sodium and cholesterol restrictions

● maintain a balance between activity and rest by trying to sleep at least 8 hours each night, scheduling a short rest period each afternoon, and resting frequently when engaging in tiring physical activity

● participate in an exercise program or cardiac rehabilitation if prescribed

● follow lifestyle modifications (no smoking, improved diet, and regular exercise) to reduce atherosclerotic progression

● contact a local chapter of the Mended Hearts Club and the American Heart Association for information and support

● make sure he understands the dose, frequency of administration, and adverse effects of prescribed drugs.

Advantages of MIDCAB include shorter hospital stays, use of shorter-acting anesthetic agents, fewer postoperative complications, earlier extubation, reduced cost, smaller incisions, and earlier return to work. Patients eligible for MIDCAB include those with proximal left anterior descending lesions and some lesions of the right coronary and circumflex arteries. (See *Comparing types of CABGs*.)

PREPARING THE PATIENT

■ Review the procedure with the patient, and answer his questions. Tell the patient that he'll be extubated in the operating room or within 2 to 4 hours after surgery.

■ Teach the patient to cough and breathe deeply through use of an incentive spirometer.

■ Explain the use of drugs for pain after surgery as well as nonpharmacologic methods to control pain.

■ Let the patient know that he should be able to walk with assistance the first postoperative day and be discharged within 48 hours.

■ Make sure that the patient or a responsible family member has signed a consent form.

COMPARING TYPES OF CABGs

FEATURES	ON-PUMP CORONARY ARTERY BYPASS GRAFT (CABG)	OFF-PUMP CABG	MINIMALLY INVASIVE DIRECT CABG
Access site	● Breastbone severed for heart access	● Breastbone severed for heart access	● Incision made between ribs for anterior heart access, no bones cut
Indications	● Suitable for multivessel disease, any coronary artery	● Suitable for multivessel disease, any coronary artery	● Only used for one-vessel diseases in anterior portions of heart, such as left anterior descending artery, or some portions of the right coronary and circumflex arteries
Graft types	● Combination of artery and vein grafts	● Combination of artery and vein grafts	● Arterial grafts (better long-term results)
Complications	● Highest risk of postoperative complications	● Reduced blood usage, fewer rhythm problems, less kidney dysfunction than on-pump CABG	● Reduced blood usage, fewest complications, fastest recovery
Intubation	● Up to 24 hours	● Up to 24 hours	● Usually for 2 to 4 hours
Incisions	● Leg incisions for vein grafting, possibly arm incision for radial artery grafting	● Leg incisions for vein grafting, possibly arm incision for radial artery grafting	● No leg incisions, possibly arm incision for radial artery grafting

(continued)

	COMPARING TYPES OF CABGs *(continued)*		
FEATURES	**ON-PUMP CORONARY ARTERY BYPASS GRAFT (CABG)**	**OFF-PUMP CABG**	**MINIMALLY INVASIVE DIRECT CABG**
Heart and lung function	● Heart and lung circulation bypassed mechanically, affecting blood cells	● Drugs and special equipment used to slow heart and immobilize it; cardiopulmonary and systemic circulation still function	● Drugs used to slow heart; cardiopulmonary and systemic circulation still function

MONITORING AND AFTERCARE

■ After a MIDCAB, look for signs of hemodynamic compromise, such as severe hypotension, decreased cardiac output, and shock.

■ Keep emergency resuscitative equipment immediately available.

■ Check and record vital signs and hemodynamic parameters every 5 to 15 minutes until the patient's condition stabilizes. Give drugs as indicated, and adjust according to the patient's response.

■ Monitor ECGs continuously for disturbances in heart rate and rhythm. If you detect serious abnormalities, notify the physician, and be prepared to assist with epicardial pacing or, if necessary, cardioversion or defibrillation.

■ To ensure adequate myocardial perfusion, keep arterial pressure within the limits set by the physician. Usually, MAP less than 70 mm Hg results in inadequate tissue perfusion; pressure greater than 110 mm Hg can cause hemorrhage and graft rupture. Monitor PAP, CVP, left atrial pressure, and cardiac output if a pulmonary artery (PA) catheter was inserted.

■ Frequently evaluate the patient's peripheral pulses, capillary refill time, and skin temperature and color and auscultate for heart sounds; report abnormalities.

■ Evaluate tissue oxygenation by assessing breath sounds, chest excursion, and symmetry of chest expansion.

- Monitor the patient's intake and output, and assess for electrolyte imbalance, especially hypokalemia and hypomagnesemia. Assess urine output at least hourly during the immediate postoperative period and then less frequently as the patient's condition stabilizes.
- Provide analgesia, or encourage the use of patient-controlled analgesia if appropriate.
- Throughout the recovery period, assess for symptoms of stroke, pulmonary embolism, and impaired renal perfusion.
- Provide chest physiotherapy and incentive spirometry, and encourage the patient to cough, turn frequently, and deep-breathe. Assist with ROM exercises to enhance peripheral circulation and prevent thrombus formation.
- Explain that postpericardiotomy syndrome commonly develops after open-heart surgery. Instruct the patient about signs and symptoms, such as fever, muscle and joint pain, weakness, and chest discomfort.
- Prepare the patient for the possibility of postoperative depression, which may not develop until weeks after discharge. Reassure him that this depression is normal and should pass quickly.
- Maintain nothing-by-mouth status until bowel sounds return. Then begin the patient on clear liquids, and advance his diet as tolerated. Tell the patient to expect sodium and cholesterol restrictions, and explain that this diet can help reduce the risk of recurrent arterial occlusion.
- Gradually allow the patient to increase activities as indicated.
- Monitor the incision site for signs of infection or drainage.
- Provide support to the patient and his family to help them cope with recovery and lifestyle changes. (See *Teaching the patient after a MIDCAB,* page 186.)

Heart transplantation

Heart transplantation involves the replacement of a person's heart with a donor heart. It's the treatment of choice for patients with end-stage cardiac disease who have a poor prognosis, estimated survival of 6 to 12 months, and poor quality of life. A heart transplant candidate typically has uncontrolled symptoms and no other surgical options.

Transplantation doesn't guarantee a cure. Serious postoperative complications include infection and tissue rejection. Most patients experience one or both of these complications postoperatively.

Heart transplantation may be either orthotopic or heterotopic. Orthotopic is the most common type of heart transplantation. In this procedure, most of the patient's native heart is removed. The donor

TEACHING THE PATIENT AFTER A MIDCAB

Before discharge from the facility following a minimally invasive direct coronary artery bypass (MIDCAB), instruct the patient to:

● continue with the progressive exercise started in the facility
● perform coughing and deep-breathing exercises (while splinting the incision with a pillow to reduce pain), and use the incentive spirometer to reduce pulmonary complications
● avoid lifting objects that weigh more than 10 lb (4.5 kg) for the next 4 to 6 weeks
● wait 2 to 4 weeks before resuming sexual activity

● check the incision site daily, and immediately notify the practitioner of any signs of infection (redness, foul-smelling drainage, or swelling) or possible graft occlusion (slow, rapid, or irregular pulse; angina; dizziness; or dyspnea)
● perform any necessary incision care
● follow lifestyle modifications
● take medications as prescribed, and report adverse effects to the practitioner
● consider participation in a cardiac rehabilitation program.

heart is then attached to the atrial cusps and the aorta and pulmonary artery are anastomosed. (See *Quick guide to orthotopic heart transplantation.*) Heterotopic heart transplantation is less commonly performed. In this procedure, the donor heart is grafted to the recipient heart, and the donor heart is used to help augment the native heart's pumping ability.

Rejection typically occurs in the first 6 weeks after surgery, but it may still occur after this time. The patient is treated with monoclonal antibodies and potent immunosuppressants. The resulting immunosuppression places the patient at risk for life-threatening infection.

PREPARING THE PATIENT

■ Provide emotional support to the patient and his family. Begin to address their fears by discussing the procedure, possible complications, and the impact of transplantation and a prolonged recovery period on the patient's life.
■ Reinforce the physician's explanation of the surgery.
■ Discuss the immunosuppressant drugs that the patient will be taking. Remind the patient that these drugs increase his risk of infection
■ Explain the complex equipment and procedures used in the ICU and PACU.

QUICK GUIDE TO ORTHOTOPIC HEART TRANSPLANTATION

The following illustrations show how a heart is transplanted.

The donor's heart

The donor's heart is removed after the surgeon cuts along these dissection lines.

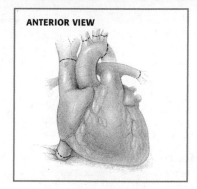

ANTERIOR VIEW

The recipient's heart

Before it can be removed, the recipient's heart is resected along these lines.

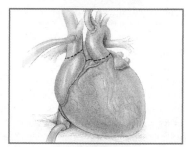

The transplanted heart

The transplanted heart is sutured.

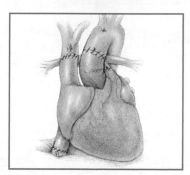

- Explain that the patient awakens from surgery with an ET tube in place and connected to a mechanical ventilator. He'll also be connected to a cardiac monitor and have in place an NG tube, a chest tube, an indwelling urinary catheter, arterial lines, epicardial pacing wires and, possibly, a PA catheter. Tell him that discomfort is minimal and that the equipment is removed as soon as possible.
- Review incentive spirometry techniques and ROM exercises with the patient.
- Make sure that the patient or a responsible family member has signed a consent form.
- Before surgery, prepare the patient's skin.
- Immediately before surgery, begin cardiac monitoring, and then assist with PA catheterization and insertion of arterial lines. Some facilities insert PA catheters and arterial lines in the operating room before surgery.

MONITORING AND AFTERCARE

- After surgery, maintain reverse isolation and strict infection control precautions.
- Administer immunosuppressants, and monitor the patient closely for signs of infection. Transplant recipients may exhibit only subtle signs because immunosuppressants mask obvious signs.
- Monitor vital signs every 15 minutes until stabilized, and assess the patient for signs of hemodynamic compromise, such as hypotension, decreased cardiac output, and shock.
- If necessary, administer nitroprusside during the first 24 to 48 hours to control blood pressure. An infusion of dopamine can improve contractility and renal perfusion.
- Volume replacement with normal saline, plasma expanders, or blood products may be necessary to maintain central venous pressure.
- Patients with elevated PAP may receive prostaglandin E to produce pulmonary vasodilation and reduced right ventricular afterload.
- Monitor ECGs for rhythm disturbances. Keep in mind that the transplanted heart's ECG waveform appears different from that of the patient's native heart. (See *Effects of cardiac transplantation on an ECG waveform.*)
- Maintain the chest tube drainage system at the prescribed negative pressure. Regularly assess for hemorrhage or sudden stop of drainage.

   RED FLAG Be alert for signs suggestive of rejection, such as a cardiac index less than 2.2, hypotension, atrial or other arrhythmias,

EFFECTS OF CARDIAC TRANSPLANTATION ON AN ECG WAVEFORM

An orthotopic heart transplantation (OHT) leads to characteristic findings on an electrocardiogram (ECG). Because the procedure provides the patient with a second functioning heart, the ECG shows two distinct cardiac rhythms—that of the native heart and that of the donor heart. These can be differentiated by analyzing the recipient's preoperative ECG. In addition, the donor heart's QRS complex usually has a higher amplitude. Remember that in OHT, the native heart's sinoatrial (SA) node remains intact. This accounts for the two P waves commonly seen on the posttransplant ECG. However, only the donor heart's SA node conducts through to the ventricles.

Initially, the atrial and ventricular rates are slow, requiring the use of a temporary pacemaker in the immediate postoperative period or therapy with such drugs as theophylline (Theo-Dur). The patient's native P waves will have a regular rhythm unrelated to the donor heart's QRS complexes. The donor atrial and ventricular rhythms are usually regular. Typically, two separate P waves are seen and the QRS complex may be widened secondary to ventricular conduction defects. Pacemaker activity should appear as long as the patient requires pacemaker support for chronotropic incompetence.

Orthotopic heart transplantation

This waveform shows two distinct types of P waves. P waves caused by the native heart's SA node are unrelated to the QRS

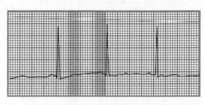

complexes (first shaded area). P waves caused by the donor heart's SA node precede each QRS complex (second shaded area).

Heterotopic heart transplantation

This waveform shows the ECG of the recipient's own heart (first shaded area) and the donor heart (second shaded area).

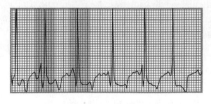

fever above 99.5° F (37.5° C), evidence of a third or fourth heart sound, peripheral edema, jugular vein distention, and crackles.

■ Be prepared to help with a myocardial biopsy at about 7 days and 14 days postoperatively.

TEACHING THE PATIENT AFTER HEART TRANSPLANTATION

Before discharge from the facility, instruct the patient to:

● continue with the progressive exercise started in the facility

● perform coughing and deep-breathing exercises (while splinting the incision with a pillow to reduce pain) and use the incentive spirometer to reduce pulmonary complications

● avoid lifting objects that weigh more than 10 lb (4.5 kg) for the next 4 to 6 weeks

● wait 2 to 4 weeks before resuming sexual activity

● check the incision site daily and immediately notify the practitioner of any signs of infection (redness, foul-smelling drainage, or swelling)

● perform any necessary incisional care

● follow lifestyle modifications

● take prescribed drugs (which will be lifelong), and report adverse effects to the practitioner

● consider participation in a cardiac rehabilitation program as advised

● immediately report any episodes of chest pain or shortness of breath

● avoid crowds and anyone with an infectious illness

● comply with follow-up visits as instructed.

■ Keep in mind that the effects of denervated heart muscle or denervation (in which the vagus nerve is cut during heart transplant surgery) makes drugs such as edrophonium (Tensilon) and anticholinergics (such as atropine) ineffective. (See *Teaching the patient after heart transplantation.*)

Vascular repair

Vascular repair includes aneurysm resection, grafting, embolectomy, vena caval filtering, endarterectomy, and vein stripping. The specific surgery used depends on the type, location, and extent of vascular occlusion or damage. (See *Types of vascular repair*, pages 192 and 193.)

Vascular repair can be used to treat:

■ vessels damaged by arteriosclerotic or thromboembolic disorders (such as aortic aneurysm or arterial occlusive disease), trauma, infections, or congenital defects

■ vascular obstructions that severely compromise circulation

■ vascular disease that doesn't respond to drug therapy or nonsurgical treatments such as balloon catheterization

■ life-threatening dissecting or ruptured aortic aneurysms

■ limb-threatening acute arterial occlusion.

All vascular surgeries carry a risk of vessel trauma, emboli, hemorrhage, infection, and other complications. Grafting carries added risks because the graft may occlude, narrow, dilate, or rupture.

PREPARING THE PATIENT

- Make sure the patient and his family understand the physician's explanation of the surgery and its possible complications.
- Make sure that the patient or a responsible family member has signed a consent form.
- Tell the patient that he'll receive a general anesthetic and will awaken from the anesthetic in the ICU or PACU. Explain that he'll have an I.V. line in place, ECG electrodes for continuous cardiac monitoring, and possibly an arterial line or a PA catheter to provide continuous pressure monitoring. He may also have a urinary catheter in place to allow accurate output measurement. If appropriate, explain that he'll be intubated and placed on mechanical ventilation.
- Before surgery, perform a complete vascular assessment. Take vital signs to provide a baseline. Evaluate the strength and sound of the blood flow and the symmetry of the pulses, and note bruits. Record the temperature of the extremities, their sensitivity to motor and sensory stimuli, and pallor, cyanosis, or redness. Rate peripheral pulse volume and strength on a scale of 0 to 4, and check capillary refill time by blanching the fingernail or toenail; normal refill time is less than 3 seconds.
- Instruct the patient to restrict food and fluids for at least 8 hours before surgery.

RED FLAG If the patient is awaiting surgery for aortic aneurysm repair, be on guard for signs and symptoms of acute dissection or rupture. Especially note sudden severe pain in the chest, abdomen, or lower back; severe weakness; diaphoresis; tachycardia; or a precipitous drop in blood pressure. If any of these occurs, notify the physician immediately.

MONITORING AND AFTERCARE

- Check and record the patient's vital signs every 15 minutes until his condition stabilizes, then every 30 minutes for 1 hour, and hourly thereafter for 2 to 4 hours. Report hypotension and hypertension immediately.
- Auscultate heart, breath, and bowel sounds, and report abnormal findings. Monitor the ECG for abnormalities in heart rate or rhythm. Also monitor other pressure readings, and carefully record intake and output.
- Check the patient's dressing regularly for excessive bleeding.

TYPES OF VASCULAR REPAIR

Several surgical options exist to repair damaged or diseased vessels. These options include aortic aneurysm repair, vena caval filter insertion, embolectomy, and bypass grafting.

Aortic aneurysm repair

Aortic aneurysm repair involves removing an aneurysmal segment of the aorta. The surgeon first makes an incision to expose the aneurysm site. If necessary, the patient is placed on a cardiopulmonary bypass machine. Next, the surgeon clamps the aorta, resects the aneurysm, and repairs the damaged portion of the aorta.

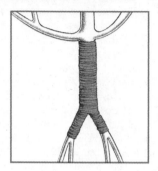

Vena caval filter insertion

A vena caval filter traps emboli in the vena cava, preventing them from reaching the pulmonary vessels. Inserted transvenously by catheter, the vena caval filter, or *umbrella*, traps emboli but allows venous blood flow.

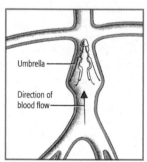

Umbrella

Direction of blood flow

- Assess the patient's neurologic and renal function, and report abnormalities.
- Provide analgesics, as indciated, for incisional pain.
- Frequently assess peripheral pulses, using Doppler ultrasonography if palpation is difficult. Check all extremities bilaterally for muscle strength and movement, color, temperature, and capillary refill time.
- Change dressings and provide incision care as indicated. Position the patient to avoid pressure on grafts and to reduce edema. Give

Embolectomy

To remove an embolism from an artery, a surgeon may perform an embolectomy. In this procedure, he inserts a balloon-tipped indwelling catheter in the artery and passes it through the thrombus (as shown below left). He then inflates the balloon and withdraws the catheter to remove the thrombus (as shown below right).

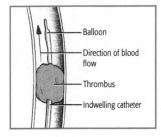

- Balloon
- Direction of blood flow
- Thrombus
- Indwelling catheter

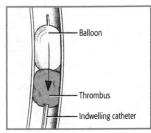

- Balloon
- Thrombus
- Indwelling catheter

Bypass grafting

Bypass grafting serves to bypass an arterial obstruction resulting from arteriosclerosis. After exposing the affected artery, the surgeon anastomoses a synthetic or autogenous graft to divert blood flow around the occluded arterial segment. The autogenous graft may be a vein or artery harvested from elsewhere in the patient's body. This illustration shows a femoropopliteal bypass.

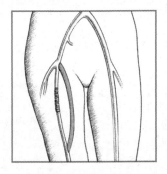

antithrombotics, as indciated, and monitor appropriate laboratory values to evaluate effectiveness.

- Assess for complications, and immediately report relevant signs and symptoms. (See *Complications of vascular repair,* page 194.)
- As the patient's condition improves, take steps to wean him from the ventilator if appropriate. To promote good pulmonary hygiene, encourage the patient to cough, turn, and deep breathe frequently.
- Assist the patient with ROM exercises to prevent thrombus formation. Assist with early ambulation to prevent complications of immobility.

COMPLICATIONS OF VASCULAR REPAIR

After a patient has undergone vascular repair surgery, monitor for these potential complications.

COMPLICATIONS	SIGNS AND SYMPTOMS
Pulmonary infection	<ul><li>Fever</li><li>Cough</li><li>Congestion</li><li>Dyspnea</li></ul>
Infection	<ul><li>Redness</li><li>Warmth</li><li>Drainage</li><li>Pain</li><li>Fever</li></ul>
Renal dysfunction	<ul><li>Low urine output</li><li>Elevated blood urea nitrogen and serum creatinine levels</li></ul>
Occlusion	<ul><li>Reduced or absent peripheral pulses</li><li>Paresthesia</li><li>Severe pain</li><li>Cyanosis</li></ul>
Hemorrhage	<ul><li>Hypotension</li><li>Tachycardia</li><li>Restlessness and confusion</li><li>Shallow respirations</li><li>Abdominal pain</li><li>Increased abdominal girth</li></ul>

■ Provide support to the patient and his family to help them cope with recovery and lifestyle changes. (See *Teaching the patient after vascular repair.*)

Valve surgery

To prevent heart failure, a patient with valvular stenosis or insufficiency accompanied by severe, unmanageable symptoms may require valve replacement (with a mechanical or prosthetic valve), valvular repair, or commissurotomy. (See *Types of valve surgery, page 196.*)

TEACHING THE PATIENT AFTER VASCULAR REPAIR

Before discharge from the facility, instruct the patient to:

● check his pulse (or have a family member do it) in the affected extremity before rising from bed each morning and to notify the practitioner if he can't palpate his pulse or if he develops coldness, pallor, numbness, tingling, or pain in his extremities

● continue with the progressive exercise started in the facility

● perform coughing and deep-breathing exercises (while splinting the incision with a pillow to reduce pain)

and use the incentive spirometer to reduce pulmonary complications

● avoid lifting objects that weigh more than 10 lb (4.5 kg) for the next 4 to 6 weeks

● check the incision site daily and immediately notify the practitioner of any signs and symptoms of infection

● take medications as prescribed and report adverse effects to the practitioner

● comply with the laboratory schedule for monitoring International Normalized Ratio if the patient is receiving warfarin (Coumadin).

Because of the high pressure generated by the left ventricle during contraction, stenosis and insufficiency most commonly affect the mitral and aortic valves. Other indications for valve surgery depend on the patient's symptoms and on the affected valve:

■ aortic insufficiency—valve replacement indicated after symptoms (palpitations, dizziness, dyspnea on exertion, angina, and murmurs) have developed or the chest X-ray and ECG reveal left ventricular hypertrophy

■ aortic stenosis—may not produce symptoms; valve replacement (or balloon valvuloplasty) recommended if cardiac catheterization reveals significant stenosis

■ mitral stenosis—valvuloplasty or commissurotomy indicated if the patient develops fatigue, dyspnea, hemoptysis, arrhythmias, pulmonary hypertension, or right ventricular hypertrophy

■ mitral insufficiency—valvuloplasty or valve replacement indicated when symptoms (dyspnea, fatigue, and palpitations) interfere with patient activities or in acute insufficiency (as in papillary muscle rupture).

Although valve surgery carries a low risk of mortality, it can cause serious complications. Hemorrhage, for instance, may result from unligated vessels, anticoagulant therapy, or coagulopathy resulting from cardiopulmonary bypass during surgery. Stroke may result from thrombus formation caused by turbulent blood flow through the pros-

TYPES OF VALVE SURGERY

When a patient with valve disease develops severe symptoms, surgery may be necessary. Several surgical procedures are available.

Commissurotomy

During commissurotomy, the surgeon incises fused mitral valve leaflets and removes calcium deposits to improve valve mobility.

Valve repair

Valve repair includes resection or patching of valve leaflets, stretching or shortening of chordae tendineae, or placing a ring in a dilatated annulus (annuloplasty). Valve repair is done to avoid the complications associated with the use of prosthetic valves.

Valve replacement

Valve replacement involves replacement of the patient's diseased valve with a mechanical or biological valve.

In the Ross procedure, the patient's own pulmonic valve is excised and used to replace the diseased aortic valve. An allograft from a human cadaver is then used to replace the pulmonic valve. Advantages of this procedure include the potential for the pulmonary autograft to grow when used in children, anticoagulation isn't necessary, and increased durability.

Minimally invasive valve surgery

Minimally invasive valve surgery can be performed without a large median sternotomy incision to repair or replace aortic and mitral valves. Port access techniques may also be used for mitral valve surgery using endovascular cardiopulmonary bypass. Advantages of these types of surgery include a less invasive procedure, shorter hospital stays, fewer postoperative complications, reduced costs, and smaller incisions.

---

thetic valve or from poor cerebral perfusion during cardiopulmonary bypass. In valve replacement, bacterial endocarditis can develop within days of implantation or months later. Valve dysfunction or failure may occur as the prosthetic device wears out.

PREPARING THE PATIENT

- As necessary, reinforce and supplement the physician's explanation of the procedure.
- Tell the patient that he'll awaken from surgery in an ICU or a PACU. Mention that he'll be connected to a cardiac monitor and have I.V. lines, an arterial line and, possibly, a PA or left atrial catheter in place.
- Explain that he'll breathe through an ET tube connected to a mechanical ventilator and that he'll have a chest tube in place.

- Make sure that the patient or a responsible family member has signed a consent form.

MONITORING AND AFTERCARE

- Closely monitor the patient's hemodynamic status for signs of compromise. Watch especially for severe hypotension, decreased cardiac output, and shock. Check and record vital signs every 15 minutes until his condition stabilizes.
- Frequently assess heart sounds; report distant heart sounds or new murmurs, which may indicate prosthetic valve failure.

RED FLAG Monitor the ECG continuously for disturbances in heart rate and rhythm, such as bradycardia, ventricular tachycardia, and heart block. Such disturbances may signal injury of the conduction system, which may occur during valve replacement from proximity of the atrial and mitral valves to the atrioventricular node. Arrhythmias may also result from myocardial irritability or ischemia, fluid and electrolyte imbalance, hypoxemia, or hypothermia. If you detect serious abnormalities, notify the practitioner, and be prepared to assist with temporary epicardial pacing.

- Take steps to maintain the patient's MAP between 70 and 100 mm Hg. Also, monitor PAP and left atrial pressure as indicated.
- Frequently assess the patient's peripheral pulses, capillary refill time, and skin temperature and color, and auscultate for heart sounds. Evaluate tissue oxygenation by assessing breath sounds, chest excursion, and symmetry of chest expansion. Report any abnormalities.
- Check ABG values every 2 to 4 hours, and adjust ventilator settings as needed.
- Maintain chest tube drainage at the prescribed negative pressure (usually −10 to −40 cm H_2O for adults). Assess chest tubes frequently for signs of hemorrhage, excessive drainage (greater than 200 ml/hour), and a sudden decrease or cessation of drainage.
- As indicated, give analgesic, anticoagulant, antibiotic, antiarrhythmic, inotropic, and pressor drugs as well as I.V. fluids and blood products. Monitor intake and output, and assess for electrolyte imbalances, especially hypokalemia. When anticoagulant therapy begins, evaluate its effectiveness by monitoring prothrombin time and International Normalized Ratio daily.
- After weaning from the ventilator and removing the ET tube, promote chest physiotherapy. Start the patient on incentive spirometry, and encourage him to cough, turn frequently, and deep-breathe.
- Throughout the patient's recovery period, observe him carefully for complications. (See *Teaching the patient after valve surgery*, page 198.)

Ventricular assist device insertion

A VAD is a device that's implanted to support a failing heart. A VAD consists of a blood pump, cannulas, and a pneumatic or electrical drive console.

VADs are designed to decrease the heart's workload and increase cardiac output in patients with ventricular failure.

A VAD is commonly used while a patient waits for a heart transplant. In a surgical procedure, blood is diverted from a ventricle to an artificial pump. This pump is synchronized to the patient's ECG and then functions as the ventricle. (See *Ventricular assist device: Help for the failing heart.*) VADs are also indicated for use in patients with cardiogenic shock that doesn't respond to maximal pharmacologic therapy or with an inability to be weaned from cardiopulmonary bypass.

A VAD is used to provide systemic or pulmonary support, or both:

■ A right VAD provides pulmonary support by diverting blood from the failing right ventricle to the VAD, which then pumps the blood to the pulmonary circulation by way of the VAD connection to the pulmonary artery.
■ With a left VAD, blood flows from the left ventricle to the VAD, which then pumps blood back to the body by way of the VAD connection to the aorta.

VENTRICULAR ASSIST DEVICE: HELP FOR THE FAILING HEART

A ventricular assist device (VAD) functions like an artificial heart. The major difference is that the VAD assists the heart instead of replacing it. The VAD can aid one or both ventricles. The pumping chambers themselves aren't usually implanted in the patient.

A permanent VAD is implanted in the patient's chest cavity, although it still provides only temporary support. The device receives power through the skin by a belt of electrical transformer coils (worn externally as a portable battery pack). It can also operate off an implanted, rechargeable battery for up to 1 hour at a time.

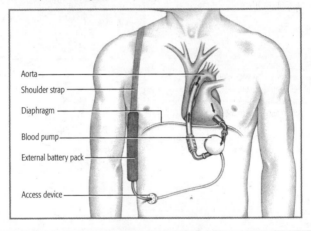

Aorta

Shoulder strap

Diaphragm

Blood pump

External battery pack

Access device

- When biventricular support is needed, both may be used. (See *A closer look at VADs,* page 200.)

PREPARING THE PATIENT
- Prepare the patient and his family for VAD insertion; be sure to explain how the device works, what its purpose is, and what to expect after insertion.
- If possible, make sure that the patient or a responsible family member has signed a consent form.
- Continue close patient monitoring, including continuous ECG monitoring, pulmonary artery and hemodynamic status monitoring, and intake and output monitoring.

A CLOSER LOOK AT VADs

There are three types of ventricular assist devices (VADs).

● A right VAD provides pulmonary support by diverting blood from the failing right ventricle to the VAD, which then pumps the blood to the pulmonary circulation via the VAD connection to the left pulmonary artery.

RIGHT VAD

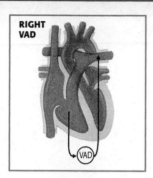

● With a left VAD, blood flows from the left ventricle to the VAD, which then pumps blood back to the body via the VAD connection to the aorta.

● When a right and left VAD are used, it's referred to as a biventricular VAD.

LEFT VAD

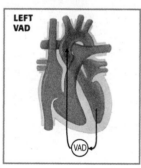

MONITORING AND AFTERCARE

Assess the patient's cardiovascular status at least every 15 minutes until stable, and then hourly. Monitor blood pressure and hemodynamic parameters, including cardiac output and cardiac index, ECG, and peripheral pulses.

■ Inspect the incision and dressing at least every hour initially, and then every 2 to 4 hours as indicated by the patient's condition.

■ Monitor urine output hourly, and maintain I.V. fluid therapy as indicated. Watch for signs of fluid overload or decreasing urine output.

■ Assess chest tube drainage and function frequently. Notify the physician if drainage is greater than 150 ml over 2 hours. Auscultate lungs for evidence of abnormal breath sounds. Evaluate oxygen

DISCHARGE TEACHING

TEACHING THE PATIENT AFTER VAD INSERTION

Before discharge following the insertion of a ventricular assist device (VAD), instruct the patient to:
● immediately report redness, swelling, or drainage at the incision site; chest pain; or fever
● immediately notify the practitioner if signs or symptoms of heart failure (weight gain, dyspnea, or edema) develop
● follow his prescribed medication regimen and report adverse effects

● follow his prescribed diet, especially sodium and fat restrictions
● maintain a balance between activity and rest
● follow his exercise or rehabilitation program (if prescribed)
● comply with the laboratory schedule for monitoring International Normalized Ratio if the patient is receiving warfarin (Coumadin).

saturation or mixed venous oxygen saturation levels, and administer oxygen as indicated.

■ Obtain hemoglobin levels, hematocrit, and coagulation studies as indicated. Administer blood component therapy as indicated.

■ Assess the incision and the cannula insertion site for signs of infection. Monitor the white blood cell count and differential daily, and take rectal or core temperatures every 4 hours.

■ Use sterile technique in dressing changes. Change the dressing site over the cannula sites daily or according to facility policy.

■ Assess for signs and symptoms of bleeding.

■ Turn the patient every 2 hours, and begin ROM exercises when he's stable.

■ Administer antibiotics prophylactically if ordered. (See *Teaching the patient after VAD insertion.*)

Balloon catheter treatments

Balloon catheter treatments for cardiovascular disorders include percutaneous balloon valvuloplasty, percutaneous transluminal coronary angioplasty (PTCA) and intra-aortic balloon pump (IABP) counterpulsation.

PERCUTANEOUS BALLOON VALVULOPLASTY

Percutaneous balloon valvuloplasty can be performed in the cardiac catheterization laboratory. It's intended to improve valvular function

PERCUTANEOUS BALLOON VALVULOPLASTY

In balloon valvuloplasty, the physician inserts a balloon-tipped catheter through the femoral vein or artery and threads it into the heart. After locating the stenotic valve, he inflates the balloon, increasing the size of the valve opening.

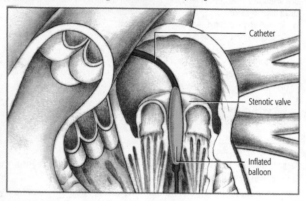

Catheter

Stenotic valve

Inflated balloon

by enlarging the orifice of a stenotic heart valve caused by congenital defect, calcification, rheumatic fever, or aging. A small balloon valvuloplasty catheter is introduced through the skin at the femoral vein. (See *Percutaneous balloon valvuloplasty*.)

Although valve surgery remains the treatment of choice for valvular heart disease, percutaneous balloon valvuloplasty offers an alternative for individuals who are considered poor candidates for surgery.

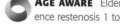 **AGE AWARE** Elderly patients with aortic disease commonly experience restenosis 1 to 2 years after undergoing valvuloplasty.

Despite the decreased risks associated with more invasive procedures, balloon valvuloplasty can lead to complications, including:
- worsening valvular insufficiency by misshaping the valve so that it doesn't close completely
- pieces breaking off of the calcified valve, which may travel to the brain or lungs and cause embolism (rare)
- severely damaging delicate valve leaflets, requiring immediate surgery to replace the valve (rare)
- bleeding and hematoma at the arterial puncture site

- MI (rare), arrhythmias, myocardial ischemia, and circulatory defects distal to the catheter entry site.

PREPARING THE PATIENT

- Describe the procedure to the patient and his family, and tell them that it takes 1 to 4 hours to complete.
- Explain that a catheter will be inserted into an artery or a vein in the patient's groin and that he may feel pressure as the catheter moves along the vessel.
- Reassure the patient that although he'll be awake during the procedure, he'll be given a sedative. Instruct him to report any angina during the procedure.
- Check the patient's history for allergies; if he has had allergic reactions to shellfish, iodine, or contrast media, notify the physician.
- Make sure that the patient or a responsible family member has signed a consent form.
- Restrict food and fluids for at least 6 hours before the procedure.
- Make sure that the results of coagulation studies, complete blood count (CBC), serum electrolyte studies, blood typing and cross-matching, blood urea nitrogen (BUN) levels, and serum creatinine levels are available.
- Obtain baseline vital signs and assess peripheral pulses.
- Apply ECG electrodes and insert an I.V. line if not already in place.
- Administer oxygen through a nasal cannula.
- Perform skin preparation according to your facility's policy.
- Give the patient a sedative as indicated.

MONITORING AND AFTERCARE

- Assess the patient's vital signs and oxygen saturation every 15 minutes for the first hour and then every 30 minutes for 4 hours, unless his condition warrants more frequent checking.
- Monitor I.V. infusions, such as heparin or nitroglycerin, as indicated.
- Assess peripheral pulses distal to the catheter insertion site as well as the affected extremity's color, sensation, temperature, and capillary refill time.
- Monitor cardiac rhythm continuously, and assess hemodynamic parameters closely for changes.
- Auscultate for murmurs, which may indicate worsening valvular insufficiency. Report changes to the physician immediately.
- Instruct the patient to remain in bed for 8 hours and to keep the affected extremity straight. Maintain sandbags in position, if used to apply pressure to the catheter site. Elevate the head of the bed 15

to 30 degrees. If a hemostatic device was used to close the catheter insertion site, anticipate that the patient may be allowed out of bed in only a few hours.

■ Assess the catheter site for hematoma, ecchymosis, and hemorrhage. If an expanding ecchymotic area appears, mark the area to help determine the pace of expansion. If bleeding occurs, locate the artery and apply manual pressure; then notify the physician.

■ Administer I.V. fluids as indicated (usually 100 ml/hour) to promote excretion of the contrast medium. Be sure to assess for signs of fluid overload.

■ Document the patient's tolerance of the procedure and status after it, including vital signs, hemodynamic parameters, appearance of the catheter site, ECG findings, condition of the extremity distal to the insertion site, complications, and necessary interventions. (See *Teaching the patient after percutaneous balloon valvuloplasty*.)

Percutaneous transluminal coronary angioplasty

PTCA offers a nonsurgical alternative to coronary artery bypass surgery. The physician uses a balloon-tipped catheter to dilate a coronary artery that has become narrowed because of atherosclerotic plaque. (See *Looking at PTCA*.)

Performed in the cardiac catheterization laboratory under local anesthesia, PTCA doesn't involve a sternotomy, so it's less costly and requires shorter hospitalization. Patients can usually walk the next day and return to work in 2 weeks.

PTCA works best when lesions are readily accessible, noncalcified, less than 10 mm, concentric, discrete, and smoothly tapered. Patients with a history of less than 1 year of disabling angina make good

LOOKING AT PTCA

Percutaneous transluminal coronary angioplasty (PTCA) can open an occluded coronary artery without opening the chest. This procedure is outlined in the steps below.

First, the cardiologist must thread the catheter into the artery. The illustration below shows the entrance of a guide catheter into the coronary artery.

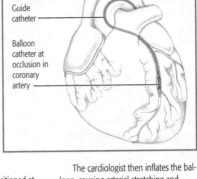

When angiography shows the guide catheter positioned at the occlusion site, the cardiologist carefully inserts a smaller double-lumen balloon catheter through the guide catheter and directs the balloon through the occlusion.

The cardiologist then inflates the balloon, causing arterial stretching and plaque fracture as shown below. The balloon may need to be inflated or deflated several times until successful arterial dilatation occurs.

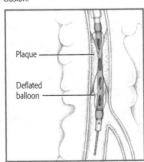

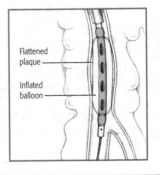

candidates because their lesions tend to be softer and more compressible.

Complications of PTCA are acute vessel closure and late restenosis. To prevent restenosis, such procedures as stenting, atherectomy, and laser angioplasty may be performed. Also, vascular brachytherapy

PREVENTING RESTENOSIS

Standard angioplasty is performed to remove the plaque blockage in the coronary artery. However, restenosis of the vessel is a frequent complication that occurs from scar tissue formation rather than plaque buildup.

Vascular brachytherapy

Vascular brachytherapy is the use of radiation in the coronary vessels to inhibit the development of this scar tissue, thus preventing restenosis of the vessel. The procedure involves a specialized radiation catheter that's inserted after angioplasty to direct beta radiation to the treated area for a few minutes. The radiation and catheter are then removed, with no radiation source being left in the body.

Coronary drug-eluting stents

Stents are used to open arteries that feed the heart, thereby improving circulation to myocardial tissue. One complication of stents is restenosis of the vessel. Drug-eluting stents open the artery and also release a drug to the implantation site that helps reduce restenosis. The drug works by blocking smooth-muscle proliferation.

Placement of drug-eluting stents during a cardiac catheterization or angioplasty procedure is the same as for regular stents. Postprocedural care is also the same.

and drug-eluting stents have been found to decrease the incidence of restenosis. (See *Preventing restenosis*.)

PREPARING THE PATIENT

- Describe the procedure to the patient and his family, and tell them that it takes 1 to 4 hours to complete.
- Explain that a catheter will be inserted into an artery or a vein in the patient's groin and that he may feel pressure as the catheter moves along the vessel.
- Reassure the patient that although he'll be awake during the procedure, he'll be given a sedative. Instruct him to report any angina during the procedure.
- Explain that the physician injects a contrast medium to outline the lesion's location. Warn the patient that he may feel a hot, flushing sensation or transient nausea during the injection.
- Check the patient's history for allergies; if he has had allergic reactions to shellfish, iodine, or contrast media, notify the practitioner.
- Make sure that the patient or a responsible family member has signed a consent form.
- Locate, mark, and record the amplitude of bilateral distal pulses.

- Restrict food and fluids for at least 6 hours before the procedure.
- Make sure that the results of coagulation studies, CBC, serum electrolyte studies, blood typing and crossmatching, BUN levels, and serum creatinine levels are available.
- Obtain baseline vital signs and assess peripheral pulses.
- Apply ECG electrodes and insert an I.V. line if not already in place.
- Administer oxygen through a nasal cannula.
- Perform skin preparation according to your facility's policy.
- Instruct the patient to tell the surgical team immediately if he has breathing difficulties, sweating, numbness, itching, nausea, vomiting, chills, or heart palpitations during the procedure.
- Give the patient a sedative as indicated.

MONITORING AND AFTERCARE

- Assess the patient's vital signs and oxygen saturation every 15 minutes for the first hour and then every 30 minutes for 4 hours, unless his condition warrants more frequent checking.
- Administer an anticoagulant, I.V. nitroglycerin, and I.V. fluids as indicated.
- Assess peripheral pulses distal to the catheter insertion site as well as the affected extremity's color, sensation, temperature, and capillary refill time.
- Monitor cardiac rhythm continuously, and assess hemodynamic parameters closely for changes.
- Monitor the 12-lead ECG results, particularly changes in ST segments indicating ischemia or infarction.

RED FLAG Immediately report signs and symptoms of angina (including chest pain), fluid overload (tachycardia, dyspnea, edema), and abrupt arterial reclosure (chest pain, ECG changes)

- Instruct the patient to remain in bed for 8 hours and to keep the affected extremity straight. Maintain sandbags in position, if used to apply pressure to the catheter site.
- Elevate the head of the bed 15 to 30 degrees. If a hemostatic device was used to close the catheter insertion site, anticipate that the patient may be allowed out of bed in only a few hours.
- Administer I.V. fluids as indicated (usually 100 ml/hour) to promote excretion of the contrast medium. Be sure to assess for signs of fluid overload.
- Assess the catheter site for hematoma, ecchymosis, and hemorrhage. If bleeding occurs, locate the artery and apply manual pressure; then notify the physician.

■ After the physician removes the catheter, apply direct pressure for at least 10 minutes, and monitor the site often.

■ Document the patient's tolerance of the procedure and status afterward, including vital signs, hemodynamic parameters, appearance of the catheter site, ECG findings, condition of the extremity distal to the insertion site, complications, and necessary interventions. (See *Teaching the patient after PTCA.*)

Intra-aortic balloon pump counterpulsation

IABP counterpulsation temporarily reduces left ventricular workload and improves coronary perfusion. (See *Understanding a balloon pump.*)

A 34-, 40-, or 50-cc balloon-tipped catheter is placed in the descending aorta between the left subclavian artery and the renal artery. The balloon is attached to a console that contains the gas for inflation (usually helium) and displays the waveforms. (See *Parts of an IABP,* page 210.)

IABP counterpulsation may benefit patients with:

■ cardiogenic shock due to acute MI

■ septic shock

■ intractable angina before surgery

■ intractable ventricular arrhythmias

■ ventricular septal or papillary muscle ruptures.

It's also used for patients who suffer pump failure before or after cardiac surgery.

The physician may perform balloon catheter insertion at the patient's bedside as an emergency procedure or in the operating room.

UNDERSTANDING A BALLOON PUMP

An intra-aortic balloon pump consists of a polyurethane balloon attached to an external pump console by means of a large-lumen catheter. It's inserted percutaneously through the femoral artery and positioned in the descending aorta just distal to the left subclavian artery and above the renal arteries.

Inflation

This external pump works in precise counterpoint to the left ventricle, inflating the balloon with helium early in diastole and deflating it just before systole. As the balloon inflates, it forces blood toward the aortic valve, thereby raising pressure in the aortic root and augmenting diastolic pressure to improve coronary perfusion. It also improves peripheral circulation by forcing blood through the brachiocephalic, common carotid, and subclavian arteries arising from the aortic trunk.

Deflation

The balloon deflates rapidly at the end of diastole, creating a vacuum in the aorta. This reduces aortic volume and pressure, thereby decreasing the resistance to left ventricular ejection (afterload). This decreased workload, in turn, reduces the heart's oxygen requirements and, combined with the improved myocardial perfusion, helps prevent or diminish myocardial ischemia.

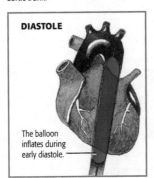

DIASTOLE

The balloon inflates during early diastole.

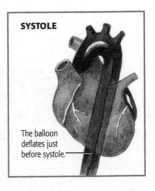

SYSTOLE

The balloon deflates just before systole.

PREPARING THE PATIENT

- Explain to the patient that the physician is going to place a catheter in the aorta to help his heart pump more easily. Tell him that, while the catheter is in place, he can't sit up, bend his knee, or flex his hip more than 30 degrees.

PARTS OF AN IABP

The following illustrations show a balloon pump and a close up of the controls and screen.

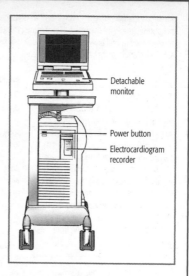

Detachable monitor

Power button

Electrocardiogram recorder

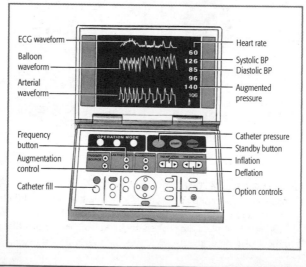

ECG waveform

Balloon waveform

Arterial waveform

Heart rate — 60
Systolic BP — 126
Diastolic BP — 85
96
Augmented pressure — 140
106

Frequency button

Augmentation control

Catheter fill

OPERATION MODE

Catheter pressure

Standby button

Inflation

Deflation

Option controls

- Attach the patient to a continuous ECG monitor, and make sure he has an arterial line, a PA catheter, and a peripheral I.V. line in place.
- Gather a surgical tray for percutaneous catheter insertion, heparin, normal saline solution, the IABP catheter, and the pump console. Connect the ECG monitor to the pump console.
- If possible, make sure the patient or a responsible family member has signed a consent form.

MONITORING AND AFTERCARE

- After the IABP catheter is inserted, select either the ECG or the arterial waveform to regulate inflation and deflation of the balloon. With the ECG waveform, the pump inflates the balloon in the middle of the T wave (diastole) and deflates with the R wave (before systole). With the arterial waveform, the upstroke of the arterial wave triggers balloon inflation. (See *Interpreting intra-aortic balloon waveforms,* pages 212 to 214.)
- Frequently assess the insertion site. Don't elevate the head of the bed more than 30 degrees, to prevent upward migration of the catheter and occlusion of the left subclavian artery. If the balloon occludes the artery, you may see a diminished left radial pulse, and the patient may report dizziness. Incorrect balloon placement may also cause flank pain or a sudden decrease in urine output.
- Asses the patient's cardiovascular and respiratory status at least every 4 hours. If possible, place the IABP on standby to eliminate extraneous sounds.
- Give anticoagulants as indicated to help prevent thrombus formation.
- Assess distal pulses, color, temperature, and capillary refill of the patient's extremities every 15 minutes for the first 4 hours after insertion. After 4 hours, assess hourly for the duration of IABP therapy.
- Watch for signs of thrombus formation, such as a sudden weakening of pedal pulses, pain, and motor or sensory loss.
- If indicated, apply antiembolism stockings.
- Encourage active ROM exercises every 2 hours for the arms, the unaffected leg, and the affected ankle.
- Maintain adequate hydration to help prevent thrombus formation.
- If bleeding occurs at the catheter insertion site, apply direct pressure and notify the physician
- An alarm on the console may indicate a gas leak from a damaged catheter or ruptured balloon. If the alarm sounds or you see blood in the catheter, shut down the pump console, and immediately

(Text continues on page 214.)

INTERPRETING INTRA-AORTIC BALLOON WAVEFORMS

During intra-aortic balloon counterpulsation, you can use electrocardiogram and arterial pressure waveforms to determine whether the balloon pump is functioning properly.

Normal inflation-deflation timing

Balloon inflation occurs after aortic valve closure; deflation, during isovolumetric contraction, occurs just before the aortic valve opens. In a properly timed waveform such as the one shown below, the inflation point lies at or slightly above the dicrotic notch. Both inflation and deflation cause a sharp V. Peak diastolic pressure exceeds peak systolic pressure; peak systolic pressure exceeds assisted peak systolic pressure.

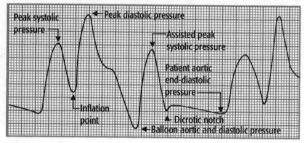

Early inflation

With early inflation, the inflation point lies before the dicrotic notch. Early inflation dangerously increases myocardial stress and decreases cardiac output.

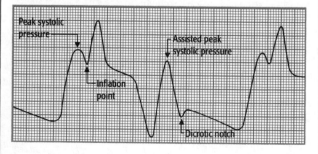

INTERPRETING INTRA-AORTIC BALLOON WAVEFORMS *(continued)*

Early deflation

With early deflation, a U shape appears, and peak systolic pressure is less than or equal to assisted peak systolic pressure. This won't decrease afterload or myocardial oxygen consumption.

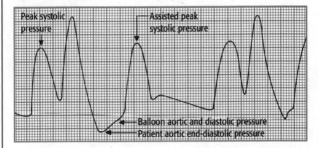

Late inflation

With late inflation, the dicrotic notch precedes the inflation point, and the notch and the inflation point create a W shape. This can lead to a reduction in peak diastolic pressure, coronary and systemic perfusion augmentation time, and augmented coronary perfusion pressure.

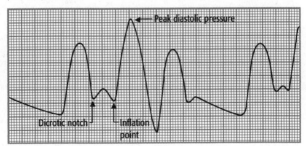

(continued)

INTERPRETING INTRA-AORTIC BALLOON WAVEFORMS *(continued)*

Late deflation

With late deflation, peak systolic pressure exceeds assisted peak systolic pressure. This threatens the patient by increasing afterload, myocardial oxygen consumption, cardiac workload, and preload. It occurs when the balloon has been inflated for too long.

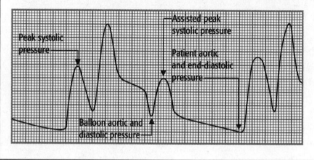

place the patient in Trendelenburg's position to prevent an embolus from reaching the brain. Then notify the physician. (See *Trouble-shooting an IABP*.)

■ After the patient's signs and symptoms of left-sided heart failure diminish, only minimal drug support is required, and the physician begins weaning the patient from IABP counterpulsation by reducing the frequency of pumping or decreasing the balloon volume. A minimum volume or pumping ratio must be maintained to prevent thrombus formation. Most consoles have a flutter function that moves the balloon to prevent clot formation. Use the flutter function when the patient has been weaned from counterpulsation but the catheter hasn't yet been removed.

■ To discontinue the IABP, the physician deflates the balloon, clips the sutures, removes the catheter, and allows the site to bleed for 5 seconds to expel clots.

■ After the physician discontinues the IABP, apply direct pressure for 30 minutes, and then apply a pressure dressing. Evaluate the site for bleeding and hematoma formation hourly for the next 4 hours. (See *Teaching the patient after IABP treatment*, page 218.)

(Text continues on page 218.)

TROUBLESHOOTING AN IABP

PROBLEM	POSSIBLE CAUSES	INTERVENTIONS
High gas leak (automatic mode only)	Balloon leakage or abrasion	● Check for blood in the tubing. ● Stop pumping. ● Notify the physician to remove the balloon.
	Condensation in extension tubing, volume limiter disk, or both	● Remove condensate from the tubing and volume limiter disk. ● Refill, autopurge, and resume pumping.
	Kink in balloon catheter or tubing	● Check the catheter and tubing for kinks and loose connections; straighten and tighten any found. ● Refill and resume pumping.
	Tachycardia	● Change wean control to 1:2 or operate on "manual" mode. ● Autopurge the balloon every 1 to 2 hours, and monitor the balloon pressure waveform closely.
	Malfunctioning or loose volume limiter disk	● Replace or tighten the disk. ● Refill, autopurge, and resume pumping.
	System leak	● Perform a leak test.
Balloon line block (in automatic mode only)	Kink in balloon or catheter	● Check the catheter and tubing for kinks and loose connections; straighten and tighten any found. ● Refill and resume pumping.
	Balloon catheter not unfurled; sheath or balloon positioned too high	● Notify the physician immediately to verify placement. ● Anticipate the need for repositioning or manual inflation of the balloon.

(continued)

TROUBLESHOOTING AN IABP *(continued)*

PROBLEM	POSSIBLE CAUSES	INTERVENTIONS
Balloon line block (in automatic mode only) *(continued)*	Condensation in tubing, volume limiter disk, or both	● Remove condensate from the tubing and volume limiter disk. ● Refill, autopurge, and resume pumping.
	Balloon too large for aorta	● Decrease volume control percentage by one notch.
	Malfunctioning volume limiter disk or incorrect volume limiter disk size	● Replace the volume limiter disk. ● Refill, autopurge, and resume pumping.
No electrocardiogram (ECG) trigger	Inadequate signal	● Adjust ECG gain, and change the lead or trigger mode.
	Lead disconnected	● Replace the lead.
	Improper ECG input mode (skin or monitor) selected	● Adjust ECG input to appropriate mode (skin or monitor).
No atrial pressure trigger	Arterial line damped	● Flush the line.
	Arterial line open to atmosphere	● Check connections on the arterial pressure line.
Trigger mode change	Trigger mode changed while pumping	● Resume pumping.
Irregular heart rhythm	Patient experiencing arrhythmia, such as atrial fibrillation or ectopic beats	● Change to R or QRS sense (if necessary to accommodate irregular rhythm). ● Notify the physician of arrhythmia.

TROUBLESHOOTING AN **IABP** *(continued)*

PROBLEM	POSSIBLE CAUSES	INTERVENTIONS
Erratic atrio-ventricular (AV) pacing	Demand for paced rhythm occurring when in AV sequential trigger mode	● Change to pacer reject trigger or QRS sense.
Noisy ECG signal	Malfunctioning leads	● Replace the leads. ● Check the ECG cable.
	Electrocautery in use	● Switch to atrial pressure trigger.
Internal trigger	Trigger mode set on internal 80 beats/minute	● Select an alternative trigger if the patient has a heartbeat or rhythm. ● Keep in mind that the internal trigger is used only during cardiopulmonary bypass or cardiac arrest.
Purge incomplete	OFF button pressed during autopurge; interrupted purge cycle	● Initiate autopurging again or initiate pumping.
High fill pressure	Malfunctioning volume limiter disk	● Replace the volume limiter disk. ● Refill, autopurge, and resume pumping.
	Occluded vent line or valve	● Attempt to resume pumping. ● If unsuccessful, notify the physician and contact the manufacturer.
No balloon drive	No volume limiter disk	● Insert the volume limiter disk, and lock it securely in place.
	Tubing disconnected	● Reconnect the tubing. ● Refill, autopurge, and pump.

(continued)

TROUBLESHOOTING AN **IABP** *(continued)*

PROBLEM	POSSIBLE CAUSES	INTERVENTIONS
Incorrect timing	INFLATE and DE-FLATE controls set incorrectly	● Place the INFLATE and DEFLATE controls at set midpoints. ● Reassess timing and readjust.
Low volume percentage	Volume control percentage not 100%	● Assess the cause of decreased volume, and reset if necessary.

DISCHARGE TEACHING

TEACHING THE PATIENT AFTER IABP TREATMENT

Before discharge from the facility, instruct the patient to:
● call his practitioner if he experiences bleeding or bruising at the insertion site
● return for follow-up testing as recommended by his practitioner
● report chest pain to the practitioner.

CARDIOVASCULAR RESYNCHRONIZATION TECHNIQUES

When the electrical conduction of the heart is disrupted, cardiac output is diminished, and perfusion of blood and oxygen to all body tissues is affected. Treatment to restore the heart's conduction needs to begin quickly. Some treatments include defibrillation, an implantable cardioverter-defibrillator (ICD), synchronized cardioversion, and pacemaker insertion.

Defibrillation

In defibrillation, electrode paddles are used to direct an electric current through the patient's heart. The current causes the myocardium to depolarize, which in turn encourages the SA node to resume control of the heart's electrical activity. (See *Biphasic defibrillators*.)

BIPHASIC DEFIBRILLATORS

Many hospital defibrillators are monophasic, delivering a single electric current that travels in one direction between the two pads or paddles on the patient's chest. A large amount of electric current is required for effective monophasic defibrillation.

Differences between monophasic and biphasic defibrillators

Biphasic defibrillators are becoming more common in hospitals. Pad or paddle placement is the same as with the monophasic defibrillator. The difference is that during biphasic defibrillation, the electric current discharged from the pads or paddles travels in a positive direction for a specified duration and then reverses and flows in a negative direction for the remaining time of the electrical discharge.

Energy usage

The biphasic defibrillator delivers two electric currents and lowers the heart muscle's defibrillation threshold, making it possible to successfully defibrillate ventricular fibrillation with smaller amounts

of energy. Instead of using 200 joules, an initial shock of 150 joules is usually effective.

Number of shocks needed

The biphasic defibrillator can adjust for differences in impedance (the resistance of the current through the chest). This reduces the number of shocks needed to terminate ventricular fibrillation.

Benefits of biphasic defibrillation

Because the biphasic defibrillator requires lower energy levels and fewer shocks, damage to the myocardial muscle is reduced. Biphasic defibrillators used at the appropriate energy level may be used for defibrillation and, in the synchronized mode, for synchronized cardioversion.

The electrode paddles delivering the current may be placed on the patient's chest or, during cardiac surgery, directly on the myocardium.

Because some arrhythmias, such as ventricular fibrillation, can cause death if not corrected, the success of defibrillation depends on early recognition and quick treatment.

In addition to treating ventricular fibrillation, defibrillation may also be used to treat ventricular tachycardia that doesn't produce a pulse, or polymorphic ventricular tachycardia with a pulse.

Automated external defibrillators

An automated external defibrillator (AED) has a cardiac rhythm analysis system. The AED interprets the patient's cardiac rhythm and gives the operator step-by-step directions on how to proceed if defibrilla-

DEFIBRILLATOR PADDLE PLACEMENT

Here's a guide to correct paddle placement for defibrillation.

Anterolateral placement

For anterolateral placement, place one paddle to the right of the upper sternum, just below the right clavicle, and the other over the fifth or sixth intercostal space at the left anterior axillary line.

Anteroposterior placement

For anteroposterior placement, place the anterior paddle directly over the heart at the precordium, to the left of the lower sternal border. Place the flat posterior paddle under the patient's body beneath the heart and immediately below the scapulae.

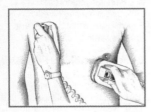
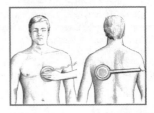

tion is indicated. Most AEDs have a "quick-look" feature that allows visualization of the rhythm with the paddles before electrodes are connected.

The AED is equipped with a microcomputer that analyzes a patient's heart rhythm at the push of a button. It then audibly or visually prompts you to deliver a shock.

PATIENT PREPARATION

- Assess the patient to determine if he lacks a pulse. Call for help, and perform cardiopulmonary resuscitation (CPR) until the defibrillator and other emergency equipment arrive.
- Connect the monitoring leads of the defibrillator to the patient, and assess his cardiac rhythm in two leads.
- Expose the patient's chest, and apply conductive pads at the paddle placement positions. (See *Defibrillator paddle placement*.)

MONITORING AND AFTERCARE

- Turn on the defibrillator and, if performing external defibrillation, set the energy level at 360 joules (J) for an adult.

- Charge the paddles by pressing the charge buttons, which are located on either the machine or the paddles.
- Place the paddles over the conductive pads, and press firmly against the patient's chest, using 25 lb (11.3 kg) of pressure.
- Reassess the patient's cardiac rhythm in two leads.
- If the patient remains in a shockable rhythm, instruct all personnel to stand clear of the patient and the bed. Also, make a visual check to make sure everyone is clear of the patient and the bed.
- Discharge the current by pressing both paddle discharge buttons simultaneously.
- Reassess the patient's pulse, and give 2 minutes of CPR. Reassess his cardiac rhythm.
- If necessary, prepare to defibrillate a second time at 360 J. Announce that you're preparing to defibrillate, and follow the procedure described above.
- Reassess the patient and continue CPR.
- If the patient still has no pulse after the first two cycles of defibrillation and CPR, give supplemental oxygen, and begin administering appropriate medications such as epinephrine. Also, consider possible causes for failure of the patient's rhythm to convert, such as acidosis and hypoxia.
- If defibrillation restores a normal rhythm, assess the patient. Obtain baseline ABG levels and a 12-lead ECG. Provide supplemental oxygen, ventilation, and medications as needed. Prepare the defibrillator for immediate reuse.
- Document the procedure, including the patient's ECG rhythms before and after defibrillation; the number of times defibrillation was performed; the voltage used during each attempt; whether a pulse returned; the dosage, route, and time of any drugs administered; whether CPR was used; how the airway was maintained; and the patient's outcome. (See *Teaching the patient after defibrillation,* page 222.)

Implantable cardioverter-defibrillator

An ICD has a programmable pulse generator and lead system that monitors the heart's activity, detects ventricular bradyarrhythmias and tachyarrhythmias, and responds with appropriate therapies. It's used for antitachycardia and bradycardia pacing, cardioversion, and defibrillation. (See *Types of ICD therapy,* page 222.) Some defibrillators also have the ability to pace the atrium and the ventricle. ICDs store information, and ECGs allow the information to be retrieved to revaluate the device's function.

TEACHING THE PATIENT AFTER DEFIBRILLATION

Before discharge:
● instruct the patient to report any episodes of chest pain to the practitioner
● encourage the family to learn cardiopulmonary resuscitation as well as how to use an automated external defibrillator
● instruct the patient to consider an implantable cardioverter-defibrillator, if recommended by his practitioner.

TYPES OF ICD THERAPY

Implantable cardioverter-defibrillators (ICDs) can deliver a range of therapies, depending on the arrhythmia detected and how the device is programmed. Therapies include antitachycardia pacing, cardioversion, defibrillation, and bradycardia pacing. Some ICDs can also provide biventricular pacing.

THERAPY	DESCRIPTION
Antitachycardia pacing	A series of small, rapid electrical pacing pulses used to interrupt atrial arrhythmias or ventricular tachycardia and return the heart to its normal rhythm. Antitachycardia pacing isn't appropriate for all patients; it's initiated by the practitioner after appropriate evaluation of electrophysiology studies.
Cardioversion	A low- or high-energy shock (up to 34 joules) that's timed to the R wave to terminate atrial fibrillation or ventricular tachycardia and return the heart to its normal rhythm.
Defibrillation	A high-energy shock (up to 34 joules) to the heart to terminate atrial fibrillation or ventricular fibrillation and return the heart to its normal rhythm.
Bradycardia pacing	Electrical pacing pulses used when the natural electrical signals are too slow. ICD systems can pace one chamber (VVI pacing) of the heart at a preset rate or sense and pace both chambers (DDD pacing).

INSERTING AN ICD

To insert an implantable cardioverter-defibrillator (ICD), the cardiologist makes a small incision near the collarbone and accesses the subclavian vein. The leadwires are inserted through the subclavian vein, threaded into the heart, and placed in contact with the endocardium.

The leads are connected to the pulse generator, which is placed under the skin in a specially prepared pocket in the right or left upper chest. (Placement is similar to that used for a pacemaker.) The cardiologist then closes the incision and programs the device.

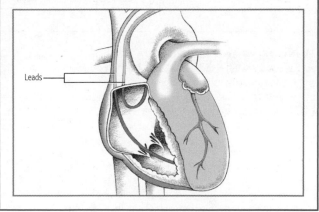

To implant an ICD, the cardiologist positions the lead (or leads) transvenously in the endocardium of the right ventricle (and the right atrium, if both chambers require pacing). The lead connects to a generator box, which is implanted in the right or left upper chest near the clavicle. (See *Inserting an ICD.*)

PATIENT PREPARATION

- Reinforce the cardiologist's instructions to the patient and his family, answering any questions they may have.
- Be sure to emphasize the need for the device, the potential complications, and ICD terminology.
- Restrict food and fluid for 12 hours before the procedure.
- Give a sedative on the morning of the procedure to help the patient relax.
- Make sure that the patient or a responsible family member has signed a consent form.

MONITORING AND AFTERCARE

■ The patient will be monitored on a telemetry unit.

■ Monitor for arrhythmias and proper device functioning.

RED FLAG Monitor for signs and symptoms of a perforated ventricle with resultant cardiac tamponade, distant heart sounds, pulsus paradoxus, hypotension accompanied by narrowed pulse pressure, bulging neck veins, increased venous pressure, cyanosis, decreased urine output, restlessness, and complaints of fullness in the chest. Notify the practitioner immediately, and prepare the patient for emergency surgery.

■ Gradually allow the patient to increase activities.

■ Monitor the incision site for signs of infection or drainage.

■ Maintain the occlusive dressing for the first 24 hours.

■ If the patient experiences cardiac arrest, initiate CPR and advanced cardiac life support.

RED FLAG For external defibrillation, use anteroposterior paddle placement; don't place paddles directly over the pulse generator.

■ Provide support to the patient and his family to help them cope with recovery and lifestyle changes.

■ Encourage family members to learn CPR. (See *Teaching the patient after ICD implantation.*)

Synchronized cardioversion

Cardioversion (synchronized countershock) is an elective or emergency procedure used to correct tachyarrhythmias (such as atrial tachycardia, atrial flutter, atrial fibrillation, and symptomatic ventricular tachycardia). It's also the treatment of choice for patients with arrhythmias that don't respond to drug therapy.

In synchronized cardioversion, an electric current is delivered to the heart to correct an arrhythmia. Compared with defibrillation, it uses much lower energy levels and is synchronized to deliver an electric charge to the myocardium at the peak R wave.

The procedure causes immediate depolarization, interrupting reentry circuits (abnormal impulse conduction that occurs when cardiac tissue is activated two or more times, causing reentry arrhythmias) and allowing the SA node to resume control.

Synchronizing the electric charge with the R wave ensures that the current won't be delivered on the vulnerable T wave and disrupt repolarization. Thus, it reduces the risk that the current will strike during the relative refractory period of a cardiac cycle and induce ventricular fibrillation.

PREPARING THE PATIENT

- Describe the procedure to the patient.
- If possible, make sure that the patient or a responsible family member has signed a consent form.
- Withhold all food and fluids for 6 to 12 hours before the procedure. If cardioversion is urgent, withhold food beginning as soon as possible.
- Obtain a baseline 12-lead ECG.
- Connect the patient to a pulse oximeter and blood pressure cuff.
- If the patient is awake, give a sedative.
- Place the leads on the patient's chest, and assess his cardiac rhythm.
- Apply conductive gel to the paddles or attach defibrillation pads to the chest wall; position the pads so that one pad is to the right of the sternum, just below the clavicle, and the other is at the fifth or sixth intercostal space in the left anterior axillary line.

MONITORING AND AFTERCARE

- Turn on the defibrillator, and select the ordered energy level, usually between 50 and 100 J. (See *Choosing the correct cardioversion energy level,* page 226.)
- Activate the synchronized mode by depressing the synchronizer switch.
- Check that the machine is sensing the R wave correctly.
- Place the paddles on the chest, and apply firm pressure.
- Charge the paddles.
- Instruct other personnel to stand clear of the patient and the bed to avoid the risk of an electric shock.
- Discharge the current by pushing both paddles' discharge buttons simultaneously.

CHOOSING THE CORRECT CARDIOVERSION ENERGY LEVEL

When choosing an energy level for cardioversion, try the lowest energy level first. If the arrhythmia isn't corrected, repeat the procedure using the next energy level. Repeat this procedure until the arrhythmia is corrected or until the highest energy level is reached. The monophasic energy doses (or equivalent biphasic energy dose) used for cardioversion are:

● 100, 200, 300, 360 joules (J) for unstable monomorphic ventricular tachycardia with a pulse
● 50, 100, 200, 300, 360 J for unstable paroxysmal supraventricular tachycardia
● 100, 200, 300, 360 J for unstable atrial fibrillation with a rapid ventricular response
● 50, 100, 200, 300, 360 J for unstable atrial flutter with a rapid ventricular response.

■ If cardioversion is unsuccessful, repeat the procedure two or three times as indicated, gradually increasing the energy with each additional countershock.
■ If normal rhythm is restored, continue to monitor the patient, and provide supplemental ventilation as long as needed.
■ If the patient's cardiac rhythm changes to ventricular fibrillation, switch the mode from synchronized to defibrillate, and defibrillate the patient immediately after charging the machine.
■ When using handheld paddles, continue to hold the paddles on the patient's chest until the energy is delivered.
■ Remember to reset the sync mode on the defibrillator after each synchronized cardioversion. Resetting this switch is necessary because most defibrillators automatically reset to an unsynchronized mode.
■ Document the use of synchronized cardioversion, the rhythm before and after cardioversion, the amperage used, and how the patient tolerated the procedure. (See *Teaching the patient after synchronized cardioversion*.)

Permanent pacemaker insertion

A permanent pacemaker is a self-contained device that's surgically implanted in a pocket under the patient's skin. This implantation is usually performed in an operating room or a cardiac catheterization laboratory.

Permanent pacemakers function in the demand mode, allowing the patient's heart to beat on its own but preventing it from falling below a preset rate.

Permanent pacemakers are indicated for patients with:
- persistent brady-arrhythmia
- complete heart block
- congenital or degenerative heart disease
- Stokes-Adams syndrome
- Wolff-Parkinson-White syndrome
- sick sinus syndrome.

Pacing electrodes can be placed in the atria, the ventricles, or both chambers (atrioventricular sequential or dual chamber). Biventricular pacemakers are also available for cardiac resynchronization therapy in some patients with heart failure. (See *Understanding pacemaker codes,* pages 228.)

The most common pacing codes are VVI for single-chamber pacing and DDD for dual-chamber pacing. To keep the patient healthy and active, some pacemakers are designed to increase the heart rate with exercise. (See *Biventricular pacemaker,* page 229.)

PREPARING THE PATIENT
- Explain the procedure to the patient.
- Before pacemaker insertion, clip the hair on the patient's chest from the axilla to the midline and from the clavicle to the nipple line on the side selected by the physician.
- Establish an I.V. line.
- Obtain baseline vital signs and a baseline 12-lead ECG.
- Make sure that the patient or a responsible family member has signed a consent form.
- Give sedation as indciated.

MONITORING AND AFTERCARE
- Monitor the patient's ECG to check for arrhythmias and to ensure correct pacemaker functioning.

UNDERSTANDING PACEMAKER CODES

The capabilities of pacemakers are described by a five-letter coding system, although typically only the first three letters are used.

First letter

The first letter identifies which heart chambers are paced. Here are the letters used to signify these options:
- V–Ventricle
- A–Atrium
- D–Dual (ventricle and atrium)
- O–None.

Second letter

The second letter signifies the heart chamber where the pacemaker senses the intrinsic activity:
- V–Ventricle
- A–Atrium
- D–Dual
- O–None.

Third letter

The third letter shows the pacemaker's response to the intrinsic electrical activity it senses in the atrium or ventricle:
- T–Triggers pacing
- I–Inhibits pacing
- D–Dual; can be triggered or inhibited depending on the mode and where intrinsic activity occurs
- O–None; the pacemaker doesn't change its mode in response to sensed activity.

Fourth letter

The fourth letter denotes the pacemaker's programmability; it tells whether the pacemaker can be modified by an external programming device:
- P–Basic functions programmable
- M–Multiprogrammable parameters
- C–Communicating functions such as telemetry
- R–Rate responsiveness (rate adjusts to fit the patient's metabolic needs and achieve normal hemodynamic status)
- O–None.

Fifth letter

The fifth letter denotes the pacemaker's response to a tachyarrhythmia:
- P–Pacing ability–pacemaker's rapid burst paces the heart at a rate above its intrinsic rate to override the tachycardia source
- S–Shock–an implantable cardioverter-defibrillator identifies ventricular tachycardia and delivers a shock to stop the arrhythmia
- D–Dual ability to shock and pace
- O–None.

- Check the dressing for signs of bleeding and infection.
- Change the dressing according to your facility's policy.
- Check vital signs and level of consciousness (LOC) every 15 minutes for the first hour, every hour for the next 4 hours, and then every 4 hours.
- Provide the patient with an identification card that lists the pacemaker type and manufacturer, serial number, pacemaker rate set-

BIVENTRICULAR PACEMAKER

A biventricular pacemaker is a type of pacemaker that's currently being used to treat heart failure.

How it works
It works by sending tiny electrical signals to the left and right ventricles at the same time, ultimately causing the walls of the left ventricle to pump together. The result is more efficient pumping of the heart, improved circulation, and decreased fluid backup in the heart muscle and lungs.

How it's placed
Insertion is similar to a regular pacemaker. However, in addition to the two leads that are used in most pacemakers, a third lead is placed into a cardiac vein and paces the left ventricle.

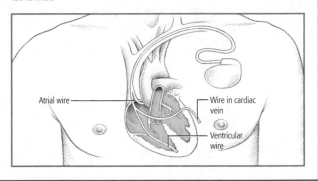

Atrial wire

Wire in cardiac vein

Ventricular wire

ting, date implanted, and the physician's name. (See *Teaching the patient after permanent pacemaker insertion*, page 230.)

Temporary pacemaker insertion

A temporary pacemaker is typically used in an emergency. The device consists of an external, battery-powered pulse generator and a lead or electrode system.

Temporary pacemakers usually come in three types:
- transcutaneous
- transvenous
- epicardial.

In a life-threatening situation, a transcutaneous pacemaker is the best choice. This device works by sending an electrical impulse from

DISCHARGE TEACHING

TEACHING THE PATIENT AFTER PERMANENT PACEMAKER INSERTION

Before discharge from the facility, instruct the patient to:
- report any chest pain or palpitations to his practitioner
- carry information regarding his pacemaker with him at all times
- wear medical alert identification regarding his pacemaker
- follow instructions from his practitioner regarding checkups on pacemaker function.

the pulse generator to the patient's heart by way of two electrodes, which are placed on the front and back of the patient's chest.

Transcutaneous pacing is quick and effective, but it's used only until the physician can institute transvenous or permanent pacing.

In addition to being more comfortable for the patient, a transvenous pacemaker is more reliable than a transcutaneous pacemaker.

Transvenous pacing involves threading an electrode catheter through a vein into the patient's right atrium or right ventricle. The electrode is attached to an external pulse generator that can provide an electrical stimulus directly to the endocardium.

Indications for a temporary transvenous pacemaker include:
- management of bradycardia
- presence of tachyarrhythmias
- other conduction system disturbances.

The purposes of temporary transvenous pacemaker insertion are:
- to maintain circulatory integrity by providing for standby pacing in case of sudden complete heart block
- to increase heart rate during periods of symptomatic bradycardia
- occasionally, to control sustained supraventricular or ventricular tachycardia.

Among the contraindications to pacemaker therapy are electromechanical dissociation and ventricular fibrillation.

Epicardial pacing is used during cardiac surgery, when the surgeon may insert electrodes through the epicardium of the right ventricle and, if he wants to institute AV sequential pacing, the right atrium. From there, the electrodes pass through the chest wall, where they remain available if temporary pacing becomes necessary.

PREPARING THE PATIENT
- Teach measures to prevent microshock; warn the patient not to use any electrical equipment that isn't grounded.

■ When using a transcutaneous pacemaker, don't place the electrodes over a bony area because bone conducts current poorly. With a female patient, place the anterior electrode under the patient's breast but not over her diaphragm.

■ If the physician inserts the transvenous pacer wire through the brachial or femoral vein, immobilize the patient's arm or leg to avoid putting stress on the pacing wires.

MONITORING AND AFTERCARE

■ After instituting use of any temporary pacemaker, assess the patient's vital signs, skin color, LOC, and peripheral pulses to determine the effectiveness of the paced rhythm. Perform a 12-lead ECG to serve as a baseline, and then perform additional ECGs daily or with clinical changes. Also, if possible, obtain a rhythm strip before, during, and after pacemaker placement; any time the pacemaker settings are changed; and whenever the patient receives treatment because of a complication due to the pacemaker.

■ Continuously monitor the ECG reading, noting capture, sensing, rate, intrinsic beats, and competition of paced and intrinsic rhythms. If the pacemaker is sensing correctly, the sense indicator on the pulse generator should flash with each beat.

■ Record the date and time of pacemaker insertion, the type of pacemaker, the reason for insertion, and the patient's response. Note the pacemaker settings. Document complications and the measures taken to resolve them.

■ If the patient has epicardial pacing wires in place, clean the insertion site and change the dressing daily. At the same time, monitor the site for signs of infection. Always keep the pulse generator nearby in case pacing becomes necessary.

■ Prepare the patient for permanent pacemaker surgery as appropriate.

Radiofrequency ablation

Radiofrequency ablation is a procedure that destroys the heart's tissue in order to treat a heartbeat that originates outside the SA node. (See *Types of cardiac ablation,* pages 232 and 233.) It's most commonly used for atrial fibrillation, atrial flutter, and supraventricular tachycardias, including AV nodal reentry and Wolff-Parkinson-White syndrome, and certain types of ventricular tachycardia.

PREPARING THE PATIENT

■ Explain the treatment and preparation to the patient and his family.

■ Make sure the patient or a responsible family member has signed a consent form.

TYPES OF CARDIAC ABLATION

Cardiac ablation therapy depends on the specific ablative method and type of medical procedure required. Here's a list of common types of cardiac ablation:

● *Surgical ablation:* This term is generally used to specify that the patient will be undergoing surgical opening of the chest. It can refer to open heart surgery with cardiopulmonary bypass or any of the newer techniques for open chest or minimally invasive chest procedures. The ablation technique itself may not involve direct surgical incision of the heart.

● *Minimally invasive ablation:* Although this term can be used as above, it generally means a procedure where peripheral access (femoral, brachial, subclavian) to a vein is obtained followed by placement of several specialized catheters that provide intracardiac rhythm monitoring and a source of energy for ablation of the cardiac tissue. This procedure generally takes place in the electrophysiology laboratory instead of the operating suite.

● *The maze or Cox-Maze III procedure:* The gold standard for arrhythmia treatment, including atrial fibrillation, this procedure was originally only done during open heart surgery with cardiopulmonary bypass. The procedure can now be done in some patients via minimally invasive access to the beating heart through a smaller chest incision where endoscopes guide the surgical treatment. However, not all arrhythmias can be treated with this more limited access.

The surgeon makes several small, specifically located cuts in the heart muscle where abnormal impulses are originating based on intracardiac monitoring leads, leaving the normal conduction pathways open. The cut areas form scar tissue that prevents the abnormal impulses from being conducted through the heart.

● *Radiofrequency ablation:* Instead of surgical incisions, radio waves are directed to the ectopic foci in the heart muscle, obliterating small portions of abnormal tissue by heat. These areas also scar, permanently blocking abnormal conduction. Newer radiofrequency ablation equipment comes with the capacity to direct cooled saline to the area to reduce excessive heat production, making the procedure safer and more comfortable. Most of these procedures are carried out with minimally invasive techniques through peripheral access sites, but they can be done during other cardiac surgery as well.

● *Microwave and ultrasound techniques:* Microwave and high-frequency sound waves are being used in several research hospitals to determine if either of these methods of tissue destruction reduces the risks of ablation, such as damage to adjacent tissues or stenosing of veins or arteries proximal to the ectopic tissue. These procedures are primarily done via peripheral access sites using specialized catheters and monitoring leads.

● *Laser ablation:* The increased technology of laser use has made delicate procedures, such as cardiac ablation, possible with small, very focused laser beams. The essential goals of the procedure remain the same. There's hope that this technique will be particularly useful for atrial fibrillation by reducing the risk

TYPES OF CARDIAC ABLATION *(continued)*

of pulmonary vein stenosis. The procedure can be done by peripheral access or during cardiac surgery.

● *Cryoablation:* This technique uses a special, extremely cold catheter tip to freeze and destroy tiny amounts of abnormally conducting cardiac tissue. Still being studied extensively, preliminary results show equal results compared with the Maze procedure, and equal complication rates. Cryoablation has been done by peripheral access and during other cardiac surgical procedures.

DISCHARGE TEACHING

TEACHING THE PATIENT AFTER RADIOFREQUENCY ABLATION

Before discharge from the facility, instruct the patient to:
● call the practitioner if redness, welling, or drainage at the incision site occurs
● report signs and symptoms that his arrhythmia is recurring
● take his pulse and keep a record for the practitioner
● remember that he may be on antibiotics for up to 12 weeks after the procedure.

■ Obtain a 12-lead ECG and laboratory studies, and make sure other tests (such as an echocardiogram and cardiac catheterization) have been completed.

■ Withhold food and fluids for 8 hours before the procedure

RED FLAG Left atrial ablation and ablation for persistent atrial flutter are contraindicated if an atrial thrombus is present. Left ventricular ablation is contraindicated if a left ventricular thrombus is found. Ablation catheters usually aren't inserted through a mechanical prosthetic heart.

MONITORING AND AFTERCARE

■ Enforce bed rest for 1 to 6 hours with the operative leg extended during this time.

■ Monitor the patient's ECG for the onset of new arrhythmias.

■ Initiate aspirin therapy to prevent thromboembolic aftereffects.

■ Review any medication changes with the patient. (See *Teaching the patient after radiofrequency ablation.*)

Arrhythmias

Cardiac arrhythmias are variations in the normal pattern of electrical stimulation of the heart. Arrhythmias vary in severity—from those that are mild, cause no symptoms, and require no treatment (such as sinus arrhythmia) to those that require emergency intervention (such as catastrophic ventricular fibrillation). Arrhythmias are generally classified according to their origin (ventricular or supraventricular). Their effects on cardiac output and blood pressure determine their significance. Lethal arrhythmias, such as pulseless ventricular tachycardia and ventricular fibrillation, are a major cause of cardiac death.

The most common types of arrhythmias include:

- sinus node arrhythmias
- atrial arrhythmias
- junctional arrhythmias
- ventricular arrhythmias
- atrioventricular (AV) blocks.

BASIC ELECTROCARDIOGRAPHY

Before you can begin to recognize arrhythmias, you need to know the parts of the electrocardiogram (ECG).

An ECG complex represents the electrical events occurring in one cardiac cycle. A complex consists of five waveforms labeled with the letters P, Q, R, S, and T. The middle three letters—Q, R, and S—are referred to as a unit, the QRS complex. ECG tracings represent the conduction of electrical impulses from the atria to the ventricles. (See *ECG waveform components.*)

ECG WAVEFORM COMPONENTS

This illustration shows the components of a normal electrocardiogram (ECG) waveform.

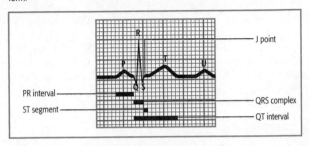

P wave

The P wave is the first component of a normal ECG waveform. It represents atrial depolarization or conduction of an electrical impulse through the atria. When evaluating a P wave, look closely at its characteristics, especially its location, configuration, and deflection.

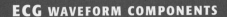

A normal P wave has these characteristics:

- *Location:* precedes the QRS complex
- *Amplitude:* 2 to 3 mm high
- *Duration:* 0.06 to 0.12 second
- *Configuration:* usually rounded and upright
- *Deflection:* positive or upright in leads I, II, aV_F, and V_2 to V_6; usually positive but may vary in leads III and aV_L; negative or inverted in lead aV_R; biphasic or variable in lead V_1.

If the deflection and configuration of a P wave are normal—for example, if the P wave is upright in lead II and is rounded and smooth—and if the P wave precedes each QRS complex, you can assume that this electrical impulse originated in the sinoatrial (SA) node. The atria start to contract partway through the P wave, but you won't see this on the ECG. Remember, the ECG records electrical activity only, not mechanical activity or contraction.

Peaked, notched, or enlarged P waves may represent atrial hypertrophy or enlargement associated with chronic obstructive pulmonary disease, pulmonary emboli, valvular disease, or heart failure. Inverted P waves may signify retrograde or reverse conduction from the AV junction toward the atria. Whenever an upright sinus P wave becomes inverted, consider possible retrograde or reverse conduction.

Varying P waves indicate that the impulse may be coming from different sites, as with a wandering pacemaker rhythm, irritable atrial tissue, or damage near the SA node. Absent P waves may signify conduction by a route other than the SA node, as with a junctional or atrial fibrillation rhythm. When a P wave doesn't precede the QRS complex, complete heart block may be present. Absence of a P wave doesn't mean that there is no atrial depolarization; the P wave may be buried or hidden in the T wave or the QRS complex.

PR interval

The PR interval tracks the atrial impulse from the atria through the AV node, bundle of His, and right and left bundle branches. When evaluating a PR interval, look especially at its duration. Changes in the PR interval indicate an altered impulse formation or a conduction delay, as seen in AV block.

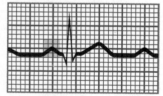 A normal PR interval has these characteristics (amplitude, configuration, and deflection aren't measured):

■ *Location:* from the beginning of the P wave to the beginning of the QRS complex

■ *Duration:* 0.12 to 0.20 second.

Short PR intervals (less than 0.12 second) indicate that the impulse originated somewhere other than the SA node. This variation is associated with junctional arrhythmias and preexcitation syndromes. Prolonged PR intervals (greater than 0.20 second) may represent a conduction delay through the atria or AV junction from digoxin toxicity, common cardiac drugs such as beta-adrenergic receptor and calcium channel blockers, or heart block—slowing related to ischemia or conduction tissue disease.

QRS complex

The QRS complex follows the P wave and represents depolarization of the ventricles, or impulse conduction. Immediately after the ventricles depolarize, as represented by the QRS complex, they contract. That contraction ejects blood from the ventricles and pumps it through the arteries, creating a pulse.

When you're monitoring cardiac rhythm, remember that the waveform you see represents the heart's electrical activity only. It doesn't guarantee a mechanical contraction of the heart and a subsequent pulse. The contraction could be weak, as happens with premature ventricular contractions, or absent, as happens with pulseless electrical activity. So, before you treat the strip, check the patient.

Pay special attention to the duration and configuration when evaluating a QRS complex.

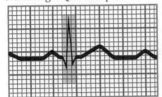

A normal complex has these characteristics:

■ *Location:* follows the PR interval
■ *Amplitude:* 5 to 30 mm high, but differs for each lead used
■ *Duration:* 0.06 to 0.10 second, or half of the PR interval. Duration is measured from the beginning of the Q wave to the end of the S wave, or from the beginning of the R wave if the Q wave is absent.

■ *Configuration:* consists of the Q wave (the first negative deflection, or deflection below the baseline, after the P wave), the R wave (the first positive deflection after the Q wave), and the S wave (the first negative deflection after the R wave). You may not always see all three waves. The ventricles depolarize quickly, minimizing contact time between the stylus and the ECG paper, so the QRS complex typically appears thinner than other ECG components. It may also look different in each lead.

■ *Deflection:* positive (with most of the complex above the baseline) in leads I, II, III, aV_L, aV_F, and V_4 to V_6, negative in leads aV_R and V_1 to V_2, and biphasic in lead V_3.

Remember that the QRS complex represents intraventricular conduction time. That's why identifying and correctly interpreting it is so crucial. If no P wave appears with the QRS complex, then the impulse may have originated in the ventricles, indicating a ventricular arrhythmia.

Deep, wide Q waves may represent myocardial infarction. In this case, the Q wave amplitude (depth) is greater than or equal to 25% of the height of the succeeding R wave, or the duration of the Q wave is 0.04 second or more. A notched R wave may signify a bundle-branch block. A widened QRS complex (greater than 0.12 second) may signi-

CHANGES IN THE ST SEGMENT

Closely monitoring the ST segment on a patient's electrocardiogram can help you detect ischemia or injury before infarction develops.

ST-segment depression

An ST segment is considered depressed when it's 0.5 mm or more below the baseline. A depressed ST segment may indicate myocardial ischemia or digoxin toxicity.

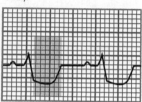

ST-segment elevation

An ST segment is considered elevated when it's 1 mm or more above the baseline. An elevated ST segment may indicate myocardial injury.

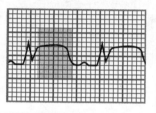

fy a ventricular conduction delay. A missing QRS complex may indicate AV block or ventricular standstill.

ST segment

The ST segment represents the end of ventricular conduction or depolarization and the beginning of ventricular recovery or repolarization. The point that marks the end of the QRS complex and the beginning of the ST segment is known as the J point.

Pay special attention to the deflection of an ST segment.

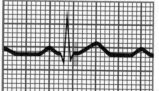

A normal ST segment has these characteristics (amplitude, duration, and configuration aren't observed):

■ *Location:* extends from the S wave to the beginning of the T wave

■ *Deflection:* usually isoelectric (neither positive nor negative); may vary from –0.5 to +1 mm in some precordial leads.

A change in the ST segment may indicate myocardial injury or ischemia. An ST segment may become either elevated or depressed. (See *Changes in the ST segment.*)

T wave

The peak of the T wave represents the relative refractory period of re-polarization or ventricular recovery. When evaluating a T wave, look at the amplitude, configuration, and deflection.

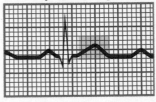

Normal T waves have these characteristics (duration isn't measured):

- *Location:* follows the ST segment
- *Amplitude:* 0.5 mm in leads I, II, and III and up to 10 mm in the precordial leads
- *Configuration:* rounded and smooth
- *Deflection:* usually positive or upright in leads I, II, and V_2 to V_6; inverted in lead aV_R; variable leads III and V_1.

The T wave's peak represents the relative refractory period of ventricular repolarization, a period during which cells are especially vulnerable to extra stimuli. Bumps in a T wave may indicate that a P wave is hidden in it. If a P wave is hidden, atrial depolarization has occurred, and the impulse has originated above the ventricles.

Tall, peaked, or "tented" T waves may indicate myocardial injury or electrolyte imbalances such as hyperkalemia. Hypokalemia can cause flattened T waves. Inverted T waves in leads I, II, aV_L, aV_F, or V_2 through V_6 may represent myocardial ischemia. Heavily notched or pointed T waves in an adult may indicate pericarditis.

QT interval

The QT interval measures the time needed for ventricular depolarization and repolarization. The length of the QT interval varies according to heart rate. The faster the heart rate, the shorter the QT interval. When checking the QT interval, look closely at the duration.

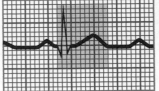

A normal QT interval has these characteristics (amplitude, configuration, and deflection aren't observed):

- *Location:* extends from the beginning of the QRS complex to the end of the T wave
- *Duration:* varies according to age, sex, and heart rate; usually lasts from 0.36 to 0.44 second; shouldn't be greater than half the distance between the two consecutive R waves (called the R-R interval) when the rhythm is regular.

CORRECTING THE QT INTERVAL

The QT interval is affected by the patient's heart rate. As the heart rate increases, the QT interval decreases; as the heart rate decreases, the QT interval increases. For this reason, evaluating the QT interval based on a standard heart rate of 60 is recommended. This corrected QT interval is known as QTc. The following formula is used to determine the QTc:

$$\frac{\text{QT interval}}{\sqrt{\text{R-R interval in seconds}}}$$

The normal QTc for women is less than 0.46 seconds and for men is less than 0.45 seconds. When the QTc is longer than 0.50 seconds in men or women, torsades de pointes is more likely to develop.

The QT interval measures the time needed for ventricular depolarization and repolarization. Prolonged QT intervals indicate that ventricular repolarization time is slowed, meaning that the relative refractory or vulnerable period of the cardiac cycle is longer. (See *Correcting the QT interval.*)

This variation is also associated with certain drugs such as class I antiarrhythmics. Prolonged QT syndrome is a congenital conduction-system defect present in certain families. Short QT intervals may result from digoxin toxicity or electrolyte imbalances such as hypercalcemia.

U wave

The U wave represents repolarization of the His-Purkinje system or ventricular conduction fibers. It isn't present on every rhythm strip. The configuration is the most important characteristic of the U wave.

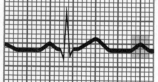

When present, a normal U wave has these characteristics (amplitude and duration aren't measured):

- *Location:* follows the T wave
- *Configuration:* typically upright and rounded
- *Deflection:* upright.

The U wave may not appear on an ECG. A prominent U wave may be from hypercalcemia, hypokalemia, or digoxin toxicity.

RECOGNIZING NORMAL SINUS RHYTHM

Normal sinus rhythm, shown below, represents normal impulse conduction through the heart.

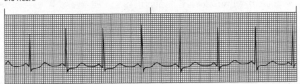

- *Rhythm:* atrial and ventricular rhythms regular
- *Rate:* atrial and ventricular rates normal; 60 beats/minute
- *P wave:* normal; precedes each QRS complex; all P waves similar in size and shape

- *PR interval:* normal; 0.10 second
- *QRS complex:* 0.06 second
- *T wave:* normal shape (upright and rounded)
- *QT interval:* normal; 0.40 second
- *Other:* no ectopic or aberrantly conducted impulses

NORMAL SINUS RHYTHM

Before you can recognize an arrhythmia, you first need to be able to recognize a normal cardiac rhythm. The term *arrhythmia* literally means an absence of rhythm. The more accurate term *dysrhythmia* means an abnormality in rhythm. These terms, however, are frequently used interchangeably.

Normal sinus rhythm (NSR) occurs when an impulse starts in the sinus node and progresses to the ventricles through a normal conduction pathway—from the sinus node to the atria and AV node, through the bundle of His, to the bundle branches, and on to the Purkinje fibers. There are no premature or aberrant contractions. NSR is the standard against which all other rhythms are compared. (See *Recognizing normal sinus rhythm.*)

Practice the 8-step method, described below, to analyze an ECG strip with NSR. The ECG characteristics of NSR are:
- *Rhythm:* atrial and ventricular rhythms are regular
- *Rate:* atrial and ventricular rates are 60 to 100 beats/minute, the sinoatrial node's normal firing rate

- *P wave:* normally shaped (round and smooth) and upright in lead II; all P waves similar in size and shape; a P wave for every QRS complex
- *PR interval:* within normal limits (0.12 to 0.20 second)
- *QRS complex:* within normal limits (0.06 to 0.10 second)
- *T wave:* normally shaped; upright and rounded in lead II
- *QT interval:* within normal limits (0.36 to 0.44 second)
- *Other:* no ectopic or aberrant beats.

AGE AWARE Always keep the patient's age in mind when interpreting the ECG. Changes that might be seen in the ECG of an older adult include increased PR, QRS, and QT intervals, decreased amplitude of the QRS complex, and a shift of the QRS axis to the left.

THE 8-STEP METHOD

Analyzing a rhythm strip is a skill developed through practice. You can use several methods, as long as you're consistent. Rhythm strip analysis requires a sequential and systematic approach such as the 8 steps outlined here.

Step 1: Determine rhythm

To determine the heart's atrial and ventricular rhythms, use either the paper-and-pencil method or the caliper method. (See *Methods of measuring rhythm.*)

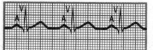

For atrial rhythm, measure the P-P intervals; that is, the intervals between consecutive P waves. These intervals should occur regularly, with only small variations from respirations. Then compare the P-P intervals in several cycles. Consistently similar P-P intervals indicate regular atrial rhythm; dissimilar P-P intervals indicate irregular atrial rhythm.

To determine the ventricular rhythm, measure the intervals between two consecutive R waves in the QRS complexes. If an R wave isn't present, use either the Q wave or the S wave of consecutive QRS complexes. The R-R intervals should occur regularly. Then compare R-R intervals in several cycles. As with atrial rhythms, consistently similar intervals mean a regular rhythm; dissimilar intervals point to an irregular rhythm.

After completing your measurements, ask yourself:
- Is the rhythm regular or irregular? Consider a rhythm with only slight variations, up to 0.04 second, to be regular.

METHODS OF MEASURING RHYTHM

You can use either of these methods to determine atrial or ventricular rhythm.

Paper-and-pencil method

Place the ECG strip on a flat surface. Then position the straight edge of a piece of paper along the strip's baseline. Move the paper up slightly so the straight edge is near the peak of the R wave.

With a pencil, mark the paper at the R waves of two consecutive QRS complexes, as shown below. This is the R-R interval. Next, move the paper across the strip lining up the two marks with succeeding R-R intervals. If the distance for each R-R interval is the same, the ventricular rhythm is regular. If the distance varies, the rhythm is irregular.

Use the same method to measure the distance between the P waves (the P-P interval) and determine whether the atrial rhythm is regular or irregular.

Caliper method

With the ECG on a flat surface, place one point of the calipers on the peak of the first R wave of two consecutive QRS complexes. Then adjust the caliper legs so the other point is on the peak of the next R wave, as shown below. This distance is the R-R interval.

Now pivot the first point of the calipers toward the third R wave, and note whether it falls on the peak of that wave. Check succeeding R-R intervals in the same way. If they're all the same, the ventricular rhythm is regular. If they vary, the rhythm is irregular.

Using the same method, measure the P-P intervals to determine whether the atrial rhythm is regular or irregular.

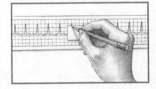

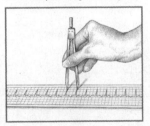

- If the rhythm is irregular, is it slightly or markedly irregular? Does the irregularity occur in a pattern?

Step 2: Calculate rate

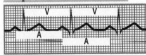

You can use one of three methods to determine atrial and ventricular heart rates from an ECG waveform. Although these methods can provide accurate information, you shouldn't rely solely on them when assessing your patient. Remember, the ECG waveform represents electrical, not mechanical, activity. Therefore, although an ECG can show you that ventricular depolarization has occurred, it doesn't mean that ventricular contraction has occurred. To calculate heart rate, you must take the patient's pulse. So remember, always check a pulse to correlate it with the heart rate on the ECG.

- *Times-ten method.* The simplest, quickest, and most common way to calculate rate is the times-ten method, especially if the rhythm is irregular. ECG paper is marked in increments of 3 seconds, or 15 large boxes. To calculate the atrial rate, obtain a 6-second strip, count the number of P waves on it, and multiply by 10. Ten 6-second strips equal 1 minute. Calculate ventricular rate the same way, using the R waves.

- *1,500 method.* If the heart rhythm is regular, use the 1,500 method, so named because 1,500 small squares equal 1 minute. Count the number of small squares between identical points on two consecutive P waves, and then divide 1,500 by that number to get the atrial rate. To obtain the ventricular rate, use the same method with two consecutive R waves.

- *Sequence method.* The third method of estimating heart rate is the sequence method, which requires memorizing a sequence of numbers. For atrial rate, find a P wave that peaks on a heavy black line, and assign the following numbers to the next six heavy black lines: 300, 150, 100, 75, 60, and 50. Then find the next P wave peak, and estimate the atrial rate based on the number assigned to the nearest heavy black line. Estimate the ventricular rate the same way, using the R wave.

Step 3: Evaluate P wave

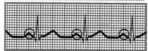

When examining a rhythm strip for P waves, ask yourself:
- Are P waves present?
- Do the P waves have a normal

configuration?
- Do all the P waves have a similar size and shape?
- Is there one P wave for every QRS complex?

Step 4: Determine PR-interval duration

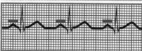

To measure the PR interval, count the small squares between the start of the P wave and the start of the QRS complex; then multiply the number of squares by 0.04 second. After performing this calculation, ask yourself:

- Does the duration of the PR interval fall within normal limits, 0.12 to 0.20 second (or 3 to 5 small squares)?
- Is the PR interval constant?

Step 5: Determine QRS complex duration

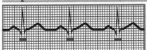

When determining QRS complex duration, make sure you measure straight across from the end of the PR interval to the end of the S wave, not just to the peak. Remember, the QRS complex has no horizontal components. To calculate duration, count the number of small squares between the beginning and end of the QRS complex, and multiply this number by 0.04 second. Then ask yourself:

- Does the duration of the QRS complex fall within normal limits, 0.06 to 0.10 second?
- Are all QRS complexes the same size and shape? (If not, measure each one and describe them individually.)
- Does a QRS complex appear after every P wave?

Step 6: Evaluate T wave

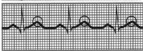

Examine the T waves on the ECG strip. Then ask yourself:
- Are T waves present?
- Do all of the T waves have a normal shape?

- Could a P wave be hidden in a T wave?
- Do all T waves have a normal amplitude?
- Do the T waves have the same deflection as the QRS complexes?

Step 7: Determine QT-interval duration

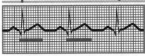

Count the number of small squares between the beginning of the QRS complex and the end of the T wave, where the T wave returns to the baseline. Multiply this number by 0.04 second. Ask yourself:

- Does the duration of the QT interval fall within normal limits, 0.36 to 0.44 second?

Step 8: Evaluate other components

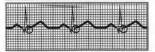

Note the presence of ectopic or aberrantly conducted beats or other abnormalities. Also check the ST segment for abnormalities, and look for the presence of a U wave.

Now, interpret your findings by classifying the rhythm strip according to one or all of the following:

- *Site of origin of the rhythm:* for example, sinus node, atria, atrioventricular node, or ventricles
- *Rate:* normal (60 to 100 beats/minute), bradycardia (less than 60 beats/minute), or tachycardia (greater than 100 beats/minute)
- *Rhythm:* normal or abnormal; for example, flutter, fibrillation, heart block, escape rhythm, or other arrhythmias.

SINUS NODE ARRHYTHMIAS

When the heart functions normally, the sinoatrial (SA) node, also called the *sinus node,* acts as the primary pacemaker. The sinus node assumes this role because its automatic firing rate exceeds that of the heart's other pacemakers. In an adult at rest, the sinus node has an inherent firing rate of 60 to 100 times/minute.

In about half of the population, the SA node's blood supply comes from the right coronary artery, and from the left circumflex artery in the other half of the population. The autonomic nervous system (ANS) richly innervates the sinus node through the vagal nerve, a parasympathetic nerve, and several sympathetic nerves. Stimulation of the vagus nerve decreases the node's firing rate, and stimulation of the sympathetic system increases it.

Changes in the automaticity of the sinus node, alterations in its blood supply, and ANS influences may all lead to sinus node arrhythmias. This chapter will help you to identify sinus node arrhythmias on an electrocardiogram (ECG). It will also help you to determine the causes, clinical significance, signs and symptoms, and interventions associated with each arrhythmia presented.

The 8-step method for analyzing the ECG strip will be used for each of the following arrhythmias.

Sinus arrhythmia

In sinus tachycardia and sinus bradycardia, the cardiac rate falls outside the normal limits. In sinus arrhythmia, the rate stays within normal limits, but the rhythm is irregular and corresponds to the respiratory cycle. Sinus arrhythmia can occur normally in athletes, children, and older adults, but it rarely occurs in infants.

CAUSES

Sinus arrhythmia, the heart's normal response to respirations, results from an inhibition of reflex vagal activity, or tone. During inspiration,

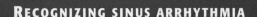

RECOGNIZING SINUS ARRHYTHMIA

The following rhythm strip illustrates sinus arrhythmia. Look for these distinguishing characteristics.

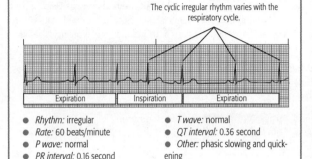

The cyclic irregular rhythm varies with the respiratory cycle.

| Expiration | Inspiration | Expiration |

- *Rhythm:* irregular
- *Rate:* 60 beats/minute
- *P wave:* normal
- *PR interval:* 0.16 second
- *QRS complex:* 0.06 second

- *T wave:* normal
- *QT interval:* 0.36 second
- *Other:* phasic slowing and quickening

an increase in the flow of blood back to the heart reduces vagal tone, which increases the heart rate. ECG complexes fall closer together, which shortens the P-P interval. During expiration, venous return decreases, which in turn increases vagal tone, slows the heart rate, and lengthens the P-P interval. (See *Recognizing sinus arrhythmia*.)

Conditions unrelated to respiration may also produce sinus arrhythmia, including:

- heart disease
- inferior wall myocardial infarction
- the use of certain drugs, such as digoxin and morphine
- conditions involving increased intracranial pressure (ICP).

CLINICAL SIGNIFICANCE

Sinus arrhythmia usually isn't significant and produces no symptoms. A marked variation in P-P intervals in an older adult, however, may indicate sick sinus syndrome—a related, but potentially more serious, phenomenon.

ECG CHARACTERISTICS

- *Rhythm:* Atrial rhythm is irregular, corresponding to the respiratory cycle. The P-P interval is shorter during inspiration, longer during expiration. The difference between the longest and shortest P-P interval exceeds 0.12 second. Ventricular rhythm is also irregular, corresponding to the respiratory cycle. The R-R interval is shorter during inspiration, longer during expiration. The difference between the longest and shortest R-R interval exceeds 0.12 second.
- *Rate:* Atrial and ventricular rates are within normal limits (60 to 100 beats/minute) and vary with respiration. Typically, the heart rate increases during inspiration and decreases during expiration.
- *P wave:* Normal size and configuration; P wave precedes each QRS complex.
- *PR interval:* May vary slightly within normal limits.
- *QRS complex:* Normal duration and configuration.
- *QT wave:* Normal size and configuration.
- *QT interval:* May vary slightly, but usually within normal limits.
- *Other:* None.

SIGNS AND SYMPTOMS

The patient's peripheral pulse rate increases during inspiration and decreases during expiration. Sinus arrhythmia is easier to detect when the heart rate is slow; it may disappear when the heart rate increases, as with exercise.

If the arrhythmia is caused by an underlying condition, you may note signs and symptoms of that condition. Marked sinus arrhythmia may cause dizziness or syncope in some cases.

INTERVENTIONS

Unless the patient is symptomatic, treatment usually isn't necessary. If sinus arrhythmia is unrelated to respirations, the underlying cause may require treatment.

When caring for a patient with sinus arrhythmia, observe the heart rhythm during respiration to determine whether the arrhythmia coincides with the respiratory cycle. Check the monitor carefully to avoid an inaccurate interpretation of the waveform.

If sinus arrhythmia is induced by drugs, such as morphine and other sedatives, the practitioner may decide to continue to give the patient those medications. If sinus arrhythmia develops suddenly in a patient taking digoxin (Lanoxin), notify the practitioner immediately. The patient may be experiencing digoxin toxicity.

RECOGNIZING SINUS BRADYCARDIA

The following rhythm strip illustrates sinus bradycardia. Look for these distinguishing characteristics.

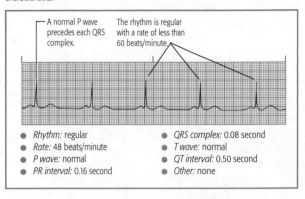

A normal P wave precedes each QRS complex.

The rhythm is regular with a rate of less than 60 beats/minute.

- *Rhythm:* regular
- *Rate:* 48 beats/minute
- *P wave:* normal
- *PR interval:* 0.16 second
- *QRS complex:* 0.08 second
- *T wave:* normal
- *QT interval:* 0.50 second
- *Other:* none

BRADYCARDIA AND TACHYCARDIA IN CHILDREN

Evaluate bradycardia and tachycardia in children in context. Bradycardia (less than 90 beats/minute) may occur in the healthy infant during sleep, and tachycardia may occur when the child is crying or otherwise upset. Because the heart rate varies considerably from the neonate to the adolescent, neither bradycardia nor tachycardia can be assigned a single definition to be used for all children.

Sinus bradycardia

Sinus bradycardia is characterized by a sinus rate below 60 beats/minute and a regular rhythm. All impulses originate in the SA node. This arrhythmia's significance depends on the symptoms and the underlying cause. Unless the patient shows symptoms of decreased cardiac output, no treatment is necessary. (See *Recognizing sinus bradycardia* and *Bradycardia and tachycardia in children.*)

CAUSES

Sinus bradycardia usually occurs as the normal response to a reduced demand for blood flow. In this case, vagal stimulation increases and sympathetic stimulation decreases. As a result, automaticity (the tendency of cells to initiate their own impulses) in the SA node diminishes. It may occur normally during sleep or in a person with a well-conditioned heart—an athlete, for example.

Sinus bradycardia may be caused by:

- noncardiac disorders, such as hyperkalemia, increased ICP, hypothyroidism, hypothermia, and glaucoma
- conditions producing excess vagal stimulation or decreased sympathetic stimulation, such as sleep, deep relaxation, the Valsalva maneuver, carotid sinus massage, and vomiting
- cardiac diseases, such as SA node disease, cardiomyopathy, myocarditis, and myocardial ischemia, can also occur immediately following an inferior wall myocardial infarction (MI) that involves the right coronary artery, which supplies blood to the SA node
- certain drugs, especially beta-adrenergic receptor blockers, digoxin, calcium channel blockers, lithium, and antiarrhythmics, such as sotalol (Betapace), amiodarone (Cordarone), propafenone (Rhythmol), and quinidine (Quinora).

CLINICAL SIGNIFICANCE

The clinical significance of sinus bradycardia depends on how low the rate is and whether the patient is symptomatic. For example, most adults can tolerate a sinus bradycardia of 45 to 59 beats/minute but are less tolerant of a rate below 45 beats/minute.

Usually, sinus bradycardia doesn't produce symptoms and is insignificant. Many athletes develop sinus bradycardia because their well-conditioned hearts can maintain a normal stroke volume with less-than-normal effort. Sinus bradycardia also occurs normally during sleep as a result of circadian variations in heart rate.

When sinus bradycardia produces symptoms, however, prompt attention is critical. The heart of a patient with underlying cardiac disease may not be able to compensate for a drop in rate by increasing its stroke volume. The resulting drop in cardiac output produces such signs and symptoms as hypotension and dizziness. Bradycardia may also predispose some patients to more serious arrhythmias, such as ventricular tachycardia and ventricular fibrillation.

In a patient with acute inferior wall MI, sinus bradycardia is considered a favorable prognostic sign, unless it's accompanied by hypotension. Because sinus bradycardia rarely affects children, it's considered a poor prognostic sign in ill children.

ECG CHARACTERISTICS

- *Rhythm:* Atrial and ventricular rhythms are regular.
- *Rate:* Atrial and ventricular rates are less than 60 beats/minute.
- *P wave:* Normal size and configuration; P wave precedes each QRS complex.
- *PR interval:* Within normal limits and constant.
- *QRS complex:* Normal duration and configuration.
- *T wave:* Normal size and configuration.
- *QT interval:* Within normal limits, but may be prolonged.
- *Other:* None.

SIGNS AND SYMPTOMS

The patient will have a pulse rate of less than 60 beats/minute, with a regular rhythm. As long as he's able to compensate for the decreased cardiac output, he's likely to remain asymptomatic. If compensatory mechanisms fail, however, signs and symptoms of declining cardiac output usually appear, including:

- hypotension
- cool, clammy skin
- altered mental status
- dizziness
- blurred vision
- crackles, dyspnea, and an S_3 heart sound, indicating heart failure
- chest pain
- syncope.

Palpitations and pulse irregularities may occur if the patient experiences ectopy such as premature atrial, junctional, or ventricular contractions. This is because the SA node's increased relative refractory period permits ectopic firing. Bradycardia-induced syncope (Stokes-Adams attack) may also occur.

INTERVENTIONS

If the patient is asymptomatic and his vital signs are stable, treatment generally isn't necessary. Continue to observe his heart rhythm, monitoring the progression and duration of the bradycardia. Evaluate his tolerance of the rhythm at rest and with activity. Review the medications he's taking. Check with the practitioner about stopping medications that may be depressing the SA node, such as digoxin, beta-adrenergic receptor blockers, or calcium channel blockers. Before giving these drugs, make sure the heart rate is within a safe range.

If the patient is symptomatic, treatment aims to identify and correct the underlying cause. Meanwhile, the heart rate must be maintained with transcutaneous pacemaker. Use such drugs as atropine,

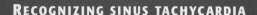

RECOGNIZING SINUS TACHYCARDIA

The following rhythm strip illustrates sinus tachycardia. Look for these distinguishing characteristics.

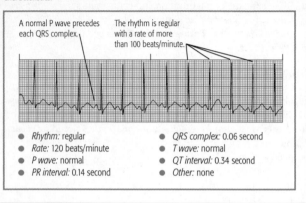

A normal P wave precedes each QRS complex.

The rhythm is regular with a rate of more than 100 beats/minute.

- *Rhythm:* regular
- *Rate:* 120 beats/minute
- *P wave:* normal
- *PR interval:* 0.14 second

- *QRS complex:* 0.06 second
- *T wave:* normal
- *QT interval:* 0.34 second
- *Other:* none

epinephrine, or dobutamine (Dobutrex) while awaiting a pacemaker or if pacing is ineffective. For the complete ACLS algorithm, see pages 328 and 329.

Keep in mind that a patient with a transplanted heart won't respond to atropine and may require pacing for emergency treatment. Treatment of chronic, symptomatic sinus bradycardia requires insertion of a permanent pacemaker.

Sinus tachycardia

Sinus tachycardia is an acceleration of the firing of the SA node beyond its normal discharge rate. Sinus tachycardia in an adult is characterized by a sinus rate of more than 100 beats/minute. The rate rarely exceeds 180 beats/minute except during strenuous exercise; the maximum rate achievable with exercise decreases with age. (See *Recognizing sinus tachycardia.*)

CAUSES

Sinus tachycardia may be a normal response to exercise, pain, stress, fever, or strong emotions, such as fear and anxiety. Other causes of sinus tachycardia include:

■ certain cardiac conditions, such as heart failure, cardiogenic shock, and pericarditis

■ other conditions, such as shock, anemia, respiratory distress, pulmonary embolism, sepsis, and hyperthyroidism where the increased heart rate serves as a compensatory mechanism

■ drugs, such as atropine, isoproterenol (Isuprel), aminophylline, dopamine (Intropin), dobutamine, epinephrine, alcohol, caffeine, nicotine, and amphetamines.

CLINICAL SIGNIFICANCE

The clinical significance of sinus tachycardia depends on the underlying cause. The arrhythmia may be the body's response to exercise or high emotional states and of no clinical significance. It may also occur with hypovolemia, hemorrhage, or pain. When the stimulus for the tachycardia is removed, the arrhythmia generally resolves spontaneously.

Although sinus tachycardia commonly occurs without serious adverse effects, persistent sinus tachycardia can also be serious, especially if it occurs in the setting of an acute MI. Tachycardia can lower cardiac output by reducing ventricular filling time and stroke volume. Normally, ventricular volume reaches 120 to 130 ml during diastole. In tachycardia, decreased ventricular volume leads to decreased cardiac output with subsequent hypotension and decreased peripheral perfusion.

Tachycardia worsens myocardial ischemia by increasing the heart's demand for oxygen and reducing the duration of diastole, the period of greatest coronary blood flow. Sinus tachycardia occurs in about 30% of patients after an acute MI and is considered a poor prognostic sign because it may be associated with massive heart damage.

An increase in heart rate can also be detrimental for patients with obstructive types of heart conditions, such as aortic stenosis and hypertrophic cardiomyopathy. Persistent tachycardia may also signal impending heart failure or cardiogenic shock. Sinus tachycardia can also cause angina in patients with coronary artery disease.

ECG CHARACTERISTICS

■ *Rhythm:* Atrial and ventricular rhythms are regular.

■ *Rate:* Atrial and ventricular rates are greater than 100 beats/minute, usually between 100 and 160 beats/minute.

■ *P wave:* Normal size and configuration, but it may increase in amplitude. The P wave precedes each QRS complex, but as the heart rate increases, the P wave may be superimposed on the preceding T wave and difficult to identify.

■ *PR interval:* Within normal limits and constant.

■ *QRS complex:* Normal duration and configuration.
■ *T wave:* Normal size and configuration.
■ *QT interval:* Within normal limits, but commonly shortened.
■ *Other:* None.

SIGNS AND SYMPTOMS

The patient will have a peripheral pulse rate above 100 beats/minute, but with a regular rhythm. Usually, he'll be asymptomatic. However, if his cardiac output falls and compensatory mechanisms fail, he may experience hypotension, syncope, and blurred vision. He may report chest pain and palpitations, commonly described as a pounding chest or a sensation of skipped heartbeats. He may also report a sense of nervousness or anxiety. If heart failure develops, he may exhibit crackles, an extra heart sound (S_3), and jugular vein distention.

INTERVENTIONS

When treating the asymptomatic patient, focus on determining the cause of the tachycardia. The focus of treatment in the symptomatic patient with sinus tachycardia is to maintain adequate cardiac output and tissue perfusion and to identify and correct the underlying cause. For example, if the tachycardia is caused by hemorrhage, treatment includes stopping the bleeding and replacing blood and fluid losses.

If tachycardia leads to cardiac ischemia, treatment may include medications to slow the heart rate. The most commonly used drugs include beta-adrenergic receptor blockers, such as metoprolol and atenolol, and calcium channel blockers, such as verapamil and diltiazem.

Check the patient's medication history. Over-the-counter sympathomimetic agents, which mimic the effects of the sympathetic nervous system, may contribute to the sinus tachycardia. Sympathomimetic agents may be contained in nose drops and cold formulas.

Also question the patient about the use of caffeine, nicotine, and alcohol, each of which can trigger tachycardia. Advise him to avoid these substances. Ask about the use of illicit drugs, such as cocaine and amphetamines, which can also cause tachycardia.

Here are other steps you should take for the patient with sinus tachycardia:
■ Because sinus tachycardia can lead to injury of the heart muscle, assess the patient for signs and symptoms of angina. Also assess for signs and symptoms of heart failure, including crackles, an S_3 heart sound, and jugular vein distention.
■ Monitor intake and output, along with daily weight.

- Check the patient's level of consciousness to assess cerebral perfusion.
- Provide the patient with a calm environment. Help to reduce fear and anxiety, which can aggravate the arrhythmia.
- Teach about procedures and treatments. Include relaxation techniques in the information you provide.
- Be aware that a sudden onset of sinus tachycardia after an MI may signal extension of the infarction. Prompt recognition is vital so treatment can be started.
- Keep in mind that tachycardia is frequently the initial sign of pulmonary embolism. Maintain a high index of suspicion, especially if your patient has predisposing risk factors for thrombotic emboli.

Sinus arrest and sinoatrial exit block

Although sinus arrest and SA or sinus exit block are two separate arrhythmias with different etiologies, they're discussed together because distinguishing the two can be difficult. In addition, there's no difference in their clinical significance and treatment.

In sinus arrest, the normal sinus rhythm is interrupted by an occasional, prolonged failure of the SA node to initiate an impulse. Therefore, sinus arrest is caused by episodes of failure in the automaticity or impulse formation of the SA node. The atria aren't stimulated, and an entire PQRST complex is missing from the ECG strip. Except for this missing complex, or pause, the ECG usually remains normal. (See *Recognizing sinus arrest,* page 256.)

In sinus exit block, the SA node discharges at regular intervals, but some impulses are delayed or blocked from reaching the atria, resulting in long sinus pauses. Blocks result from failure to conduct impulses, whereas sinus arrest results from failure to form impulses in the SA node. Both arrhythmias cause atrial activity to stop. In sinus arrest, the pause often ends with a junctional escape beat. In sinus exit block, the pause occurs for an indefinite period and ends with a sinus rhythm. (See *Recognizing sinoatrial exit block,* page 257.)

CAUSES

Causes of sinus arrest and sinus exit block include:
- acute infection
- sick sinus syndrome
- sinus node diseases, such as fibrosis and idiopathic degeneration
- increased vagal tone, such as with Valsalva's maneuver, carotid sinus massage, and vomiting
- digoxin, quinidine, procainamide (Procan SR), and salicylate toxicity

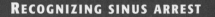

RECOGNIZING SINUS ARREST

The following rhythm strip illustrates sinus arrest. Look for these distinguishing characteristics.

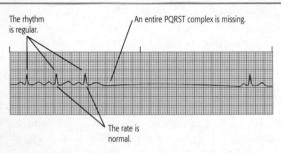

The rhythm is regular.

An entire PQRST complex is missing.

The rate is normal.

- *Rhythm:* regular, except for the missing PQRST complexes
- *Rate:* 40 beats/minute
- *P wave:* normal; missing during pause
- *PR interval:* 0.20 second

- *QRS complex:* 0.08 second, absent during pause
- *T wave:* normal, absent during pause
- *QT interval:* 0.40 second, absent during pause
- *Other:* none

- excessive doses of beta-adrenergic receptor blockers, such as metoprolol (Lopressor) and propranolol (Inderal)
- cardiac disorders, such as coronary artery disease (CAD), acute myocarditis, cardiomyopathy, hypertensive heart disease, and acute inferior wall myocardial infarction.

CLINICAL SIGNIFICANCE

The clinical significance of these two arrhythmias depends on the patient's symptoms. If the pauses are short and infrequent, the patient will most likely be asymptomatic and won't require treatment. He may have a normal sinus rhythm for days or weeks between episodes of sinus arrest or sinus exit block, and he may be totally unaware of the arrhythmia. Pauses of 2 to 3 seconds normally occur in healthy adults during sleep and occasionally in patients with increased vagal tone or hypersensitive carotid sinus disease.

RECOGNIZING SINOATRIAL EXIT BLOCK

This rhythm strip illustrates sinoatrial (SA) exit block.

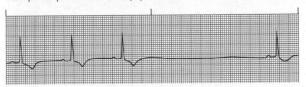

- *Rhythm:* regular, except for pauses
- *Rate:* underlying rhythm, 60 beats/minute before SA block; length or frequency of the pause may result in bradycardia
- *P wave:* periodically absent
- *PR interval:* 0.16 second
- *QRS complex:* 0.08 second; missing during pause
- *T wave:* normal; missing during pause
- *QT interval:* 0.40 second; missing during pause
- *Other:* entire PQRST complex missing; pause ends with sinus rhythm

If either of the arrhythmias is frequent or prolonged, however, the patient will most likely experience symptoms related to low cardiac output. The arrhythmias can produce syncope or near-syncopal episodes usually within 7 seconds of asystole.

During a prolonged pause, the patient may fall and injure himself. Other situations are potentially just as serious. For example, a symptom-producing arrhythmia that occurs while the patient is driving a car could result in a fatal accident. Extremely slow rates can also give rise to other arrhythmias.

ECG CHARACTERISTICS

Sinus arrest and SA exit block share these ECG characteristics:

- *Rhythm:* Atrial and ventricular rhythms are usually regular except when sinus arrest or SA exit block occurs.
- *Rate:* The underlying atrial and ventricular rates are usually within normal limits (60 to 100 beats/minute) before the arrest or SA exit block occurs. The length or frequency of the pause may result in bradycardia.
- *P wave:* Periodically absent, with entire PQRST complex missing. However, when present, the P wave is normal in size and configuration and precedes each QRS complex.

- *PR interval:* Within normal limits and constant when a P wave is present.
- *QRS complex:* Normal duration and configuration, but absent during a pause.
- *T wave:* Normal size and configuration, but absent during a pause.
- *QT interval:* Usually within normal limits, but absent during a pause.

To differentiate between these two rhythms, compare the length of the pause with the underlying P-P or R-R interval. If the underlying rhythm is regular, determine if the underlying rhythm resumes on time following the pause. With sinus exit block, because the regularity of the SA node discharge is blocked, not interrupted, the underlying rhythm will resume on time following the pause. In addition, the length of the pause will be a multiple of the underlying P-P or R-R interval.

In sinus arrest, the timing of the SA node discharge is interrupted by the failure of the SA node to initiate an impulse. The result is that the underlying rhythm doesn't resume on time after the pause and the length of the pause is not a multiple of the previous R-R intervals.

SIGNS AND SYMPTOMS

You won't be able to detect a pulse or heart sounds when sinus arrest or sinus exit block occurs. Short pauses usually produce no symptoms. Recurrent or prolonged pauses may cause signs of decreased cardiac output, such as low blood pressure; altered mental status; cool, clammy skin; or syncope. The patient may also complain of dizziness or blurred vision.

INTERVENTIONS

An asymptomatic patient needs no treatment. Symptomatic patients are treated following the guidelines for patients with symptom-producing bradycardia. Treatment will also focus on the cause of the sinus arrest or sinus exit block. This may involve discontinuation of medications that contribute to SA node discharge or conduction, such as digoxin, beta-adrenergic receptor blockers, and calcium channel blockers.

Examine the circumstances under which the pauses occur. Both SA arrest and SA exit block may be insignificant if detected while the patient is sleeping. If the pauses are recurrent, assess the patient for evidence of decreased cardiac output, such as altered mental status, low blood pressure, and cool, clammy skin.

Ask him whether he's dizzy or light-headed or has blurred vision. Does he feel as if he has passed out? If so, he may be experiencing syncope from a prolonged sinus arrest or sinus exit block.

Document the patient's vital signs and how he feels during pauses as well as the activities he was involved in at the time. Activities that increase vagal stimulation, such as Valsalva's maneuver or vomiting, increase the likelihood of sinus pauses.

Assess for a progression of the arrhythmia. Notify the practitioner immediately if the patient becomes unstable. If appropriate, be alert for signs of digoxin, quinidine, or procainamide toxicity. Obtain a serum digoxin level and a serum electrolyte level.

Sick sinus syndrome

Also known as *sinoatrial (SA) syndrome, sinus nodal dysfunction,* and *Stokes-Adams syndrome,* sick sinus syndrome (SSS) refers to a wide spectrum of SA node arrhythmias. This syndrome is caused by disturbances in the way impulses are generated or in the ability to conduct impulses to the atria. These disturbances may be either intrinsic or mediated by the autonomic nervous system (ANS).

SSS usually shows up as bradycardia, with episodes of sinus arrest and SA block interspersed with sudden, brief periods of rapid atrial fibrillation. Patients are also prone to paroxysms of other atrial tachyarrhythmias, such as atrial flutter and ectopic atrial tachycardia, a condition sometimes referred to as bradycardia-tachycardia (or "brady-tachy") syndrome.

Most patients with SSS are over age 60, but anyone can develop the arrhythmia. It's rare in children except after open-heart surgery that results in SA node damage. The arrhythmia affects men and women equally. The onset is progressive, insidious, and chronic. (See *Recognizing sick sinus syndrome,* page 260.)

CAUSES

SSS results either from a dysfunction of the sinus node's automaticity or from abnormal conduction or blockages of impulses coming out of the nodal region. These conditions, in turn, stem from a degeneration of the area's ANS and partial destruction of the sinus node, as may occur with an interrupted blood supply after an inferior wall myocardial infarction.

In addition, certain conditions can affect the atrial wall surrounding the SA node and cause exit blocks. Conditions that cause inflammation or degeneration of atrial tissue can also lead to SSS. In many patients, though, the exact cause is never identified.

Causes of SSS include:

RECOGNIZING SICK SINUS SYNDROME

The following rhythm strip illustrates sick sinus syndrome. Look for these distinguishing characteristics.

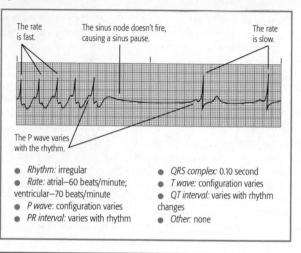

The rate is fast.

The sinus node doesn't fire, causing a sinus pause.

The rate is slow.

The P wave varies with the rhythm.

- *Rhythm:* irregular
- *Rate:* atrial—60 beats/minute; ventricular—70 beats/minute
- *P wave:* configuration varies
- *PR interval:* varies with rhythm

- *QRS complex:* 0.10 second
- *T wave:* configuration varies
- *QT interval:* varies with rhythm changes
- *Other:* none

- conditions leading to fibrosis of the SA node, such as increased age, atherosclerotic heart disease, hypertension, and cardiomyopathy
- trauma to the SA node caused by open heart surgery (especially valvular surgery), pericarditis, or rheumatic heart disease
- autonomic disturbances affecting autonomic innervation, such as hypervagotonia or degeneration of the autonomic system
- cardioactive medications, such as digoxin, beta-adrenergic receptor blockers, and calcium channel blockers.

CLINICAL SIGNIFICANCE

The significance of SSS depends on the patient's age, the presence of other diseases, and the type and duration of the specific arrhythmias that occur. If atrial fibrillation is involved, the prognosis is worse, most likely because of the risk of thromboembolic complications.

If prolonged pauses are involved with SSS, syncope may occur. The length of a pause needed to cause syncope varies with the patient's age, posture at the time, and cerebrovascular status. Any pause that lasts 2 to 3 seconds or more should be considered significant.

A significant part of the diagnosis is whether the patient experiences symptoms while the disturbance occurs. Because the syndrome is progressive and chronic, a symptomatic patient will need lifelong treatment. In addition, thromboembolism may develop as a complication of SSS, possibly resulting in stroke or peripheral embolization.

ECG CHARACTERISTICS

SSS encompasses several potential rhythm disturbances that may be intermittent or chronic. SSS may include one, or a combination, of these rhythm disturbances:

- sinus bradycardia
- SA block
- sinus arrest
- sinus bradycardia alternating with sinus tachycardia
- episodes of atrial tachyarrhythmias, such as atrial fibrillation and atrial flutter
- failure of the sinus node to increase heart rate with exercise.

SSS displays these ECG characteristics:

- *Rhythm:* atrial and ventricular rhythms irregular because of sinus pauses and abrupt rate changes
- *Rate:* atrial and ventricular rates are fast or slow or alternate between fast and slow; and interrupted by a long sinus pause
- *P wave:* varies with the prevailing rhythm; may be normal size and configuration or may be absent; when present, a P wave usually precedes each QRS complex
- *PR interval:* usually within normal limits; varies with change in rhythm
- *QRS complex:* duration usually within normal limits; may vary with changes in rhythm; usually normal configuration
- *T wave:* usually normal size and configuration
- *QT interval:* usually within normal limits; varies with rhythm changes
- *Other:* usually more than one arrhythmia on a 6-second strip.

SIGNS AND SYMPTOMS

The patient's pulse rate may be fast, slow, or normal, and the rhythm may be regular or irregular. You can usually detect an irregularity on the monitor or when palpating the pulse, which may feel inappropriately slow, then rapid.

If you monitor the patient's heart rate during exercise or exertion, you may observe an inappropriate response to exercise, such as a failure of the heart rate to increase. You may also detect episodes of brady-tachy syndrome, atrial flutter, atrial fibrillation, SA block, or sinus arrest on the monitor.

Other assessment findings depend on the patient's condition. For example, he may have crackles in the lungs, S_3, or a dilated and displaced left ventricular apical impulse if he has underlying cardiomyopathy. The patient may also show signs and symptoms of decreased cardiac output, such as fatigue, hypotension, blurred vision, and syncope, a common experience with this arrhythmia. Syncopal episodes, when related to SSS, are referred to as Stokes-Adams attacks.

When caring for a patient with SSS, be alert for signs and symptoms of thromboembolism, especially if the patient has atrial fibrillation. Blood clots or thrombi forming in the heart can dislodge and travel through the bloodstream, resulting in decreased blood supply to the lungs, heart, brain, kidneys, intestines, or other organs. Assess the patient for:

- neurologic changes (such as confusion)
- vision disturbances
- weakness
- chest pain
- dyspnea
- tachypnea
- tachycardia
- acute onset of pain.

Early recognition allows for prompt treatment.

AGE AWARE Because the older adult with SSS may have mental status changes, be sure to perform a thorough assessment to rule out other disorders, such as stroke, delirium, or dementia.

INTERVENTIONS

As with other sinus node arrhythmias, no treatment is generally necessary if the patient is asymptomatic. If the patient is symptomatic, however, treatment aims to alleviate signs and symptoms and correct the underlying cause of the arrhythmia.

Atropine or epinephrine may be given initially for symptom-producing bradycardia. A temporary pacemaker may be required until the underlying disorder resolves. Tachyarrhythmias may be treated with antiarrhythmic medications, such as metoprolol and digoxin. Unfortunately, medications used to suppress tachyarrhythmias may worsen underlying SA node disease and bradyarrhythmias.

The patient may need anticoagulants if he develops sudden bursts, or paroxysms, of atrial fibrillation. The anticoagulants help prevent thromboembolism and stroke, a complication of the condition.

When caring for a patient with SSS, monitor and document all arrhythmias as well as signs or symptoms experienced. Note changes in heart rate and rhythm related to changes in the patient's level of activity.

Watch the patient carefully after starting beta-adrenergic receptor blockers, calcium channel blockers, or other antiarrhythmic medications. If treatment includes anticoagulant therapy and pacemaker insertion, make sure the patient and his family receive appropriate instructions.

ATRIAL ARRHYTHMIAS

Atrial arrhythmias, the most common cardiac rhythm disturbances, result from impulses originating in the atrial tissue in areas outside the SA node. These arrhythmias can affect ventricular filling time and diminish atrial kick. The term *atrial kick* refers to the complete filling of the ventricles during atrial systole and normally contributes about 25% to ventricular end-diastolic volume.

Atrial arrhythmias are thought to result from three mechanisms: altered automaticity, reentry, and afterdepolarization.

- *Altered automaticity.* The term *automaticity* refers to the ability of cardiac cells to initiate electrical impulses spontaneously. An increase in the automaticity of the atrial fibers can trigger abnormal impulses. Causes of increased automaticity include extracellular factors, such as hypoxia, hypocalcemia, and digoxin toxicity as well as conditions in which the function of the heart's normal pacemaker, the SA node, is diminished. For example, increased vagal tone or hypokalemia can increase the refractory period of the SA node and allow atrial fibers to initiate impulses.
- *Reentry.* In reentry, an impulse is delayed along a slow conduction pathway. Despite the delay, the impulse remains active enough to produce another impulse during myocardial repolarization. Reentry may occur with CAD, cardiomyopathy, or MI.
- *Afterdepolarization.* Afterdepolarization can occur as a result of cell injury, digoxin toxicity, and other conditions. An injured cell sometimes only partially repolarizes. Partial repolarization can lead to repetitive ectopic firing called triggered activity. The depolarization produced by triggered activity, known as afterdepolarization, can lead to atrial or ventricular tachycardia.

Premature atrial contractions

Premature atrial contractions (PACs) originate in the atria, outside the sinoatrial (SA) node. They arise from either a single ectopic focus or from multiple atrial foci that supersede the SA node as pacemaker for

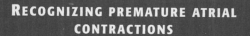

RECOGNIZING PREMATURE ATRIAL CONTRACTIONS

The following rhythm strip illustrates premature atrial contraction (PAC). Look for these distinguishing characteristics.

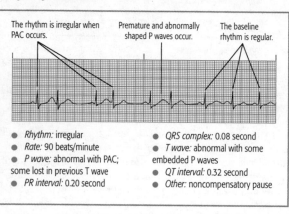

The rhythm is irregular when PAC occurs.

Premature and abnormally shaped P waves occur.

The baseline rhythm is regular.

- *Rhythm:* irregular
- *Rate:* 90 beats/minute
- *P wave:* abnormal with PAC; some lost in previous T wave
- *PR interval:* 0.20 second

- *QRS complex:* 0.08 second
- *T wave:* abnormal with some embedded P waves
- *QT interval:* 0.32 second
- *Other:* noncompensatory pause

one or more beats. PACs are generally caused by enhanced automaticity in the atrial tissue. (See *Recognizing premature atrial contractions.*)

PACs may be conducted or nonconducted (blocked) through the atrioventricular (AV) node and the rest of the heart, depending on the status of the AV and intraventricular conduction system. If the atrial ectopic pacemaker discharges too soon after the preceding QRS complex, the AV junction or bundle branches may still be refractory from conducting the previous electrical impulse. If they're still refractory, they may not be sufficiently repolarized to conduct the premature electrical impulse into the ventricles normally.

When a PAC is conducted, ventricular conduction is usually normal. Nonconducted, or blocked, PACs aren't followed by a QRS complex.

CAUSES

Alcohol, cigarettes, anxiety, fatigue, fever, and infectious diseases can trigger PACs, which commonly occur in a normal heart. Patients who eliminate or control those factors can usually correct the arrhythmia.

PACs may be associated with:

- hyperthyroidism
- coronary or valvular heart disease
- acute respiratory failure
- hypoxia
- chronic pulmonary disease
- digoxin toxicity
- certain electrolyte imbalances.

PACs may also be caused by drugs that prolong the absolute refractory period of the SA node, including quinidine and procainamide.

CLINICAL SIGNIFICANCE

PACs are rarely dangerous in patients free from heart disease. They usually cause no symptoms and can go unrecognized for years. Patients may perceive PACs as normal palpitations or skipped beats.

However, in patients with heart disease, PACs may lead to more serious arrhythmias, such as atrial fibrillation or atrial flutter. In a patient with acute myocardial infarction, PACs can serve as an early sign of heart failure or electrolyte imbalance. PACs can also result from endogenous catecholamine release during episodes of pain or anxiety.

ECG CHARACTERISTICS

- *Rhythm:* Atrial and ventricular rhythms are irregular as a result of PACs, but the underlying rhythm may be regular.
- *Rate:* Atrial and ventricular rates vary with the underlying rhythm.
- *P wave:* The hallmark characteristic of a PAC is a premature P wave with an abnormal configuration, when compared with a sinus P wave. Varying configurations of the P wave indicate more than one ectopic site. PACs may be hidden in the preceding T wave.
- *PR interval:* Usually within normal limits but may be either shortened or slightly prolonged for the ectopic beat, depending on the origin of the ectopic focus.
- *QRS complex:* Duration and configuration are usually normal when the PAC is conducted. If no QRS complex follows the PAC, the beat is called a nonconducted PAC.
- *T wave:* Usually normal; however, if the P wave is hidden in the T wave, the T wave may appear distorted.
- *QT interval:* Usually within normal limits.
- *Other:* PACs may occur as a single beat, in a bigeminal (every other beat is premature), trigeminal (every third beat), or quadrigeminal (every fourth beat) pattern, or in couplets (pairs). Three or more PACs in a row is called atrial tachycardia.

PACs are commonly followed by a pause as the SA node resets. The PAC depolarizes the SA node early, causing it to reset itself and disrupting the normal cycle. The next sinus beat occurs sooner than it normally would, causing a P-P interval between normal beats interrupted by a PAC to be shorter than three consecutive sinus beats, an occurrence referred to as noncompensatory.

SIGNS AND SYMPTOMS

The patient may have an irregular peripheral or apical pulse rhythm when the PACs occur. Otherwise, the pulse rhythm and rate will reflect the underlying rhythm. Patients may complain of palpitations, skipped beats, or a fluttering sensation. In a patient with heart disease, signs and symptoms of decreased cardiac output, such as hypotension and syncope, may occur.

INTERVENTIONS

Most asymptomatic patients don't need treatment. If the patient is symptomatic, however, treatment may focus on eliminating the cause, such as caffeine and alcohol. People with frequent PACs may be treated with drugs that prolong the refractory period of the atria. Those drugs include beta-adrenergic receptor blockers and calcium channel blockers.

When caring for a patient with PACs, assess him to help determine factors that trigger ectopic beats. Tailor patient teaching to help the patient correct or avoid underlying causes. For example, the patient may need to avoid caffeine or learn stress-reduction techniques to lessen anxiety.

If the patient has ischemic or valvular heart disease, monitor for signs and symptoms of heart failure, electrolyte imbalance, and more severe atrial arrhythmias.

Atrial tachycardia

Atrial tachycardia is a supraventricular tachycardia, which means that the impulses driving the rapid rhythm originate above the ventricles. Atrial tachycardia has an atrial rate from 150 to 250 beats/minute. The rapid rate shortens diastole, resulting in a loss of atrial kick, reduced cardiac output, reduced coronary perfusion, and the potential for myocardial ischemia. (See *Recognizing atrial tachycardia*.)

There are three forms of atrial tachycardia: atrial tachycardia with block, multifocal atrial tachycardia (MAT, or chaotic atrial rhythm), and paroxysmal atrial tachycardia (PAT). In MAT, the tachycardia originates from multiple foci. PAT is generally a transient event in which the tachycardia appears and disappears suddenly.

RECOGNIZING ATRIAL TACHYCARDIA

The following rhythm strip illustrates atrial tachycardia. Look for these distinguishing characteristics.

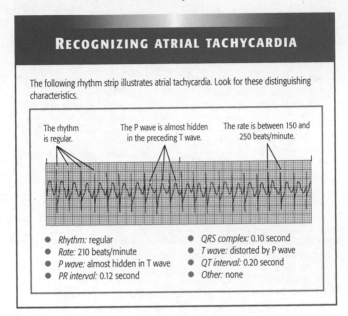

The rhythm is regular.

The P wave is almost hidden in the preceding T wave.

The rate is between 150 and 250 beats/minute.

- *Rhythm:* regular
- *Rate:* 210 beats/minute
- *P wave:* almost hidden in T wave
- *PR interval:* 0.12 second
- *QRS complex:* 0.10 second
- *T wave:* distorted by P wave
- *QT interval:* 0.20 second
- *Other:* none

CAUSES

Atrial tachycardia can occur in patients with a normal heart. In those cases, it's commonly related to excessive use of caffeine or other stimulants, marijuana use, electrolyte imbalance, hypoxia, or physical or psychological stress. Typically, however, atrial tachycardia is associated with primary or secondary cardiac disorders, including myocardial infarction (MI), cardiomyopathy, congenital anomalies, Wolff-Parkinson-White syndrome, and valvular heart disease.

This rhythm may be a component of sick sinus syndrome. Other problems resulting in atrial tachycardia include cor pulmonale, hyperthyroidism, systemic hypertension, and digoxin toxicity, the most common cause of atrial tachycardia. (See *Signs of digoxin toxicity,* page 268.)

CLINICAL SIGNIFICANCE

In a healthy person, nonsustained atrial tachycardia is usually benign. However, this rhythm may be a forerunner of more serious ventricular arrhythmias, especially if it occurs in a patient with underlying heart disease.

The increased ventricular rate that occurs in atrial tachycardia results in decreased ventricular filling time, increased myocardial oxy-

SIGNS OF DIGOXIN TOXICITY

With digoxin (Lanoxin) toxicity be alert for the following signs and symptoms, especially if the patient is taking digoxin and his potassium level is low or he's also taking amiodarone (Cordarone) (because both combinations can increase the risk of digoxin toxicity):

● *CNS:* fatigue, general muscle weakness, agitation, hallucinations
● *EENT:* yellow-green halos around visual images, blurred vision

● *GI:* anorexia, nausea, vomiting
● *CV:* arrhythmias (most commonly, conduction disturbances with or without AV block, premature ventricular contractions, and supraventricular arrhythmias), increased severity of heart failure, hypotension. (Digoxin's toxic effects on the heart may be life-threatening and always require immediate attention.)

gen consumption, and decreased oxygen supply to the myocardium. Heart failure, myocardial ischemia, and MI can result.

ECG CHARACTERISTICS

■ *Rhythm:* The atrial rhythm is usually regular. The ventricular rhythm is regular or irregular, depending on the atrioventricular (AV) conduction ratio and the type of atrial tachycardia. (See *Recognizing types of atrial tachycardia,* pages 270 and 271.)

■ *Rate:* The atrial rate is characterized by three or more consecutive ectopic atrial beats occurring at a rate between 150 and 250 beats/ minute. The rate rarely exceeds 250 beats/minute. The ventricular rate depends on the AV conduction ratio.

■ *P wave:* The P wave may be aberrant (deviating from normal appearance) or hidden in the preceding T wave. If visible, it's usually upright and precedes each QRS complex.

■ *PR interval:* The PR interval may be unmeasurable if the P wave can't be distinguished from the preceding T wave.

■ *QRS complex:* Duration and configuration are usually normal, unless the impulses are being conducted abnormally through the ventricles.

■ *T wave:* Usually distinguishable but may be distorted by the P wave; may be inverted if ischemia is present.

■ *QT interval:* Usually within normal limits but may be shorter because of the rapid rate.

■ *Other:* None.

SIGNS AND SYMPTOMS

The patient with atrial tachycardia will have a rapid apical and peripheral pulse rate. The rhythm may be regular or irregular, depending on the type of atrial tachycardia. A patient with PAT may complain that his heart suddenly starts to beat faster or that he suddenly feels palpitations. Persistent tachycardia and rapid ventricular rate cause decreased cardiac output, resulting in hypotension and syncope.

INTERVENTIONS

Treatment depends on the type of tachycardia and the severity of the patient's symptoms. Because one of the most common causes of atrial tachycardia is digoxin toxicity, assess the patient for signs and symptoms of digoxin toxicity and monitor digoxin blood levels.

Valsalva's maneuver or carotid sinus massage may be used to treat PAT. (See *Understanding carotid sinus massage,* page 272.) These maneuvers increase the parasympathetic tone, which results in a slowing of the heart rate. They also allow the sinoatrial (SA) node to resume function as the primary pacemaker.

If vagal maneuvers are used, make sure resuscitative equipment is readily available. Keep in mind that vagal stimulation can result in bradycardia, ventricular arrhythmias, and asystole.

AGE AWARE Older adults may have undiagnosed carotid atherosclerosis and carotid bruits may be absent, even with significant disease. As a result, cardiac sinus massage shouldn't be performed in late-middle-age and older patients.

Drug therapy (pharmacologic cardioversion) may be used to increase the degree of AV block and decrease ventricular response rate. Appropriate drugs include adenosine (Adenocard), amiodarone, beta-adrenergic receptor blockers, calcium channel blockers, and digoxin. When other treatments fail, or if the patient is clinically unstable, synchronized electrical cardioversion may be used. For the complete ACLS algorithm, see pages 332 and 333.

Atrial overdrive pacing (also called rapid atrial pacing or overdrive suppression) may also be used to stop the arrhythmia. This technique involves suppression of spontaneous depolarization of the ectopic pacemaker by a series of paced electrical impulses at a rate slightly higher than the intrinsic ectopic atrial rate. The pacemaker cells are depolarized prematurely and, following termination of the paced electrical impulses, the SA node resumes its normal role as the pacemaker.

Radiofrequency ablation can be used to treat PAT. The ectopic focus is mapped during the electrophysiology study, and then the area is
(*Text continues on page 272.*)

RECOGNIZING TYPES OF ATRIAL TACHYCARDIA

Atrial tachycardia comes in three varieties. Here's a quick rundown of each.

Atrial tachycardia with block

Atrial tachycardia with block is caused by increased automaticity of the atrial tissue. As the atrial rate speeds up and atrioventricular (AV) conduction becomes impaired, a 2:1 block typically occurs. Occasionally a type I (Wenckebach) second-degree AV block may be seen. Look for these distinguishing characteristics.

Two P waves occur for each QRS complex.

The ventricular rhythm is regular; the block is constant.

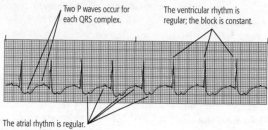

The atrial rhythm is regular.

- *Rhythm:* atrial—regular; ventricular—regular if block is constant, irregular if block is variable
- *Rate:* atrial—140 to 250 beats/minute, multiple of ventricular rate; ventricular—varies with block

- *P wave:* slightly abnormal
- *PR interval:* usually normal; may be hidden
- *QRS complex:* usually normal
- *Other:* more than one P wave for each QRS complex

Multifocal atrial tachycardia (MAT)

In MAT, atrial tachycardia occurs with numerous atrial foci firing intermittently. MAT produces varying P waves on the strip and occurs most commonly in patients with chronic pulmonary disease. The irregular baseline in this strip is caused by movement of the chest wall. Look for these distinguishing characteristics.

- *Rhythm:* both irregular
- *Rate:* atrial—100 to 250 beats/minute, usually under 160; ventricular—101 to 250 beats/minute

- *P wave:* configuration varies; must see at least three different P wave shapes
- *PR interval:* varies
- *Other:* none

Paroxysmal atrial tachycardia (PAT)

A type of paroxysmal supraventricular tachycardia, PAT features brief periods of tachycardia that alternate with periods of normal sinus rhythm. PAT starts and stops suddenly as a result of rapid firing of an ectopic focus. It commonly follows frequent premature atrial contractions, one of which initiates the tachycardia. Look for these distinguishing characteristics.

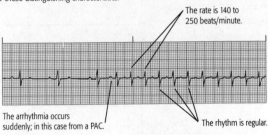

The rate is 140 to 250 beats/minute.

The arrhythmia occurs suddenly; in this case from a PAC.

The rhythm is regular.

- *Rhythm:* regular
- *Rate:* 140 to 250 beats/minute
- *P wave:* abnormal, possibly hidden in previous T wave
- *PR interval:* identical for each cycle

- *QRS complex:* can be aberrantly conducted
- *Other:* one P wave for each QRS complex

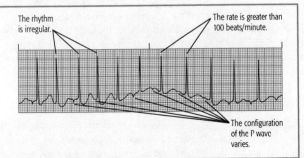

The rhythm is irregular.

The rate is greater than 100 beats/minute.

The configuration of the P wave varies.

UNDERSTANDING CAROTID SINUS MASSAGE

Carotid sinus massage may be used to interrupt paroxysmal atrial tachycardia. Massaging the carotid sinus stimulates the vagus nerve, which inhibits firing of the sinoatrial (SA) node and slows atrioventricular (AV) node conduction. As a result, the SA node can resume its function as primary pacemaker.

Carotid sinus massage involves a firm massage that lasts no longer than 5 to 10 seconds. The patient's head is turned to the left to massage the right carotid sinus, as shown below. Remember that simultaneous, bilateral massage should never be attempted.

Carotid sinus massage is contraindicated in patients with carotid bruits. Risks of the procedure include decreased heart rate, syncope, sinus arrest, increased degree of AV block, cerebral emboli, stroke, and asystole.

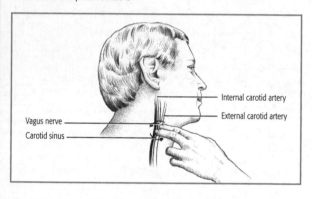

Internal carotid artery
External carotid artery
Vagus nerve
Carotid sinus

ablated. Because MAT commonly occurs in patients with chronic pulmonary disease, the rhythm may not respond to treatment.

When caring for a patient with atrial tachycardia, carefully monitor the patient's rhythm strips. Doing so may provide information about the cause of atrial tachycardia, which in turn can facilitate treatment. Monitor the patient for chest pain, indications of decreased cardiac output, and signs and symptoms of heart failure or myocardial ischemia.

Atrial flutter

Atrial flutter, a supraventricular tachycardia, is characterized by a rapid atrial rate of 250 to 350 beats/minute, although it's generally around 300 beats/minute. Originating in a single atrial focus, this

RECOGNIZING ATRIAL FLUTTER

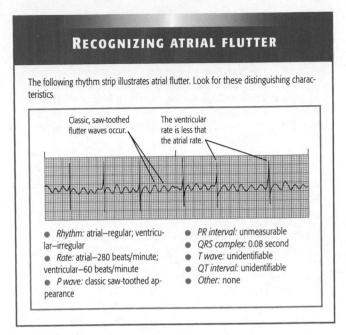

The following rhythm strip illustrates atrial flutter. Look for these distinguishing characteristics.

Classic, saw-toothed flutter waves occur.

The ventricular rate is less that the atrial rate.

- *Rhythm:* atrial—regular; ventricular—irregular
- *Rate:* atrial—280 beats/minute; ventricular—60 beats/minute
- *P wave:* classic saw-toothed appearance
- *PR interval:* unmeasurable
- *QRS complex:* 0.08 second
- *T wave:* unidentifiable
- *QT interval:* unidentifiable
- *Other:* none

rhythm results from circus reentry and possibly increased automaticity.

On an ECG, the P waves lose their normal appearance due to the rapid atrial rate. The waves blend together in a sawtooth configuration called flutter waves, or F waves. These waves are the hallmark of atrial flutter. (See *Recognizing atrial flutter.*)

CAUSES

Atrial flutter may be caused by conditions that enlarge atrial tissue and elevate atrial pressures. The arrhythmia is commonly found in patients with:

- mitral or tricuspid valvular disease
- hyperthyroidism
- pericardial disease
- digoxin toxicity
- primary myocardial disease.

The rhythm is sometimes encountered in patients following cardiac surgery or in patients with acute myocardial infarction, chronic pulmonary disease, or systemic arterial hypoxia. Atrial flutter rarely occurs in healthy people. When it does, it may indicate intrinsic cardiac disease.

Clinical significance

The clinical significance of atrial flutter is determined by the number of impulses conducted through the atrioventricular (AV) node. That number is expressed as a conduction ratio, such as 2:1 or 4:1, and the resulting ventricular rate. If the ventricular rate is too slow (below 40 beats/minute) or too fast (above 150 beats/minute), cardiac output can be seriously compromised.

Usually the faster the ventricular rate, the more dangerous the arrhythmia. Rapid ventricular rates reduce ventricular filling time and coronary perfusion, which can cause angina, heart failure, pulmonary edema, hypotension, and syncope.

ECG characteristics

- *Rhythm:* Atrial rhythm is regular. Ventricular rhythm depends on the AV conduction pattern; it's typically regular, although cycles may alternate. An irregular pattern may signal atrial fibrillation or indicate development of a block.
- *Rate:* Atrial rate is 250 to 350 beats/minute. Ventricular rate depends on the degree of AV block; usually it's 60 to 100 beats/minute, but it may accelerate to 125 to 150 beats/minute.

Varying degrees of AV block produce ventricular rates that are usually one-half to one-fourth of the atrial rate. These are expressed as ratios, for example, 2:1 or 4:1. Usually, the AV node won't accept more than 180 impulses/minute and allows every second, third, or fourth impulse to be conducted. These impulses account for the ventricular rate. At the time atrial flutter is initially recognized, the ventricular response is typically above 100 beats/minute. One of the most common ventricular rates is 150 beats/minute with an atrial rate of 300, known as 2:1 block.

- *P wave:* Atrial flutter is characterized by abnormal P waves that produce a sawtooth appearance, referred to as flutter or F waves.
- *PR interval:* Unmeasurable.
- *QRS complex:* Duration is usually within normal limits, but the complex may be widened if flutter waves are buried within the complex.
- *T wave:* Not identifiable.
- *QT interval:* Unmeasurable because the T wave isn't identifiable.
- *Other:* The patient may develop an atrial rhythm that commonly varies between a fibrillatory line and flutter waves. This variation is referred to as atrial fib-flutter. The ventricular response is irregular.

SIGNS AND SYMPTOMS

When caring for a patient with atrial flutter, you may note that the peripheral and apical pulses are normal in rate and rhythm. That's because the pulse reflects the number of ventricular contractions, not the number of atrial impulses.

If the ventricular rate is normal, the patient may be asymptomatic. If the ventricular rate is rapid, however, the patient may experience a feeling of palpitations and may exhibit signs and symptoms of reduced cardiac output.

INTERVENTIONS

If the patient is hemodynamically unstable, synchronized electrical cardioversion or countershock should be administered immediately. Cardioversion delivers electrical current to the heart to correct an arrhythmia, but unlike defibrillation, it usually uses much lower energy levels and is synchronized to discharge at the peak of the R wave. This causes immediate depolarization, interrupting reentry circuits and allowing the sinoatrial (SA) node to resume control as pacemaker. Synchronizing the energy current delivery with the R wave ensures that the current won't be delivered on the vulnerable T wave, which could initiate ventricular tachycardia or ventricular fibrillation.

The focus of treatment for hemodynamically stable patients with atrial flutter includes controlling the rate and converting the rhythm. Specific interventions depend on the patient's cardiac function, whether preexcitation syndromes are involved, and the duration (less than or greater than 48 hours) of the arrhythmia. For example, in atrial flutter with normal cardiac function and duration of rhythm less than 48 hours, electrical cardioversion may be considered; for duration greater than 48 hours, don't use electrical cardioversion because it increases the risk of thromboembolism unless the patient has been adequately anticoagulated.

Because atrial flutter may be an indication of intrinsic cardiac disease, monitor the patient closely for signs and symptoms of low cardiac output. Be alert to the effects of digoxin, which depresses the SA node.

If electrical cardioversion is indicated, prepare the patient for I.V. administration of a sedative or anesthetic as ordered. Keep resuscitative equipment at the bedside. Be alert for bradycardia because cardioversion can decrease the heart rate.

Atrial fibrillation

Atrial fibrillation, sometimes called *AFib,* is defined as chaotic, asynchronous, electrical activity in atrial tissue. It results from the firing of multiple impulses from numerous ectopic pacemakers in the atria. Atrial fibrillation is characterized by the absence of P waves and an irregularly irregular ventricular response.

When a number of ectopic sites in the atria initiate impulses, depolarization can't spread in an organized manner. Small sections of the atria are depolarized individually, resulting in the atrial muscle quivering instead of contracting. On an ECG, uneven baseline fibrillatory waves, or f waves, appear rather than clearly distinguishable P waves.

The atrioventricular (AV) node protects the ventricles from the 350 to 600 erratic atrial impulses that occur each minute by acting as a filter and blocking some of the impulses. The ventricles respond only to impulses conducted through the AV node, hence the characteristic, wide variation in R-R intervals. When the ventricular response rate drops below 100, atrial fibrillation is considered controlled. When the ventricular rate exceeds 100, the rhythm is considered uncontrolled.

Like atrial flutter, atrial fibrillation results in a loss of atrial kick. The rhythm may be sustained or paroxysmal, meaning that it occurs suddenly and ends abruptly. It can either be preceded by or be the result of premature atrial contractions. (See *Recognizing atrial fibrillation*.)

CAUSES

Atrial fibrillation occurs more commonly than atrial flutter or atrial tachycardia. Atrial fibrillation can occur following cardiac surgery. Other causes of atrial fibrillation include:

- rheumatic heart disease
- valvular heart disease (especially mitral valve disease)
- hyperthyroidism
- pericarditis
- coronary artery disease
- acute myocardial infarction
- hypertension
- cardiomyopathy
- atrial septal defects
- chronic obstructive pulmonary disease.

The rhythm may also occur in a healthy person who smokes or drinks coffee or alcohol or who is fatigued and under stress. Certain drugs, such as aminophylline and digoxin, may contribute to the development of atrial fibrillation. Endogenous catecholamine released during exercise may also trigger the arrhythmia.

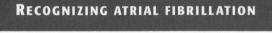

RECOGNIZING ATRIAL FIBRILLATION

The following rhythm strip illustrates atrial fibrillation. Look for these distinguishing characteristics.

The sinus P wave is replaced by erratic fibrillatory waves.

The rhythm is irregularly irregular.

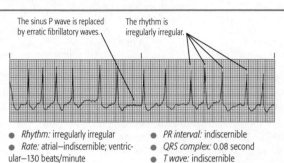

- *Rhythm:* irregularly irregular
- *Rate:* atrial—indiscernible; ventricular—130 beats/minute
- *P wave:* absent; replaced by fine fibrillation waves
- *PR interval:* indiscernible
- *QRS complex:* 0.08 second
- *T wave:* indiscernible
- *QT interval:* unmeasurable
- *Other:* none

CLINICAL SIGNIFICANCE

The loss of atrial kick from atrial fibrillation can result in the subsequent loss of approximately 20% of normal end-diastolic volume. Combined with the decreased diastolic filling time associated with a rapid heart rate, clinically significant reductions in cardiac output can result. In uncontrolled atrial fibrillation, the patient may develop heart failure, myocardial ischemia, or syncope.

Patients with preexisting cardiac disease, such as hypertrophic cardiomyopathy, mitral stenosis, rheumatic heart disease, or those with mitral prosthetic valves, tend to tolerate atrial fibrillation poorly and may develop severe heart failure.

Left untreated, atrial fibrillation can lead to cardiovascular collapse, thrombus formation, and systemic arterial or pulmonary embolism. (See *Risk of restoring sinus rhythm,* page 278.)

ECG CHARACTERISTICS

- *Rhythm:* Atrial and ventricular rhythms are grossly irregular, typically described as irregularly irregular.
- *Rate:* The atrial rate is almost indiscernible and usually exceeds 350 beats/minute. The atrial rate far exceeds the ventricular rate

RISK OF RESTORING SINUS RHYTHM

A patient with atrial fibrillation is at increased risk for developing atrial thrombus and subsequent systemic arterial embolism. In atrial fibrillation, neither atrium contracts as a whole. As a result, blood may pool on the atrial wall, and thrombi may form. Thrombus formation places the patient at higher risk for emboli and stroke.

If normal sinus rhythm is restored and the atria contract normally, clots may break away from the atrial wall and travel through the pulmonary or systemic circulation with potentially disastrous results, such as stroke, pulmonary embolism, or arterial occlusion.

because most impulses aren't conducted through the AV junction. The ventricular rate usually varies, typically from 100 to 150 beats/ minute but can be below 100 beats/minute.

- *P wave:* The P wave is absent. Erratic baseline f waves appear in place of P waves. These chaotic waves represent atrial tetanization from rapid atrial depolarizations.
- *PR interval:* Indiscernible.
- *QRS complex:* Duration and configuration are usually normal.
- *T wave:* Indiscernible.
- *QT interval:* Unmeasurable.
- *Other:* The patient may develop an atrial rhythm that commonly varies between a fibrillatory line and flutter waves, a phenomenon called atrial fib-flutter.

SIGNS AND SYMPTOMS

When caring for a patient with atrial fibrillation, you may find that the radial pulse rate is slower than the apical rate. The weaker contractions that occur in atrial fibrillation don't produce a palpable peripheral pulse; only the stronger ones do.

The pulse rhythm will be irregularly irregular, with a normal or abnormal heart rate. Patients with a new onset of atrial fibrillation and a rapid ventricular rate may demonstrate signs and symptoms of decreased cardiac output, including hypotension and light-headedness. Patients with chronic atrial fibrillation may be able to compensate for the decreased cardiac output. Although these patients may be asymptomatic, they face a greater-than-normal risk of the development of pulmonary, cerebral, or other thromboembolic events.

INTERVENTIONS

Treatment of atrial fibrillation aims to reduce the ventricular response rate to below 100 beats/minute. This may be accomplished either by

HOW SYNCHRONIZED CARDIOVERSION WORKS

A patient experiencing an arrhythmia that leads to reduced cardiac output may be a candidate for synchronized cardioversion. This procedure may be done electively or as an emergency. For example, it may be an elective procedure in a patient with recurrent atrial fibrillation or an emergency procedure in a patient with ventricular tachycardia and a pulse.

Synchronized cardioversion is similar to defibrillation, also called *unsynchronized cardioversion*, except that synchronized cardioversion generally requires lower energy levels. Synchronizing the energy delivered to the patient reduces the risk that the current will strike during the relative refractory period of a cardiac cycle and induce ventricular fibrillation (VF).

In synchronized cardioversion, the R wave on the patient's electrocardiogram is synchronized with the cardioverter (defibrillator). After the firing buttons have been pressed, the cardioverter discharges energy when it senses the next R wave.

Keep in mind that a slight delay occurs between the time the discharge buttons are depressed and the moment the energy is actually discharged. When using handheld paddles, continue to hold the paddles on the patient's chest until the energy is delivered.

Remember to reset the "sync mode" on the defibrillator after each synchronized cardioversion. Resetting this switch is necessary because most defibrillators will automatically reset to an unsynchronized mode.

If VF occurs during the procedure, turn off sync button, and immediately deliver an unsynchronized defibrillation to terminate the arrhythmia. Be aware that synchronized cardioversion carries the risk of lethal arrhythmia when used in patients with digoxin (Lanoxin) toxicity.

---

drugs that control the ventricular response or by a combination of electrical cardioversion and drug therapy, to convert the arrhythmia to normal sinus rhythm. When the onset of atrial fibrillation is acute and the patient can cooperate, vagal maneuvers or carotid sinus massage may slow the ventricular response but won't convert the arrhythmia.

If the patient is hemodynamically unstable, synchronized electrical cardioversion should be administered immediately. Electrical cardioversion is most successful if used within the first 48 hours after onset and less successful the longer the duration of the arrhythmia. Conversion to normal sinus rhythm will cause forceful atrial contractions to resume abruptly. If a thrombus forms in the atria, the resumption of contractions can result in systemic emboli. (See *How synchronized cardioversion works*.)

The focus of treatment for hemodynamically stable patients with atrial fibrillation includes:

- controlling the rate
- converting the rhythm
- providing anticoagulation if indicated.

Specific interventions depend on the patient's cardiac function, whether preexcitation syndromes are involved, and the duration of the arrhythmia.

Beta-adrenergic receptor blockers and calcium channel blockers are the drugs of choice to control the ventricular rate. Patients with reduced left ventricular function typically receive digoxin. Anticoagulation is crucial in reducing the risk of thromboembolism. Heparin and warfarin (Coumadin) are used for anticoagulation and to prepare the patient for electrical cardioversion. Symptomatic atrial fibrillation that doesn't respond to routine treatment may be treated with radiofrequency ablation therapy.

When assessing a patient with atrial fibrillation, assess the peripheral and apical pulses. If the patient isn't on a cardiac monitor, be alert for an irregular pulse and differences in the radial and apical pulse rates.

Assess for symptoms of decreased cardiac output and heart failure. If drug therapy is used, monitor serum drug levels, and observe the patient for evidence of toxicity. Tell the patient to report pulse rate changes, syncope or dizziness, chest pain, and signs of heart failure, such as dyspnea and peripheral edema.

Wandering pacemaker

Wandering pacemaker, also called *wandering atrial pacemaker,* is an atrial arrhythmia that results when the site of impulse formation shifts from the sinoatrial (SA) node to another area above the ventricles. The origin of the impulse may wander beat to beat from the SA node to ectopic sites in the atria or to the atrioventricular (AV) junctional tissue. The P wave and PR interval vary from beat to beat as the pacemaker site changes. (See *Recognizing wandering pacemaker.*)

CAUSES

In most cases, wandering pacemaker is caused by increased parasympathetic (vagal) influences on the SA node or AV junction. It can also be caused by chronic pulmonary disease, valvular heart disease, digoxin toxicity, and inflammation of the atrial tissue.

RECOGNIZING WANDERING PACEMAKER

The following rhythm strip illustrates wandering pacemaker. Look for these distinguishing characteristics.

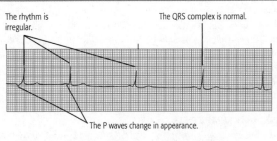

The rhythm is irregular.

The QRS complex is normal.

The P waves change in appearance.

- *Rhythm:* irregular atrial and ventricular rhythms
- *Rate:* atrial and ventricular rates of 50 beats/minute
- *P wave:* changes in size and shape; first P wave inverted, second upright

- *PR interval:* varies
- *QRS complex:* 0.08 second
- *T wave:* normal
- *QT interval:* 0.44 second
- *Other:* none

CLINICAL SIGNIFICANCE

The arrhythmia may be normal in young patients and is common in athletes who have slow heart rates. The arrhythmia may be difficult to identify because it's often transient. Although wandering pacemaker is rarely serious, chronic arrhythmias are a sign of heart disease and should be monitored.

ECG CHARACTERISTICS

- *Rhythm:* The atrial rhythm varies slightly, with an irregular P-P interval. The ventricular rhythm varies slightly, with an irregular R-R interval.
- *Rate:* Atrial and ventricular rates vary but are usually within normal limits, or below 60 beats/minute.
- *P wave:* Altered size and configuration are due to the changing pacemaker site (SA node, atria, or AV junction). The P wave may also be absent, inverted, or may follow the QRS complex if the impulse originates in the AV junction. A combination of these varia-

tions may appear, with at least three different P-wave shapes visible.

- *PR interval:* The PR interval varies from beat to beat as the pacemaker site changes but usually less than 0.20 second. If the impulse originates in the AV junction, the PR interval will be less than 0.12 second. This variation in PR interval will cause a slightly irregular R-R interval. When the P wave is present, the PR interval may be normal or shortened.
- *QRS complex:* Ventricular depolarization is normal, so duration of the QRS complex is usually within normal limits and is of normal configuration.
- *T wave:* Normal size and configuration.
- *QT interval:* Usually within normal limits, but may vary.
- *Other:* None.

SIGNS AND SYMPTOMS

Patients are generally asymptomatic and unaware of the arrhythmia. The pulse rate may be normal or below 60 beats/minute, and the rhythm may be regular or slightly irregular.

INTERVENTIONS

Usually, no treatment is needed for asymptomatic patients. If the patient is symptomatic, however, the patient's medications should be reviewed and the underlying cause investigated and treated. Monitor the patient's heart rhythm, and assess for signs of hemodynamic instability, such as hypotension and changes in mental status.

JUNCTIONAL ARRHYTHMIAS

Junctional arrhythmias originate in the atrioventricular (AV) junction—the area in and around the AV node and the bundle of His. The specialized pacemaker cells in the AV junction take over as the heart's pacemaker if the sinoatrial (SA) node fails to function properly or if the electrical impulses originating in the SA node are blocked. These junctional pacemaker cells have an inherent firing rate of 40 to 60 beats/minute.

In normal impulse conduction, the AV node slows transmission of the impulse from the atria to the ventricles, which allows the ventricles to fill as much as possible before they contract. However, these impulses don't always follow the normal conduction pathway. (See *Conduction in Wolff-Parkinson-White syndrome.*)

Because of the location of the AV junction within the conduction pathway, electrical impulses originating in this area cause abnormal

CONDUCTION IN WOLFF-PARKINSON-WHITE SYNDROME

Electrical impulses in the heart don't always follow normal conduction pathways. In preexcitation syndromes, electrical impulses enter the ventricles from the atria through an accessory pathway that bypasses the atrioventricular junction. Wolff-Parkinson-White (WPW) syndrome is a common type of preexcitation syndrome.

WPW syndrome commonly occurs in young children and in adults ages 20 to 35. The syndrome causes the PR interval to shorten and the QRS complex to lengthen as a result of a delta wave. Delta waves, which in WPW occur just before normal ventricular depolarization, are produced as a result of the premature depolarization or preexcitation of a portion of the ventricles.

WPW is clinically significant because the accessory pathway–in this case, Kent's bundle–may result in paroxysmal tachyarrhythmias by reentry and rapid conduction mechanisms.

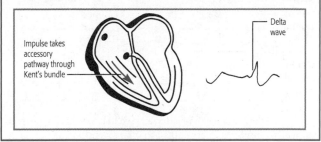

Impulse takes accessory pathway through Kent's bundle

Delta wave

depolarization of the heart. The impulse is conducted in a retrograde (backward) fashion to depolarize the atria, and antegrade (forward) to depolarize the ventricles.

Depolarization of the atria can precede depolarization of the ventricles, or the ventricles can be depolarized before the atria. Depolarization of the atria and ventricles can also occur simultaneously. (See *Locating the P wave,* page 284.)

Retrograde depolarization of the atria results in inverted P waves in leads II, III, and aV$_F$, leads in which you would normally see upright P waves appear.

Remember that arrhythmias causing inverted P waves on an ECG may originate in the atria or AV junction. Atrial arrhythmias are sometimes mistaken for junctional arrhythmias because impulses are generated so low in the atria that they cause retrograde depolarization and inverted P waves. Looking at the PR interval will help you determine whether an arrhythmia is atrial or junctional.

LOCATING THE P WAVE

When the specialized pacemaker cells in the atrioventricular junction take over as the dominant pacemaker of the heart:

- depolarization of the atria can precede depolarization of the ventricles
- the ventricles can be depolarized before the atria
- simultaneous depolarization of the atria and ventricles can occur.

The rhythm strips shown here demonstrate the various locations of the P waves in junctional arrhythmias, depending on the direction of depolarization.

Inverted P wave
If the atria are depolarized first, the P wave will occur before the QRS complex.

Inverted P wave
If the ventricles are depolarized first, the P wave will occur after the QRS complex.

Inverted P wave (hidden)
If the ventricles and atria are depolarized simultaneously, the P wave will be hidden in the QRS complex.

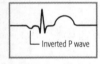

Inverted P wave

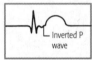

Inverted P wave

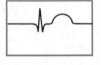

An arrhythmia with an inverted P wave before the QRS complex and with a normal PR interval (0.12 to 0.20 second) originates in the atria. An arrhythmia with a PR interval less than 0.12 second originates in the AV junction.

Premature junctional contractions

A premature junctional contraction (PJC) is a junctional beat that comes from the AV junction before the next expected sinus beat; it interrupts the underlying rhythm and causes an irregular rhythm. These ectopic beats commonly occur as a result of enhanced automaticity in the junctional tissue or bundle of His. As with all impulses generated in the atrioventricular (AV) junction, the atria are depolarized in a retrograde fashion, causing an inverted P wave. The ventricles are depolarized normally. (See *Recognizing a PJC*.)

CAUSES

PJCs may be caused by digoxin toxicity, excessive caffeine intake, amphetamine ingestion, excessive alcohol intake, excessive nicotine intake, stress, coronary artery disease, myocardial ischemia, valvular

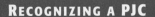

RECOGNIZING A PJC

The following rhythm strip illustrates premature junctional contraction (PJC). Look for these distinguishing characteristics.

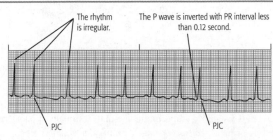

The rhythm is irregular.

The P wave is inverted with PR interval less than 0.12 second.

PJC

PJC

- *Rhythm:* irregular atrial and ventricular rhythms
- *Rate:* 100 beats/minute
- *P wave:* inverted and precedes the QRS complex

- *PR interval:* 0.14 second for the underlying rhythm and 0.06 second for the PJC
- *QRS complex:* 0.06 second
- *T wave:* normal configuration
- *QT interval:* 0.36 second
- *Other:* pause after PJC

heart disease, pericarditis, heart failure, chronic obstructive pulmonary disease, hyperthyroidism, electrolyte imbalances, or inflammatory changes in the AV junction after heart surgery.

CLINICAL SIGNIFICANCE

PJCs are generally considered harmless unless they occur frequently—typically defined as more than six/minute. Frequent PJCs indicate junctional irritability and can precipitate a more serious arrhythmia, such as junctional tachycardia. In patients taking digoxin, PJCs are a common early sign of toxicity.

ECG CHARACTERISTICS

- *Rhythm:* Atrial and ventricular rhythms are irregular during PJCs; the underlying rhythm may be regular.
- *Rate:* Atrial and ventricular rates reflect the underlying rhythm.
- *P wave:* The P wave is usually inverted. It may occur before or after the QRS complex or may appear absent when hidden in the QRS

complex. Look for an inverted P wave in leads II, III, and aV$_F$. Depending on the initial direction of depolarization, the P wave may fall before, during, or after the QRS complex.

■ *PR interval:* If the P wave precedes the QRS complex, the PR interval is shortened (less than 0.12 second); otherwise, it can't be measured.

■ *QRS complex:* Because the ventricles are usually depolarized normally, the QRS complex usually has a normal configuration and a normal duration of less than 0.12 second.

■ *T wave:* Usually has a normal configuration.

■ *QT interval:* Usually within normal limits.

■ *Other:* A compensatory pause reflecting retrograde atrial conduction may follow the PJC.

SIGNS AND SYMPTOMS

The patient is usually asymptomatic. He may complain of palpitations or a feeling of "skipped heart beats." You may be able to palpate an irregular pulse when PJCs occur. If PJCs are frequent enough, the patient may experience hypotension from a transient decrease in cardiac output.

INTERVENTIONS

PJCs don't usually require treatment unless the patient is symptomatic. In those cases, the underlying cause should be treated. For example, in digoxin toxicity, the medication should be discontinued and serum drug levels monitored.

Monitor the patient for hemodynamic instability as well. If ectopic beats occur frequently, the patient should decrease or eliminate his caffeine intake.

Junctional escape rhythm

A junctional escape rhythm, also referred to as junctional rhythm, is an arrhythmia originating in the atrioventricular (AV) junction. In this arrhythmia, the AV junction takes over as a secondary, or "escape" pacemaker. This usually occurs only when a higher pacemaker site in the atria, usually the sinoatrial (SA) node, fails as the heart's dominant pacemaker.

Remember that the AV junction can take over as the heart's dominant pacemaker if the firing rate of the higher pacemaker sites falls below the AV junction's intrinsic firing rate, if the pacemaker fails to generate an impulse, or if the conduction of the impulses is blocked.

In a junctional escape rhythm, as in all junctional arrhythmias, the atria are depolarized by means of retrograde conduction. The

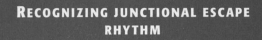

RECOGNIZING JUNCTIONAL ESCAPE RHYTHM

The following rhythm strip illustrates junctional escape rhythm. Look for these distinguishing characteristics.

The P wave is inverted.

The rhythm is regular with a rate of 40 to 60 beats/minute.

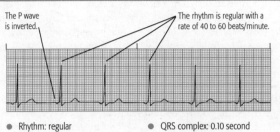

- Rhythm: regular
- Rate: 60 beats/minute
- P wave: inverted and preceding each QRS complex
- PR interval: 0.10 second

- QRS complex: 0.10 second
- T wave: normal
- QT interval: 0.44 second
- Other: none

P waves are inverted, and impulse conduction through the ventricles is normal. The normal intrinsic firing rate for cells in the AV junction is 40 to 60 beats/minute. (See *Recognizing junctional escape rhythm*.)

CAUSES
A junctional escape rhythm can be caused by a condition that disturbs normal SA node function or impulse conduction. Causes of the arrhythmia include:

- SA node ischemia
- hypoxia
- electrolyte imbalances
- valvular heart disease
- heart failure
- cardiomyopathy
- myocarditis
- sick sinus syndrome
- increased parasympathetic (vagal) tone.

Drugs, such as digoxin, calcium channel blockers, and beta-adrenergic receptor blockers, can also cause a junctional escape rhythm.

CLINICAL SIGNIFICANCE

The clinical significance of junctional escape rhythm depends on how well the patient tolerates a decreased heart rate (40 to 60 beats/minute) and associated decrease in cardiac output. In addition to a decreased cardiac output from a slower heart rate, depolarization of the atria either after or simultaneously with ventricular depolarization results in loss of atrial kick. Remember that junctional escape rhythms protect the heart from potentially life-threatening ventricular escape rhythms.

ECG CHARACTERISTICS

- *Rhythm:* Atrial and ventricular rhythms are regular.
- *Rate:* The atrial and ventricular rates are 40 to 60 beats/minute.
- *P wave:* The P wave is inverted (look for inverted P waves in leads II, III, and aV_F). The P wave may occur before or after the QRS complex or may appear absent when hidden within QRS complex.
- *PR interval:* If the P wave precedes the QRS complex, the PR interval is shortened (less than 0.12 second); otherwise, it can't be measured.
- *QRS complex:* Duration is usually within normal limits; configuration is usually normal.
- *T wave:* Usually normal configuration.
- *QT interval:* Usually within normal limits.
- *Other:* None.

SIGNS AND SYMPTOMS

A patient with a junctional escape rhythm will have a slow, regular pulse rate of 40 to 60 beats/minute. The patient may be asymptomatic. However, pulse rates under 60 beats/minute may lead to inadequate cardiac output, causing hypotension, syncope, or blurred vision.

INTERVENTIONS

Treatment for a junctional escape rhythm involves identification and correction of the underlying cause, whenever possible. If the patient is symptomatic, atropine may be used to increase the heart rate, or a temporary (transcutaneous or transvenous) or permanent pacemaker may be inserted. Because junctional escape rhythm can prevent ventricular standstill, it should never be suppressed.

RECOGNIZING ACCELERATED JUNCTIONAL RHYTHM

The following rhythm strip illustrates accelerated junctional rhythm. Look for these distinguishing characteristics.

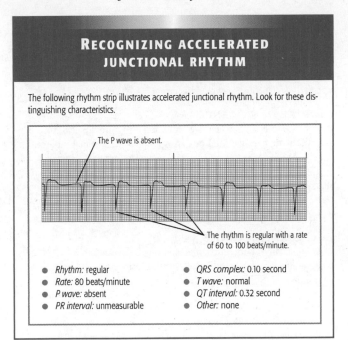

The P wave is absent.

The rhythm is regular with a rate of 60 to 100 beats/minute.

- *Rhythm:* regular
- *Rate:* 80 beats/minute
- *P wave:* absent
- *PR interval:* unmeasurable
- *QRS complex:* 0.10 second
- *T wave:* normal
- *QT interval:* 0.32 second
- *Other:* none

Monitor the patient's serum digoxin and electrolyte levels, and watch for signs of decreased cardiac output, such as hypotension, syncope, and blurred vision.

Accelerated junctional rhythm

An accelerated junctional rhythm is an arrhythmia that originates in the atrioventricular (AV) junction and is usually caused by enhanced automaticity of the AV junctional tissue. It's called accelerated because it occurs at a rate of 60 to 100 beats/minute, exceeding the inherent junctional escape rate of 40 to 60 beats/minute.

Because the rate is below 100 beats/minute, the arrhythmia isn't classified as junctional tachycardia. The atria are depolarized by means of retrograde conduction, and the ventricles are depolarized normally. (See *Recognizing accelerated junctional rhythm*.)

CAUSES

Digoxin toxicity is a common cause of accelerated junctional rhythm. Other causes include:

■ electrolyte disturbances

- valvular heart disease
- rheumatic heart disease
- heart failure
- myocarditis
- cardiac surgery
- inferior- or posterior-wall myocardial infarction.

CLINICAL SIGNIFICANCE

Patients experiencing accelerated junctional rhythm are generally asymptomatic because the rate corresponds to the normal inherent firing rate of the sinoatrial node (60 to 100 beats/minute). However, symptoms of decreased cardiac output, including hypotension and syncope, can occur if atrial depolarization occurs after or simultaneously with ventricular depolarization, which causes the subsequent loss of atrial kick.

ECG CHARACTERISTICS

- *Rhythm:* Atrial and ventricular rhythms are regular.
- *Rate:* Atrial and ventricular rates range from 60 to 100 beats/minute.
- *P wave:* If the P wave is present, it will be inverted in leads II, III, and aV_F. It may precede, follow, or be hidden in the QRS complex.
- *PR interval:* If the P wave occurs before the QRS complex, the PR interval is shortened (less than 0.12 second). Otherwise, it can't be measured.
- *QRS complex:* Duration is usually within normal limits. Configuration is usually normal.
- *T wave:* Usually within normal limits.
- *QT interval:* Usually within normal limits.
- *Other:* None.

SIGNS AND SYMPTOMS

The pulse rate will be normal with a regular rhythm. The patient may be asymptomatic because accelerated junctional rhythm has the same rate as sinus rhythm. However, if cardiac output is decreased, the patient may exhibit symptoms, such as hypotension, changes in mental status, and weak peripheral pulses.

INTERVENTIONS

Treatment for accelerated junctional rhythm involves identifying and correcting the underlying cause. Assessing the patient for signs and symptoms related to decreased cardiac output and hemodynamic instability is key, as is monitoring serum digoxin and electrolyte levels.

RECOGNIZING JUNCTIONAL TACHYCARDIA

The following rhythm strip illustrates junctional tachycardia. Look for these distinguishing characteristics.

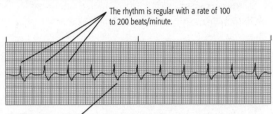

The rhythm is regular with a rate of 100 to 200 beats/minute.

The P wave is inverted.

- *Rhythm:* regular atrial and ventricular rhythms
- *Rate:* atrial and ventricular rates of 115 beats/minute
- *P wave:* inverted; follows QRS complex

- *PR interval:* unmeasurable
- *QRS complex:* 0.08 second
- *T wave:* normal
- *QT interval:* 0.36 second
- *Other:* none

Junctional tachycardia

In junctional tachycardia, three or more premature junctional contractions (PJCs) occur in a row. This supraventricular tachycardia generally occurs as a result of enhanced automaticity of the atrioventricular (AV) junction, which causes the AV junction to override the sinoatrial node as the dominant pacemaker.

In junctional tachycardia, the atria are depolarized by retrograde conduction. Conduction through the ventricles is normal. (See *Recognizing junctional tachycardia*.)

CAUSES

Digoxin toxicity is the most common cause of junctional tachycardia. In such cases, the arrhythmia can be aggravated by hypokalemia. Other causes of junctional tachycardia include:

- inferior- or posterior-wall infarction or ischemia
- inflammation of the AV junction after heart surgery
- heart failure

- electrolyte imbalances
- valvular heart disease.

CLINICAL SIGNIFICANCE

The clinical significance of junctional tachycardia depends on the rate and underlying cause. At higher ventricular rates, junctional tachycardia may reduce cardiac output by decreasing ventricular filling time. A loss of atrial kick also occurs with atrial depolarization that follows or occurs simultaneously with ventricular depolarization.

ECG CHARACTERISTICS

- *Rhythm:* Atrial and ventricular rhythms are usually regular. The atrial rhythm may be difficult to determine if the P wave is hidden in the QRS complex or preceding T wave.
- *Rate:* Atrial and ventricular rates exceed 100 beats/minute (usually between 100 and 200 beats/minute). The atrial rate may be difficult to determine if the P wave is hidden in the QRS complex or the preceding T wave.
- *P wave:* The P wave is usually inverted in leads II, III, and aV$_F$. It may occur before or after the QRS complex or be hidden in the QRS complex.
- *PR interval:* If the P wave precedes the QRS complex, the PR interval is shortened (less than 0.12 second); otherwise, the PR interval can't be measured.
- *QRS complex:* Duration is within normal limits; configuration is usually normal.
- *T wave:* Configuration is usually normal but may be abnormal if the P wave is hidden in the T wave. The fast rate may make T waves indiscernible.
- *QT interval:* Usually within normal limits.
- *Other:* None.

SIGNS AND SYMPTOMS

The patient's pulse rate will be above 100 beats/minute and have a regular rhythm. Patients with a rapid heart rate may experience signs and symptoms of decreased cardiac output and hemodynamic instability including hypotension.

INTERVENTIONS

The underlying cause should be identified and treated. If the cause is digoxin toxicity, the drug should be discontinued. In some cases of digoxin toxicity, a digoxin-binding drug may be used to reduce serum digoxin levels. Vagal maneuvers and drugs, such as adenosine, may slow the heart rate for symptomatic patients. Patients with recurrent junctional tachycardia may be treated with ablation therapy, followed by permanent pacemaker insertion.

Monitor patients with junctional tachycardia for signs of decreased cardiac output. In addition, check digoxin and potassium levels, and administer potassium supplements as ordered.

VENTRICULAR ARRHYTHMIAS

Ventricular arrhythmias originate in the ventricles below the bifurcation of the bundle of His. These arrhythmias occur when electrical impulses depolarize the myocardium using a different pathway from normal impulse conduction.

Ventricular arrhythmias appear on an ECG in characteristic ways. The QRS complex in most of these arrhythmias is wider than normal because of the prolonged conduction time through, and abnormal depolarization of, the ventricles. The deflections of the T wave and the QRS complex are in opposite directions because ventricular repolarization, as well as ventricular depolarization, is abnormal. The P wave in many ventricular arrhythmias is absent because atrial depolarization doesn't occur. If the P wave does occur, it usually doesn't have any relationship to the QRS complex.

When electrical impulses come from the ventricles instead of the atria, atrial kick is lost and cardiac output can decrease by as much as 30%. This is one reason why patients with ventricular arrhythmias may show signs and symptoms of heart failure, including hypotension, angina, syncope, and respiratory distress.

Although ventricular arrhythmias may be benign, they're generally considered the most serious arrhythmias, because the ventricles are ultimately responsible for cardiac output. Rapid recognition and treatment of ventricular arrhythmias increase the chances of successful resuscitation.

Premature ventricular contractions

Premature ventricular contractions (PVCs) are ectopic beats that originate in the ventricles and occur earlier than expected. PVCs may occur in healthy people without being clinically significant.

When PVCs occur in patients with underlying heart disease, however, they may herald the development of lethal ventricular arrhythmias, including ventricular tachycardia (VT) and ventricular fibrillation (VF).

RECOGNIZING PVCs

The following rhythm strip illustrates premature ventricular contraction (PVC) on beats 1, 6, and 11. Look for these distinguishing characteristics.

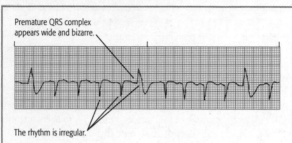

Premature QRS complex appears wide and bizarre.

The rhythm is irregular.

- *Rhythm:* irregular
- *Rate:* 120 beats/minute
- *P wave:* absent with PVC, but present with other QRS complexes
- *PR interval:* 0.12 second in underlying rhythm
- *QRS complex:* early with bizarre configuration and duration of 0.14 second in PVC; 0.08 second in underlying rhythm
- *T wave:* normal; opposite direction from QRS complex with PVC
- *QT interval:* 0.28 second with underlying rhythm
- *Other:* underlying rhythm sinus tachycardia

PVCs may occur singly, in pairs (couplets), or in clusters. PVCs may also appear in patterns, such as bigeminy or trigeminy. (See *Recognizing PVCs.*)

In many cases, PVCs are followed by a compensatory pause. (See *Compensatory pause.*) PVCs may be uniform in appearance, arising from a single ectopic ventricular pacemaker site, or multiform, originating from different sites or originating from a single pacemaker site but having QRS complexes that differ in size, shape, and direction.

PVCs may also be described as unifocal or multifocal. Unifocal PVCs originate from the same ventricular ectopic pacemaker site, whereas multifocal PVCs originate from different ectopic pacemaker sites in the ventricles.

CAUSES

PVCs are usually caused by enhanced automaticity in the ventricular conduction system or muscle tissue. The irritable focus results from a

COMPENSATORY PAUSE

You can determine if a compensatory pause exists by using calipers to mark off two normal P-P intervals. Place one leg of the calipers on the sinus P wave that comes just before the premature ventricular contraction. If the pause is compensatory, the other leg of the calipers will fall precisely on the P wave that comes after the pause.

disruption of the normal electrolyte shifts during cellular depolarization and repolarization. Possible causes of PVCs include:

- anesthetics
- electrolyte imbalances, such as hypokalemia, hyperkalemia, hypomagnesemia, and hypocalcemia
- enlargement or hypertrophy of the ventricular chambers
- hypoxia
- increased sympathetic stimulation
- infection
- irritation of the ventricles by pacemaker electrodes or a pulmonary artery catheter
- metabolic acidosis
- mitral valve prolapse
- myocardial ischemia and infarction
- myocarditis
- sympathomimetic drugs, such as epinephrine and isoproterenol (Isuprel)
- tobacco use
- caffeine or alcohol ingestion
- drug intoxication, particularly with cocaine, amphetamines, digoxin (Lanoxin), phenothiazines, and tricyclic antidepressants.

CLINICAL SIGNIFICANCE

PVCs are significant for two reasons. First, they can lead to more serious arrhythmias, such as VT or VF. The risk of developing a more serious arrhythmia increases in patients with ischemic or damaged hearts.

PVCs also decrease cardiac output, especially if ectopic beats are frequent or sustained. The decrease in cardiac output with a PVC stems from reduced ventricular diastolic filling time and the loss of atrial kick for that beat. The clinical impact of PVCs hinges on the body's ability to maintain adequate perfusion and the duration of the abnormal rhythm.

PATTERNS OF POTENTIALLY DANGEROUS PVCs

Some premature ventricular contractions (PVCs) are more dangerous than others. Here are examples of patterns of potentially dangerous PVCs.

Paired PVCs

Two PVCs in a row, called *paired PVCs* or a *ventricular couplet* (see shaded areas), can produce ventricular tachycardia (VT). That's because the second contraction usually meets refractory tissue. A burst, or a salvo, of three or more PVCs in a row is considered a run of VT.

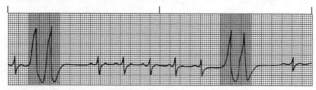

Multiform PVCs

Multiform PVCs, which look different from one another, arise from different sites or from the same site with abnormal conduction (see shaded areas). Multiform PVCs may indicate severe heart disease or digoxin toxicity.

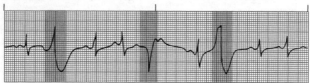

To help determine the seriousness of PVCs, ask these questions:
- How often do they occur? In patients with chronic PVCs, an increase in frequency or a change in the pattern of PVCs from the baseline rhythm may signal a more serious condition.
- What's the pattern of PVCs? If the ECG shows a dangerous pattern—such as paired PVCs, PVCs with more than one focus, a bigeminal rhythm, or R-on-T phenomenon (when a PVC strikes on the down slope of the preceding normal T wave)—the patient may require immediate treatment. (See *Patterns of potentially dangerous PVCs.*)
- Are they really PVCs? Make sure the complex is a PVC, not another, less dangerous arrhythmia. PVCs may be mistaken for ventricular escape beats or normal impulses with aberrant ventricular con-

Bigeminy and trigeminy

PVCs that occur every other beat (bigeminy) or every third beat (trigeminy) may indicate increased ventricular irritability, which can result in VT or ventricular fibrillation (see shaded areas). The rhythm strip shown below illustrates ventricular bigeminy.

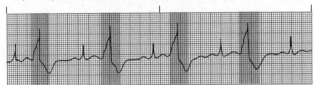

R-on-T phenomenon

In R-on-T phenomenon, a PVC occurs so early that it falls on the T wave of the preceding beat (see shaded area). Because the cells haven't fully repolarized, VT or ventricular fibrillation can result.

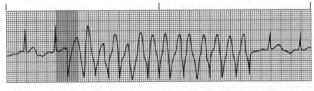

duction. Ventricular escape beats serve as a safety mechanism to protect the heart from ventricular standstill. Some supraventricular impulses may follow an abnormal (aberrant) conduction pathway causing an abnormal appearance to the QRS complex. In any event, never delay treatment if the patient is unstable.

ECG CHARACTERISTICS

- *Rhythm:* Atrial and ventricular rhythms are irregular during PVCs; the underlying rhythm may be regular.
- *Rate:* Atrial and ventricular rates reflect the underlying rhythm.
- *P wave:* Usually absent in the ectopic beat, but with retrograde conduction to the atria, the P wave may appear after the QRS complex. It's usually normal if present in the underlying rhythm.
- *PR interval:* Not measurable except in the underlying rhythm.

- *QRS complex:* Occurrence is earlier than expected. Duration exceeds 0.12 second, with a bizarre and wide configuration. Configuration of the QRS complex is usually normal in the underlying rhythm.
- *T wave:* Occurrence is in opposite direction to QRS complex. When a PVC strikes on the down slope of the preceding normal T wave—the R-on-T phenomenon—it can trigger more serious rhythm disturbances such as ventricular fibrillation.
- *QT interval:* Not usually measured, except in the underlying rhythm.
- *Other:* A PVC may be followed by a compensatory pause, which can be full or incomplete. The sum of a full compensatory pause and the preceding R-R interval is equal to the sum of two R-R intervals of the underlying rhythm. If the sinoatrial (SA) node is depolarized by the PVC, the timing of the SA node is reset, and the compensatory pause is called incomplete. In this case, the sum of an incomplete compensatory pause and the preceding R-R interval is less than the sum of two R-R intervals of the underlying rhythm. A PVC occurring between two normally conducted QRS complexes without greatly disturbing the underlying rhythm is referred to as interpolated. A full compensatory pause, usually accompanying PVCs, is absent with interpolated PVCs.

Sometimes it's difficult to distinguish PVCs from aberrant ventricular conduction.

SIGNS AND SYMPTOMS

The patient experiencing PVCs usually has a normal pulse rate with a momentarily irregular pulse rhythm when a PVC occurs.

With PVCs, the patient will have a weaker pulse wave after the premature beat and a longer-than-normal pause between pulse waves. If the carotid pulse is visible, however, you may see a weaker arterial wave after the premature beat. When auscultating for heart sounds, you'll hear an abnormally early heart sound with each PVC.

A patient with PVCs may be asymptomatic; however, patients with frequent PVCs may complain of palpitations. The patient may also exhibit signs and symptoms of decreased cardiac output, including hypotension and syncope.

INTERVENTIONS

If the PVCs are infrequent and the patient has normal heart function and is asymptomatic, the arrhythmia probably won't require treatment. If symptoms or a dangerous form of PVCs occur, the type of treatment given will depend on the cause of the problem. If PVCs have a purely cardiac origin, drugs to suppress ventricular irritability, such as procainamide (Procan SR), amiodarone (Cardarone), or lidocaine, may be used. When PVCs have a noncardiac origin, treatment is aimed at correcting the cause. For example, drug therapy may be adjusted because of the patient's acidosis, or an electrolyte imbalance may be corrected.

Patients who have recently developed PVCs need prompt assessment, especially if they have underlying heart disease or complex medical problems. Patients with chronic PVCs should be closely observed for the development of more frequent PVCs or more dangerous PVC patterns.

Until effective treatment is begun, patients with PVCs accompanied by serious symptoms should have continuous ECG monitoring and ambulate only with assistance. If the patient is discharged on antiarrhythmic medications, family members should know how to contact the emergency medical system and perform cardiopulmonary resuscitation.

Idioventricular rhythm

Idioventricular rhythm, also referred to as *ventricular escape rhythm,* originates in an escape pacemaker site in the ventricles. The inherent firing rate of this ectopic pacemaker is usually 20 to 40 beats/minute. The rhythm acts as a safety mechanism by preventing ventricular standstill, or asystole—the absence of electrical activity in the ventricles. When fewer than three QRS complexes arising from the escape pacemaker occur, they're called ventricular escape beats or complexes. (See *Recognizing idioventricular rhythm,* page 300.)

When the rate of an ectopic pacemaker site in the ventricles is less than 100 beats/minute but exceeds the inherent ventricular escape rate of 20 to 40 beats/minute, it's called accelerated idioventricular rhythm (AIVR). (See *Recognizing AIVR,* page 301.) The rate of AIVR isn't fast enough to be considered ventricular tachycardia. The rhythm is usually related to enhanced automaticity of the ventricular tissue. AIVR and idioventricular rhythm share the same ECG characteristics, differing only in heart rate.

CAUSES

Idioventricular rhythms occur when all of the heart's higher pacemakers fail to function or when supraventricular impulses can't reach the ventricles because of a block in the conduction system. Idioventricular

RECOGNIZING IDIOVENTRICULAR RHYTHM

The following rhythm strip illustrates idioventricular rhythm. Look for these distinguishing characteristics.

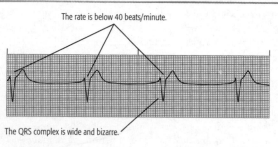

The rate is below 40 beats/minute.

The QRS complex is wide and bizarre.

- *Rhythm:* regular
- *Rate:* unable to determine atrial rate; ventricular rate of 35 beats/minute
- *P wave:* absent
- *PR interval:* unmeasurable
- *QRS complex:* wide and bizarre
- *T wave:* deflection opposite QRS complex
- *QT interval:* 0.60 second
- *Other:* none

rhythms may accompany third-degree heart block. Possible causes of the rhythm include:

- myocardial ischemia
- myocardial infarction
- digoxin toxicity, beta-adrenergic receptor blockers, calcium channel blockers, and tricyclic antidepressants
- pacemaker failure
- metabolic imbalances
- sick sinus syndrome
- successful reperfusion therapy.

CLINICAL SIGNIFICANCE

Idioventricular rhythm may be transient or continuous. Transient ventricular escape rhythm is usually related to increased parasympathetic effect on the higher pacemaker sites and isn't generally clinically significant. Although idioventricular rhythms act to protect the heart

RECOGNIZING AIVR

An accelerated idioventricular rhythm (AIVR) has the same characteristics as an idioventricular rhythm except that it's faster. The rate shown here varies between 40 and 100 beats/minute.

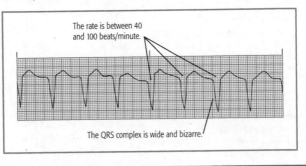

The rate is between 40 and 100 beats/minute.

The QRS complex is wide and bizarre.

from ventricular standstill, a continuous idioventricular rhythm presents a clinically serious situation.

The slow ventricular rate of this arrhythmia and the associated loss of atrial kick markedly reduce cardiac output. If not rapidly identified and appropriately managed, idioventricular arrhythmias can cause death.

ECG CHARACTERISTICS

- *Rhythm:* Usually, atrial rhythm can't be determined. Ventricular rhythm is usually regular.
- *Rate:* Usually, atrial rate can't be determined. Ventricular rate is 20 to 40 beats/minute.
- *P wave:* Absent.
- *PR interval:* Not measurable because of the absent P wave.
- *QRS complex:* Because of abnormal ventricular depolarization, the QRS complex has a duration longer than 0.12 second, with a wide and bizarre configuration.
- *T wave:* The T wave is abnormal. Deflection usually occurs in the opposite direction from that of the QRS complex.
- *QT interval:* Usually prolonged.
- *Other:* Idioventricular rhythm commonly occurs with third-degree atrioventricular block.

TRANSCUTANEOUS PACEMAKER

Transcutaneous pacing, also referred to as *external pacing* or *noninvasive pacing*, involves the delivery of electrical impulses through externally applied cutaneous electrodes. The electrical impulses are conducted through an intact chest wall using skin electrodes placed either in anterior-posterior or sternal-apex positions. (An anterior-posterior placement is shown here.)

Transcutaneous pacing is the initial pacing method of choice in emergency situations because it's the least invasive technique and can be instituted quickly.

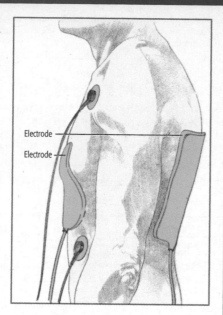

Electrode

Electrode

SIGNS AND SYMPTOMS
The patient with continuous idioventricular rhythm is generally symptomatic because of the marked reduction in cardiac output that occurs with the arrhythmia. Blood pressure may be difficult or impossible to auscultate or palpate. The patient may experience dizziness, lightheadedness, syncope, or loss of consciousness.

INTERVENTIONS
Treatment should be initiated immediately to increase the patient's heart rate, improve cardiac output, and establish a normal rhythm. Atropine may be administered to increase the heart rate.

If atropine isn't effective or if the patient develops hypotension or other signs of clinical instability, a pacemaker may be needed to reestablish a heart rate that provides enough cardiac output to perfuse organs properly. A transcutaneous pacemaker may be used in an emergency until a temporary or transvenous pacemaker can be inserted. (See *Transcutaneous pacemaker.*)

Remember that the goal of treatment doesn't include suppressing the idioventricular rhythm because it acts as a safety mechanism to protect the heart from ventricular standstill. Idioventricular rhythm should never be treated with lidocaine or other antiarrhythmics that would suppress the escape beats.

Patients with idioventricular rhythm need continuous ECG monitoring and constant assessment until treatment restores hemodynamic stability. Keep atropine and pacemaker equipment available at the bedside. Enforce bed rest until an effective heart rate has been maintained and the patient is clinically stable.

Be sure to tell the patient and his family about the serious nature of this arrhythmia and the treatment it requires. If the patient needs a permanent pacemaker, teach the patient and family how it works, how to recognize problems, when to contact the practitioner, and how pacemaker function will be monitored.

Ventricular tachycardia

Ventricular tachycardia (VT), also called *V-tach,* occurs when three or more premature ventricular contractions (PVCs) strike in a row and the ventricular rate exceeds 100 beats/minute. This life-threatening arrhythmia may precede ventricular fibrillation and sudden cardiac death, especially in patients who aren't in a health care facility.

VT is an extremely unstable rhythm and may be sustained or non-sustained. When it occurs in short, paroxysmal bursts lasting less than 30 seconds and causing few or no symptoms, it's called non-sustained. When the rhythm is sustained, however, it requires immediate treatment to prevent death, even in patients initially able to maintain adequate cardiac output. (See *Recognizing ventricular tachycardia,* page 304.)

CAUSES

This arrhythmia usually results from increased myocardial irritability, which may be triggered by enhanced automaticity, reentry within the Purkinje system, or by PVCs occurring during the downstroke of the preceding T wave.

Other causes of VT include:
- myocardial ischemia
- myocardial infarction
- coronary artery disease
- valvular heart disease

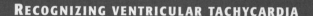

RECOGNIZING VENTRICULAR TACHYCARDIA

The following rhythm strip illustrates ventricular tachycardia. Look for these distinguishing characteristics.

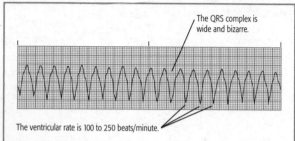

The QRS complex is wide and bizarre.

The ventricular rate is 100 to 250 beats/minute.

- *Rhythm:* regular
- *Rate:* 187 beats/minute
- *P wave:* absent
- *PR interval:* unmeasurable
- *QRS complex:* 0.24 second; wide and bizarre

- *T wave:* opposite direction of QRS complex
- *QT interval:* unmeasurable
- *Other:* none

- heart failure
- cardiomyopathy
- electrolyte imbalances such as hypokalemia
- drug intoxication from digoxin (Lanoxin), procainamide, quinidine (Quinora), or cocaine
- proarrhythmic effects of some antiarrhythmics.

CLINICAL SIGNIFICANCE

VT is significant because of its unpredictability and potential for causing death. A patient may be hemodynamically stable, with a normal pulse and blood pressure; clinically unstable, with hypotension and poor peripheral pulses; or unconscious, without respirations or pulse.

Because of the reduced ventricular filling time and the drop in cardiac output that occurs with this arrhythmia, the patient's condition can quickly deteriorate to ventricular fibrillation (VF) and complete cardiovascular collapse.

ECG CHARACTERISTICS

- *Rhythm:* Atrial rhythm can't be determined. Ventricular rhythm is usually regular but may be slightly irregular.
- *Rate:* Atrial rate can't be determined. Ventricular rate is usually rapid (100 to 250 beats/minute).
- *P wave:* The P wave is usually absent. It may be obscured by the QRS complex; P waves are dissociated from the QRS complexes. Retrograde P waves may be present.
- *PR interval:* Not measurable because the P wave can't be seen in most cases.
- *QRS complex:* Duration is greater than 0.12 second; it usually has a bizarre appearance with increased amplitude. QRS complexes in monomorphic VT have a uniform shape. In polymorphic VT, the shape of the QRS complex constantly changes.
- *T wave:* If the T wave is visible, it occurs in the opposite direction of the QRS complex.
- *QT interval:* Not measurable.
- *Other:* Ventricular flutter and torsades de pointes are two variations of this arrhythmia. Torsades de pointes is a special variation of polymorphic VT. (See *Torsades de pointes,* page 306.)

SIGNS AND SYMPTOMS

Although some patients have only minor symptoms initially, they still require rapid intervention to prevent cardiovascular collapse. Most patients with VT have weak or absent pulses. Low cardiac output will cause hypotension and a decreased level of consciousness (LOC), quickly leading to unresponsiveness if left untreated. VT may prompt angina, heart failure, or a substantial decrease in organ perfusion.

INTERVENTIONS

Treatment depends on the patient's clinical status. Is the patient conscious? Does the patient have spontaneous respirations? Is a palpable carotid pulse present?

Patients with pulseless VT are treated the same as those with VF and require immediate defibrillation and cardiopulmonary resuscitation (CPR). Treatment for patients with a detectable pulse depends on whether they're unstable or stable.

Unstable patients generally have ventricular rates greater than 150 beats/minute and have serious signs and symptoms related to the tachycardia, which may include hypotension, shortness of breath, chest pain, or altered LOC. These patients are usually treated with immediate synchronized cardioversion.

TORSADES DE POINTES

Torsades de pointes, which means "twisting about the points," is a special form of polymorphic ventricular tachycardia. The hallmark characteristics of this rhythm, shown below, are QRS complexes that rotate about the baseline, deflecting downward and upward for several beats.

The rate is 150 to 250 beats/minute, usually with an irregular rhythm, and the QRS complexes are wide with changing amplitude. The P wave is usually absent.

Paroxysmal rhythm

This arrhythmia may be paroxysmal, starting and stopping suddenly, and may deteriorate into ventricular fibrillation. It should be considered when ventricular tachycardia doesn't respond to antiarrhythmic therapy or other treatments.

Reversible causes

The cause of this form of ventricular tachycardia is usually reversible. The most common causes are drugs that lengthen the QT interval, such as amiodarone (Cordarone), ibutilide (Covert), erythromycin (E-Mycin), haloperidol (Haldol), droperidol, and sotalol (Betapace). Other causes include myocardial ischemia and electrolyte abnormalities, such as hypokalemia, hypomagnesemia, and hypocalcemia.

Cause-based treatment

Torsades de pointes is treated by correcting the underlying cause, especially if the cause is related to specific drug therapy. The practitioner may order mechanical overdrive pacing, which overrides the ventricular rate and breaks the triggered mechanism for the arrhythmia. Magnesium sulfate may also be effective. Electrical cardioversion may be used when torsades de pointes doesn't respond to other treatment.

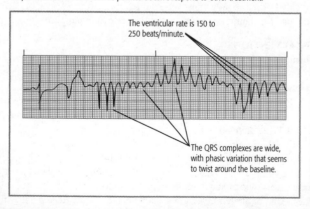

The ventricular rate is 150 to 250 beats/minute.

The QRS complexes are wide, with phasic variation that seems to twist around the baseline.

A clinically stable patient with VT and no signs of heart failure is treated differently.

Treatment for these patients is determined by whether the rhythm is regular or irregular. If the rhythm is regular (monomorphic), the patient is treated with amiodarone and possible synchronized cardioversion. If the rate is irregular (polymorphic), look at the length of the T interval when the rhythm is in sinus rhythm. If the QT interval is long, the polymorphic rhythm is most likely torsades de pointes. The treatment for polymorphic VT is to stop medications that may cause a long QT, correct electrolyte imbalances, and administer antiarrhythmics, such as magnesium or amiodarone. If at any point the patient becomes clinically unstable, immediate synchronized cardioversion is the best treatment. For the complete ACLS algorithms, see pages 332 and 333.

Patients with VT or VF not from a transient or reversible cause may need an implanted cardioverter-defibrillator (ICD). This device is a permanent solution to recurrent episodes of VT.

A 12-lead ECG and all other available clinical information is critical for establishing a specific diagnosis in a stable patient with wide QRS complex tachycardia of unknown type but regular rate. If a definitive diagnosis of SVT or VT can't be established, use amiodarone to control the rate and elective synchronized cardioversion.

Be sure to teach patients and families about the serious nature of this arrhythmia and the need for prompt treatment. If your stable patient is undergoing electrical cardioversion, inform him that he'll be given a sedative, and possibly an analgesic, prior to the procedure.

If a patient will be discharged with an ICD or a prescription for long-term antiarrhythmics, make sure that family members know how to use the emergency medical system and how to perform CPR.

Ventricular fibrillation

Ventricular fibrillation, commonly called *V-fib* or *VF*, is characterized by a chaotic, disorganized pattern of electrical activity. The pattern arises from electrical impulses coming from multiple ectopic pacemakers in the ventricles.

The arrhythmia produces no effective ventricular mechanical activity or contractions and no cardiac output. Untreated VF is the most common cause of sudden cardiac death in people outside of a health care facility. (See *Recognizing ventricular fibrillation,* page 308.)

CAUSES

Causes of VF include:

RECOGNIZING VENTRICULAR FIBRILLATION

The following rhythm strips illustrate coarse ventricular fibrillation (first strip) and fine ventricular fibrillation (second strip). Look for these distinguishing characteristics.

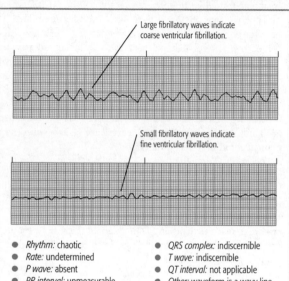

Large fibrillatory waves indicate coarse ventricular fibrillation.

Small fibrillatory waves indicate fine ventricular fibrillation.

- *Rhythm:* chaotic
- *Rate:* undetermined
- *P wave:* absent
- *PR interval:* unmeasurable

- *QRS complex:* indiscernible
- *T wave:* indiscernible
- *QT interval:* not applicable
- *Other:* waveform is a wavy line

- coronary artery disease
- myocardial ischemia
- myocardial infarction
- untreated ventricular tachycardia
- underlying heart disease such as dilated cardiomyopathy
- acid-base imbalance
- electric shock
- severe hypothermia
- drug toxicity, including digoxin, quinidine, and procainamide
- electrolyte imbalances, such as hypokalemia, hyperkalemia, and hypercalcemia
- environmental.

CLINICAL SIGNIFICANCE

With VF, the ventricular muscle quivers, replacing effective muscular contraction with completely ineffective contraction. Cardiac output falls to zero and, if allowed to continue, leads to ventricular standstill and death.

ECG CHARACTERISTICS

- *Rhythm:* Atrial rhythm can't be determined. Ventricular rhythm has no pattern or regularity. Ventricular electrical activity appears as fibrillatory waves with no recognizable pattern.
- *Rate:* Atrial and ventricular rates can't be determined.
- *P wave:* Can't be determined.
- *PR interval:* Can't be determined.
- *QRS complex:* Duration can't be determined.
- *T wave:* Can't be determined.
- *QT interval:* Not applicable.
- *Other:* Coarse fibrillatory waves are generally associated with greater chances of successful electrical defibrillation than smaller amplitude waves. Fibrillatory waves become finer as hypoxemia and acidosis progress, making the VF more resistant to defibrillation.

SIGNS AND SYMPTOMS

The patient in VF is in full cardiac arrest, unresponsive, and without a detectable blood pressure or central pulses. Whenever you see an ECG pattern resembling VF, check the patient immediately and initiate definitive treatment.

INTERVENTIONS

When faced with a rhythm that appears to be VF, always assess the patient first. Other events can mimic VF on an ECG strip, including interference from an electric razor, shivering, or seizure activity.

Immediate defibrillation and cardiopulmonary resuscitation (CPR) are the most effective treatments for VF. CPR must be performed until the defibrillator arrives to preserve oxygen supply to the brain and other vital organs. Drugs such as epinephrine and vasopressin (Pitressin) may be used for persistent VF if the first two attempts at electrical defibrillation fail to correct the arrhythmia. Antiarrhythmic agents, such as amiodarone, lidocaine, and magnesium, may also be considered. For the complete ACLS algorithm, see pages 330 and 331.

In defibrillation, two electrode pads are applied to the chest wall. Current is then directed through the pads and, subsequently, the patient's chest and heart. The current causes the myocardium to completely depolarize, which, in turn, encourages the sinoatrial node to resume normal control of the heart's electrical activity.

One electrode pad is placed to the right of the upper sternum, and one is placed over the fifth or sixth intercostal space at the left anterior axillary line. During cardiac surgery, internal paddles are placed directly on the myocardium.

Automated external defibrillators (AEDs) are increasingly being used, especially in the out-of-hospital setting, to provide early defibrillation. After a patient is confirmed to be unresponsive, breathless, and pulseless, the AED power is turned on and the electrode pads and cables attached. The AED can analyze the patient's cardiac rhythm and provide the caregiver with step-by-step instructions on how to proceed. These defibrillators can be used by people without medical experience as long as they're trained in the proper use of the device.

For the patient in VF, successful resuscitation requires rapid recognition of the problem and prompt defibrillation. Many health care facilities and emergency medical systems have established protocols so that health care workers can initiate prompt treatment. Make sure you know the location of your facility's emergency equipment and that you know how to use it.

You'll also need to teach the patient and family how to use the emergency medical system following discharge from the facility. Family members may need instruction in CPR and in how to use the AED. Teach them about long-term therapies that help prevent recurrent episodes of VF, including antiarrhythmic drug therapy and implantable cardioverter-defibrillators.

Asystole

Ventricular asystole, also called *asystole* and *ventricular standstill,* is the absence of discernible electrical activity in the ventricles. Although some electrical activity may be evident in the atria, these impulses aren't conducted to the ventricles. (See *Recognizing asystole.*)

Asystole usually results from a prolonged period of cardiac arrest without effective resuscitation. It's important to distinguish asystole from fine ventricular fibrillation, which is managed differently. Therefore, asystole must be confirmed in more than one ECG lead.

CAUSES

Possible reversible causes of asystole include:

- hypovolemia
- myocardial infarction (coronary thrombosis)

RECOGNIZING ASYSTOLE

The following rhythm strip illustrates asystole, the absence of electrical activity in the ventricles. Except for a few P waves or pacer spikes, nothing appears on the waveform, and the line is almost flat.

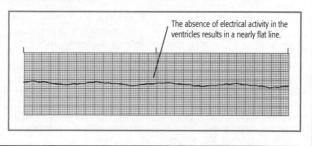

The absence of electrical activity in the ventricles results in a nearly flat line.

- severe electrolyte disturbances, especially hyperkalemia and hypo-kalemia
- massive pulmonary embolism
- hypoxia
- severe, uncorrected acid-base disturbances, especially metabolic acidosis
- drug overdose
- hypothermia
- cardiac tamponade
- tension pneumothorax.

CLINICAL SIGNIFICANCE

Without ventricular electrical activity, ventricular contractions can't occur. As a result, cardiac output drops to zero, and vital organs are no longer perfused. Asystole has been called the arrhythmia of death and is typically considered to be a confirmation of death, rather than an arrhythmia to be treated.

The patient with asystole is completely unresponsive, without spontaneous respirations or pulse (cardiopulmonary arrest). Without immediate initiation of cardiopulmonary resuscitation (CPR) and rapid identification and treatment of the underlying cause, the condition quickly becomes irreversible.

PULSELESS ELECTRICAL ACTIVITY

Pulseless electrical activity (PEA) defines a group of arrhythmias characterized by the presence of some type of electrical activity without a detectable pulse. Although organized electrical depolarization occurs, no synchronous shortening of the myocardial fibers occurs. As a result, no mechanical activity or contractions take place.

Causes

The most common causes of PEA include hypovolemia, hypoxia, acidosis, tension pneumothorax, cardiac tamponade, massive pulmonary embolism, hypothermia, hyperkalemia and hypo-kalemia, massive acute myocardial infarction, and overdoses of drugs such as tricyclic antidepressants.

Treatment

Rapid identification and treatment of underlying reversible causes is critical for treating PEA. For example, hypovolemia is treated with volume expansion. Tension pneumothorax is treated with needle decompression.

Institute cardiopulmonary resuscitation, tracheal intubation, and I.V. administration of epinephrine or atropine.

ECG CHARACTERISTICS

- *Rhythm:* Atrial rhythm is usually indiscernible; no ventricular rhythm is present.
- *Rate:* Atrial rate is usually indiscernible; no ventricular rate is present.
- *P wave:* May be present.
- *PR interval:* Not measurable.
- *QRS complex:* Absent or occasional escape beats.
- *T wave:* Absent.
- *QT interval:* Not measurable.
- *Other:* On a rhythm strip, asystole looks like a nearly flat line (except for changes caused by chest compressions during CPR). In a patient with a pacemaker, pacer spikes may be evident on the strip, but no P wave or QRS complex occurs in response to the stimulus.

SIGNS AND SYMPTOMS

The patient will be unresponsive and have no spontaneous respirations, discernible pulse, or blood pressure.

INTERVENTIONS

Immediate treatment for asystole includes effective CPR and supplemental oxygen. Resuscitation should be attempted unless evidence exists that these efforts shouldn't be initiated, such as when a do-not-resuscitate order is in effect.

Remember to verify the presence of asystole by checking more than one ECG lead. Priority must also be given to searching for and treating identified potentially reversible causes, such as hypovolemia, cardiac tamponade, and tension pneumothorax. Early CPR is vital, and I.V. or intraosseous epinephrine or a one-time dose of vasopressin and atropine is given. For the complete ACLS algorithm, see pages 330 and 331.

Be aware that pulseless electrical activity can appear as any cardiac rhythm, including asystole. Know how to recognize this problem and treat it. (See *Pulseless electrical activity*.)

With persistent asystole (despite appropriate management), consider terminating resuscitation.

ATRIOVENTRICULAR BLOCKS

Atrioventricular (AV) heart block refers to an interruption or delay in the conduction of electrical impulses between the atria and the ventricles. The block can occur at the AV node, the bundle of His, or the bundle branches. When the site of the block is the bundle of His or the bundle branches, the block is referred to as infranodal AV block. AV block can be partial, where some or all of the P waves are conducted to the ventricle (first or second degree), or complete, where no P waves conduct to the ventricle (third degree).

The heart's electrical impulses normally originate in the sinoatrial node, so when those impulses are blocked at the AV node, atrial rates are usually normal (60 to 100 beats/minute). The clinical significance of the block depends on the number of impulses completely blocked and the resulting ventricular rate. A slow ventricular rate can decrease cardiac output and cause symptoms such as light-headedness, hypotension, and confusion.

Causes
A variety of factors may lead to AV block, including underlying heart conditions, use of certain drugs, congenital anomalies, and conditions that disrupt the cardiac conduction system.

Typical causes of AV block include:
■ myocardial ischemia, which impairs cellular function so that cells repolarize more slowly or incompletely. The injured cells, in turn,

may conduct impulses slowly or inconsistently. Relief of the ischemia may restore normal function to the AV node.

- myocardial infarction, in which cellular necrosis or death occurs. If the necrotic cells are part of the conduction system, they may no longer conduct impulses, and a permanent AV block occurs.

- excessive serum levels of, or an exaggerated response to, a drug. This response can cause AV block or increase the likelihood that a block will develop. The drugs may increase the refractory period of a portion of the conduction system. Although many antiarrhythmics can have this effect, the drugs more commonly known to cause or exacerbate AV blocks include digoxin (Lanoxin), amiodarone (Cordarone), beta-adrenergic receptor blockers, and calcium channel blockers.

- lesions, including calcium and fibrotic, along the conduction pathway.

- congenital anomalies such as congenital ventricular septal defects that involve cardiac structures and affect the conduction system. Anomalies of the conduction system, such as an AV node that doesn't conduct impulses, can also occur in the absence of structural defects.

AV block can also be caused by inadvertent damage to the heart's conduction system during surgery. Damage is most likely to occur in operations involving the aortic, mitral, or tricuspid valve or in the closure of a ventricular septal defect. If the injury involves tissues adjacent to the surgical site and the conduction system isn't physically disrupted, the block may be temporary. If a portion of the conduction system is severed, permanent block results.

Similar disruption of the conduction system can occur from a procedure called radiofrequency ablation. In this invasive procedure, a transvenous catheter is used to locate the area in the heart that participates in initiating or perpetuating certain tachyarrhythmias. Radiofrequency energy is then delivered to the myocardium through this catheter to produce a small area of necrosis at that spot. The damaged tissue can no longer cause or participate in the tachyarrhythmia. If the energy is delivered close to the AV node, bundle of His, or bundle branches, however, AV block can result, and the patient may need a permanent pacemaker.

Classification of atrioventricular block

Atrioventricular (AV) blocks are classified according to the site of block and the severity of the conduction abnormality. The sites of AV block include the AV node, bundle of His, and bundle branches.

Severity of AV block is classified in degrees: first-degree AV block; second-degree AV block, type I (Wenckebach or Mobitz I); second-degree AV block, type II (Mobitz II) AV block; and third-degree (complete) AV block. The classification system for AV blocks aids in the determination of the patient's treatment and prognosis.

First-degree atrioventricular block

First-degree atrioventricular (AV) block occurs when there's a delay in the conduction of electrical impulses from the atria to the ventricles. This delay usually occurs at the level of the AV node, or bundle of His. First-degree AV block is characterized by a PR interval greater than 0.20 second. This interval remains constant beat to beat. After the impulse is slowed down, it is then conducted through the normal conduction pathway.

CAUSES

First-degree AV block may result from:

■ myocardial ischemia or myocardial infarction (MI)
■ myocarditis
■ hyperkalemia
■ rheumatic fever
■ degenerative changes in the heart associated with aging.

The condition may also be caused by such drugs as digoxin (Lanoxin), calcium channel blockers, and beta-adrenergic receptor blockers.

CLINICAL SIGNIFICANCE

First-degree AV block may cause no symptoms in a healthy person. The arrhythmia may be transient, especially if it occurs secondary to drugs or ischemia early in the course of an MI. The presence of first-degree block, the least dangerous type of AV block, indicates a delay in the conduction of electrical impulses through the normal conduction pathway. In general, a rhythm strip with this block looks like normal sinus rhythm except that the PR interval is longer than normal.

RECOGNIZING FIRST-DEGREE AV BLOCK

The following rhythm strip illustrates first-degree atrioventricular (AV) block. Look for these distinguishing characteristics.

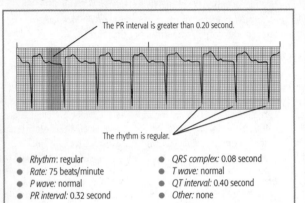

The PR interval is greater than 0.20 second.

The rhythm is regular.

- *Rhythm:* regular
- *Rate:* 75 beats/minute
- *P wave:* normal
- *PR interval:* 0.32 second
- *QRS complex:* 0.08 second
- *T wave:* normal
- *QT interval:* 0.40 second
- *Other:* none

Because first-degree AV block can progress to a more severe type of AV block, the patient's cardiac rhythm should be monitored for changes. (See *Recognizing first-degree AV block.*)

ECG CHARACTERISTICS

- *Rhythm:* Atrial and ventricular rhythms are regular.
- *Rate:* Atrial and ventricular rates are the same and within normal limits.
- *P wave:* Normal size and configuration; each P wave followed by a QRS complex.
- *PR interval:* Prolonged (greater than 0.20 second) but constant.
- *QRS complex:* Duration usually remains within normal limits if the conduction delay occurs in the AV node. If the QRS duration exceeds 0.12 second, the conduction delay may be in the His-Purkinje system.
- *T wave:* Normal size and configuration unless the QRS complex is prolonged.
- *QT interval:* Usually within normal limits.

■ *Other:* None.

SIGNS AND SYMPTOMS

The patient's pulse rate will usually be normal and the rhythm will be regular. Most patients with first-degree AV block are asymptomatic because cardiac output isn't significantly affected. If the PR interval is extremely long, a longer interval between S_1 and S_2 may be noted on cardiac auscultation.

INTERVENTIONS

Treatment generally focuses on identification and correction of the underlying cause. For example, if a drug is causing the AV block, the dosage may be reduced or the drug discontinued. Close monitoring can help detect progression of first-degree AV block to a more serious form of block.

Evaluate a patient with first-degree AV block for underlying causes that can be corrected, such as drugs or myocardial ischemia. Observe the ECG for progression of the block to a more severe form. Administer digoxin (Lanoxin), calcium channel blockers, and beta-adrenergic receptor blockers cautiously.

Second-degree atrioventricular block

Second-degree atrioventricular (AV) block occurs when some of the electrical impulses from the AV node are blocked and some are conducted through normal conduction pathways. Second-degree AV block is subdivided into type I second-degree AV block and type II second-degree AV block.

TYPE I SECOND-DEGREE AV BLOCK

Also called *Wenckebach* or *Mobitz I block,* type I second-degree AV block occurs when each successive impulse from the sinoatrial (SA) node is delayed slightly longer than the previous impulse. (See *Recognizing type I second-degree AV block,* page 318.) This pattern of progressive prolongation of the PR interval continues until an impulse fails to be conducted to the ventricles.

Usually only a single impulse is blocked from reaching the ventricles, and following this nonconducted P wave or dropped beat the pattern is repeated. This repetitive sequence of two or more consecutive beats followed by a dropped beat result in "group beating." Type I second-degree AV block generally occurs at the level of the AV node.

RECOGNIZING TYPE I SECOND-DEGREE AV BLOCK

The following rhythm strip illustrates type I second-degree atrioventricular (AV) block. Look for these distinguishing characteristics.

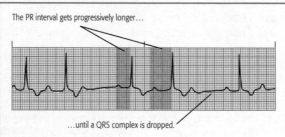

The PR interval gets progressively longer...

...until a QRS complex is dropped.

- *Rhythm:* atrial—regular; ventricular—irregular
- *Rate:* atrial—80 beats/minute; ventricular—50 beats/minute
- *P wave:* normal
- *PR interval:* progressively prolonged
- *QRS complex:* 0.08 second
- *T wave:* normal
- *QT interval:* 0.46 second
- *Other:* Wenckebach pattern of grouped beats

Causes

Type I second-degree AV block frequently results from increased parasympathetic tone or the effects of certain drugs. Coronary artery disease (CAD), inferior-wall myocardial infarction (MI), and rheumatic fever may increase parasympathetic tone and result in the arrhythmia. It may also be caused by cardiac medications, such as beta-adrenergic receptor blockers, digoxin, and calcium channel blockers.

Clinical significance

Type I second-degree AV block may occur normally in an otherwise healthy person. Almost always transient, this type of block usually resolves when the underlying condition is corrected. Although an asymptomatic patient with this block has a good prognosis, the block may progress to a more serious form, especially if it occurs early in an MI.

ECG characteristics

- *Rhythm:* Atrial rhythm is regular, and the ventricular rhythm is irregular. The R-R interval shortens progressively until a P wave appears without a QRS complex. The cycle is then repeated.
- *Rate:* The atrial rate exceeds the ventricular rate because of the nonconducted beats, but both usually remain within normal limits.
- *P wave:* Normal size and configuration; each P wave is followed by a QRS complex except for the blocked P wave.
- *PR interval:* The PR interval is progressively longer with each cycle until a P wave appears without a QRS complex. The variation in delay from cycle to cycle is typically slight. The PR interval after the nonconducted beat is shorter than the interval preceding it. The phrase commonly used to describe this pattern is long, longer, dropped.
- *QRS complex:* Duration usually remains within normal limits because the block commonly occurs at the level of the AV node. The complex is absent when the impulse isn't conducted.
- *T wave:* Normal size and configuration.
- *QT interval:* Usually within normal limits.
- *Other:* The arrhythmia is usually distinguished by "group beating," referred to as the footprints of Wenckebach. Frederik K. Wenckebach was a Dutch internist who, at the turn of the century and long before the introduction of the ECG, described the two forms of what's now known as second-degree AV block by analyzing waves in the jugular venous pulse. Following the introduction of the ECG, German cardiologist Woldemar Mobitz clarified Wenckebach's findings, identifying two types of second-degree AV block, type I and type II.

When you're trying to identify type I second-degree AV block, think of the phrase "longer, longer, drop," which describes the progressively prolonged PR intervals and the missing QRS complexes. The QRS complexes are usually normal because the delays occur in the AV node

Signs and symptoms

Usually asymptomatic, a patient with type I second-degree AV block may show signs and symptoms of decreased cardiac output, such as light-headedness or hypotension. Symptoms may be especially pronounced if the ventricular rate is slow.

Interventions

Treatment is rarely needed because the patient is generally asymptomatic. A transcutaneous pacemaker may be required for a symptomatic patient until the arrhythmia resolves.

For a patient with serious signs and symptoms related to a low heart rate, atropine may be used to improve AV node conduction.

When caring for a patient with this block, assess the tolerance for the rhythm and the need for treatment to improve cardiac output. Evaluate the patient for possible causes of the block, including the use of certain medications or the presence of myocardial ischemia.

Check the ECG frequently to see if a more severe type of AV block develops. Make sure the patient has a patent I.V. line. Provide patient teaching about a temporary pacemaker if indicated.

TYPE II SECOND-DEGREE AV BLOCK

Type II second-degree AV block (also known as *Mobitz II block*) is less common than type I, but more serious. It occurs when impulses from the SA node occasionally fail to conduct to the ventricles. This form of second-degree AV block occurs below the level of the AV node, either at the bundle of His, or more commonly at the bundle branches.

One of the hallmarks of this type of block is that, unlike type I second- degree AV block, the PR interval doesn't lengthen before a dropped beat. (See *Recognizing type II second-degree AV block.*) In addition, more than one nonconducted beat can occur in succession. (See *2:1 AV block.*)

Causes

Unlike type I second-degree AV block, type II second-degree AV block rarely results from increased parasympathetic tone or drug effect. Because the arrhythmia is usually associated with organic heart disease, it's usually associated with a poorer prognosis, and complete heart block may develop.

Type II second-degree AV block is commonly caused by
- an anterior-wall MI
- degenerative changes in the conduction system
- severe CAD.

The arrhythmia indicates a conduction disturbance at the level of the bundle of His or bundle branches.

Clinical significance

Second-degree AV block type II is more severe than type I. The patient does not tolerate this rhythm well and usually exhibits signs of de-

RECOGNIZING TYPE II SECOND-DEGREE AV BLOCK

The following rhythm strip illustrates type II second-degree atrioventricular (AV) block. Look for these distinguishing characteristics.

The atrial rhythm is regular...

...but the ventricular rhythm is irregular.

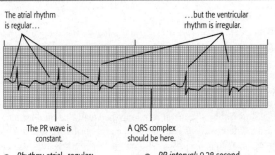

The PR wave is constant.

A QRS complex should be here.

- *Rhythm:* atrial–regular; ventricular–irregular
- *Rate:* atrial–60 beats/minute; ventricular–50 beats/minute
- *P wave:* normal

- *PR interval:* 0.28 second
- *QRS complex:* 0.10 second
- *T wave:* normal
- *QT interval:* 0.60 second
- *Other:* none

2:1 AV BLOCK

In 2:1 second-degree atrioventricular (AV) block, every other QRS complex is dropped, so there are always two P waves for every QRS complex. The resulting ventricular rhythm is regular.

To help determine whether a rhythm is type I or type II AV block, look at the width of the QRS complexes. If they're wide and a short PR interval is present, the block is probably type II.

Keep in mind that type II block is more likely to impair cardiac output, lead to symptoms such as syncope, and progress to a more severe form of block. Be sure to monitor the patient carefully.

creased cardiac output, such as hypotension and syncope. If the block is a result of an anterior wall MI, the block is likely to be permanent because of the tissue damage to the conduction system.

In type II second-degree AV block, the ventricular rate tends to be slower than in type I. In addition, cardiac output tends to be lower and symptoms are more likely to appear, particularly if the sinus rhythm is slow and the ratio of conducted beats to dropped beats is low such as 2:1.

ECG characteristics

- *Rhythm:* The atrial rhythm is regular. The ventricular rhythm can be regular or irregular. Pauses correspond to the dropped beat. When the block is intermittent or when the conduction ratio is variable, the rhythm is often irregular. When a constant conduction ratio occurs, for example, 2:1 or 3:1, the rhythm is regular.
- *Rate:* The atrial rate is usually within normal limits. The ventricular rate, slower than the atrial rate, may be within normal limits.
- *P wave:* The P wave is normal in size and configuration, but some P waves aren't followed by a QRS complex. The R-R interval containing a nonconducted P wave equals two normal R-R intervals.
- *PR interval:* The PR interval is within normal limits or prolonged but generally always constant for the conducted beats.
- *QRS complex:* Duration is within normal limits if the block occurs at the bundle of His. If the block occurs at the bundle branches, however, the QRS will be widened and display the features of bundle-branch block. The complex is absent periodically.
- *T wave:* Usually of normal size and configuration.
- *QT interval:* Usually within normal limits.
- *Other:* The PR and R-R intervals don't vary before a dropped beat, so no warning occurs. For a dropped beat to occur, there must be complete block in one bundle branch with intermittent interruption in conduction in the other bundle as well. As a result, this type of second-degree AV block is commonly associated with a wide QRS complex. However, when the block occurs at the bundle of His, the QRS may be narrow because ventricular conduction is undisturbed in beats that aren't blocked.

Signs and symptoms

Most patients who experience occasional dropped beats remain asymptomatic as long as cardiac output is maintained. As the number of dropped beats increases, the patient may experience signs and symptoms of decreased cardiac output, including fatigue, dyspnea, chest pain, or light-headedness. On physical examination, you may note hypotension and a slow pulse, with a regular or irregular rhythm.

Interventions

If the patient doesn't experience serious signs and symptoms related to the low heart rate, he may be prepared for transvenous pacemaker insertion. Alternatively, the patient may be continuously monitored, with a transcutaneous pacemaker readily available.

If the patient is experiencing serious signs and symptoms due to bradycardia, treatment goals include improving cardiac output by increasing the heart rate. Transcutaneous pacing, I.V. dopamine (Intropin), I.V. epinephrine, or I.V. atropine may be used to increase cardiac output. Use atropine cautiously because it can worsen ischemia during an MI and may induce ventricular tachycardia or fibrillation in patients with this form of second-degree AV block and complete heart block. Because this form of second-degree AV block occurs below the level of the AV node—either at the bundle of His or, more commonly, at the bundle branches—transcutaneous pacing should be initiated quickly, when indicated. For this reason, type II second-degree AV block may also require placement of a permanent pacemaker. A temporary pacemaker may be used until a permanent pacemaker can be inserted.

When caring for a patient with type II second-degree block, assess tolerance for the rhythm and the need for treatment to improve cardiac output. Evaluate for possible correctable causes such as ischemia.

Keep the patient on bed rest, if indicated, to reduce myocardial oxygen demands. Administer oxygen therapy as ordered. Observe the patient's cardiac rhythm for progression to a more severe form of AV block. Teach the patient and family about the use of pacemakers if the patient requires one.

Third-degree atrioventricular block

Also called *complete heart block,* third-degree atrioventricular (AV) block indicates the complete absence of impulse conduction between the atria and ventricles. There's no correlation between the conduction of the P waves and the QRS complex. In complete heart block, the atrial rate is generally faster than the ventricular rate.

Third-degree AV block may occur at the level of the AV node, the bundle of His, or the bundle branches. The patient's treatment and prognosis vary depending on the anatomic level of the block.

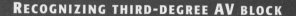

RECOGNIZING THIRD-DEGREE AV BLOCK

The following rhythm strip illustrates third-degree atrioventricular (AV) block. Look for these distinguishing characteristics.

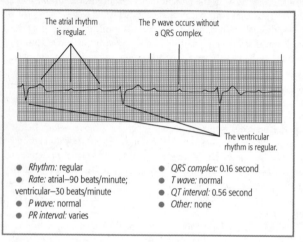

The atrial rhythm is regular.

The P wave occurs without a QRS complex.

The ventricular rhythm is regular.

- *Rhythm:* regular
- *Rate:* atrial–90 beats/minute; ventricular–30 beats/minute
- *P wave:* normal
- *PR interval:* varies
- *QRS complex:* 0.16 second
- *T wave:* normal
- *QT interval:* 0.56 second
- *Other:* none

When third-degree AV block occurs at the level of the AV node, ventricular depolarization is typically initiated by a junctional escape pacemaker. This pacemaker is usually stable with a rate of 40 to 60 beats/minute. (See *Recognizing third-degree AV block.*) The sequence of ventricular depolarization is usually normal because the block is located above the bifurcation of the bundle of His, which results in a normal-appearing QRS complex.

On the other hand, when third-degree AV block occurs at the infranodal level, a block involving the right and left bundle branches is most commonly the cause. In this case, extensive disease exists in the infranodal conduction system, and the only available escape mechanism is located distal to the site of block in the ventricle. This unstable, ventricular escape pacemaker has a slow intrinsic rate of less than 40 beats/minute. Because these depolarizations originate in the ventricle, the QRS complex will have a wide and bizarre appearance.

CAUSES

Third-degree AV block occurring at the anatomic level of the AV node can result from increased parasympathetic tone associated with inferior wall myocardial infarction (MI), AV node damage, or toxic effects of such drugs as digoxin and propranolol (Inderal).

Third-degree AV block occurring at the infranodal level is usually associated with extensive anterior MI. It generally isn't the result of increases in parasympathetic tone or drug effect.

CLINICAL SIGNIFICANCE

Third-degree AV block occurring at the AV node, with a junctional escape rhythm, is usually transient and generally associated with a favorable prognosis. In third-degree AV block at the infranodal level, however, the pacemaker is unstable and episodes of ventricular asystole are common. Third-degree AV block at this level is generally associated with a less favorable prognosis.

Because the ventricular rate in third-degree AV block can be slow and the decrease in cardiac output so significant, the arrhythmia usually results in a life-threatening situation. In addition, the loss of AV synchrony results in the loss of atrial kick, which further decreases cardiac output.

ECG CHARACTERISTICS

- *Rhythm:* Atrial and ventricular rhythms are usually regular.
- *Rate:* Acting independently, the atria, generally under the control of the sinoatrial node, tend to maintain a regular rate of 60 to 100 beats/minute. The atrial rate exceeds the ventricular rate. With intranodal block, the ventricular rate is usually 40 to 60 beats/minute (a junctional escape rhythm). With infranodal block, the ventricular rate is usually below 40 beats/minute (a ventricular escape rhythm).
- *P wave:* The P wave is normal in size and configuration. Some P waves may be buried in QRS complexes or T waves.
- *PR interval:* Not applicable or measurable because the atria and ventricles are depolarized from different pacemakers and beat independently of each other.
- *QRS complex:* Configuration depends on the location of the escape mechanism and origin of ventricular depolarization. When the block occurs at the level of the AV node or bundle of His, the QRS complex will appear normal. When the block occurs at the level of the bundle branches, the QRS complex will be widened.

- *T wave:* Normal size and configuration unless the QRS complex originates in the ventricle.
- *QT interval:* May be within normal limits.
- *Other:* None.

SIGNS AND SYMPTOMS

Most patients with third-degree AV block experience significant signs and symptoms, including severe fatigue, dyspnea, chest pain, light-headedness, changes in mental status, and changes in the level of consciousness. Hypotension, pallor, and diaphoresis may also occur. The peripheral pulse rate will be slow, but the rhythm will be regular.

A few patients will be relatively free of symptoms, complaining only that they can't tolerate exercise and that they're typically tired for no apparent reason. The severity of symptoms depends to a large extent on the resulting ventricular rate and the patient's ability to compensate for decreased cardiac output.

INTERVENTIONS

If the patient is experiencing serious signs and symptoms related to the low heart rate, or if the patient's condition seems to be deteriorating, interventions may include transcutaneous pacing or I.V. atropine, dopamine, or epinephrine. Atropine isn't indicated for third-degree AV block with new wide QRS complexes. In such cases, a permanent pacemaker is indicated because atropine rarely increases sinus rate and AV node conduction when AV block is at the His-Purkinje level.

Asymptomatic patients in third-degree AV block should be prepared for insertion of a transvenous temporary pacemaker until a decision is made about the need for a permanent pacemaker. If symptoms develop, a transcutaneous pacemaker should be used until the transvenous pacemaker is placed.

Because third-degree AV block occurring at the infranodal level is usually associated with extensive anterior MI, patients are more likely to have permanent third-degree AV block, which most likely requires insertion of a permanent pacemaker.

Third-degree AV block occurring at the anatomic level of the AV node can result from increased parasympathetic tone associated with an inferior wall MI. As a result, the block is more likely to be short-lived. In these patients, the decision to insert a permanent pacemaker is often delayed to assess how well the conduction system recovers.

When caring for a patient with third-degree AV block, immediately assess the patient's tolerance of the rhythm and the need for interventions to support cardiac output and relieve symptoms. Make sure the patient has a patent I.V. line. Administer oxygen therapy as ordered. Evaluate for possible correctable causes of the arrhythmia, such as drugs or myocardial ischemia. Minimize the patient's activity and maintain bed rest.

ACLS ALGORITHMS

Shown on the next pages are the American Heart Association ACLS algorithms for bradycardia, pulseless arrest, and tachycardia.

BRADYCARDIA

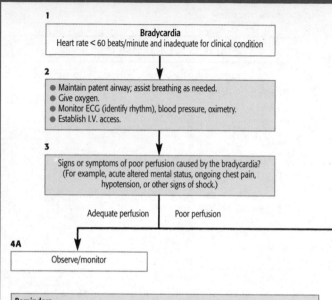

1

Bradycardia
Heart rate < 60 beats/minute and inadequate for clinical condition

2

- Maintain patent airway; assist breathing as needed.
- Give oxygen.
- Monitor ECG (identify rhythm), blood pressure, oximetry.
- Establish I.V. access.

3

Signs or symptoms of poor perfusion caused by the bradycardia?
(For example, acute altered mental status, ongoing chest pain,
hypotension, or other signs of shock.)

Adequate perfusion   Poor perfusion

4A

Observe/monitor

Reminders
- If pulseless arrest develops, go to Pulseless Arrest Algorithm.
- Search for and treat possible contributing factors, such as:
  - hypovolemia
  - hypoxia
  - hydrogen ion (acidosis)
  - hypokalemia/hyperkalemia
  - hypoglycemia
  - hypothermia
  - toxins
  - tamponade, cardiac
  - tension pneumothorax
  - thrombosis (coronary or pulmonary)
  - trauma (hypovolemia, increased intracranial pressure).

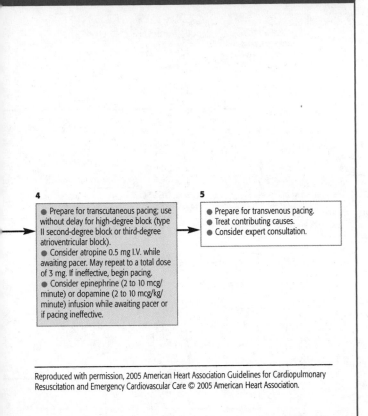

4

- Prepare for transcutaneous pacing; use without delay for high-degree block (type II second-degree block or third-degree atrioventricular block).
- Consider atropine 0.5 mg I.V. while awaiting pacer. May repeat to a total dose of 3 mg. If ineffective, begin pacing.
- Consider epinephrine (2 to 10 mcg/minute) or dopamine (2 to 10 mcg/kg/minute) infusion while awaiting pacer or if pacing ineffective.

5

- Prepare for transvenous pacing.
- Treat contributing causes.
- Consider expert consultation.

PULSELESS ARREST

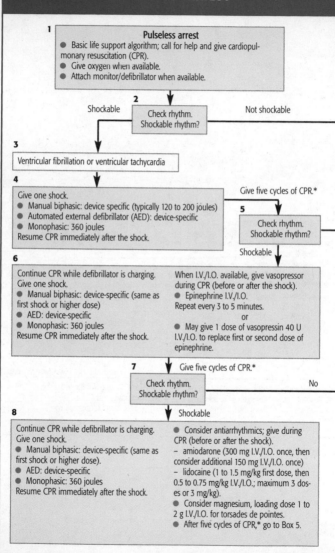

1
Pulseless arrest
● Basic life support algorithm; call for help and give cardiopul-
  monary resuscitation (CPR).
● Give oxygen when available.
● Attach monitor/defibrillator when available.

Shockable ⟶ **2** Check rhythm. Shockable rhythm? ⟵ Not shockable

3
Ventricular fibrillation or ventricular tachycardia

4
Give one shock.   Give five cycles of CPR.*
● Manual biphasic: device specific (typically 120 to 200 joules)
● Automated external defibrillator (AED): device-specific   **5**
● Monophasic: 360 joules   Check rhythm.
Resume CPR immediately after the shock.   Shockable rhythm?

                                                      Shockable ↓

6
Continue CPR while defibrillator is charging.   When I.V./I.O. available, give vasopressor
Give one shock.   during CPR (before or after the shock).
● Manual biphasic: device-specific (same as   ● Epinephrine I.V./I.O.
  first shock or higher dose)   Repeat every 3 to 5 minutes.
● AED: device-specific   or
● Monophasic: 360 joules   ● May give 1 dose of vasopressin 40 U
Resume CPR immediately after the shock.   I.V./I.O. to replace first or second dose of
                                                     epinephrine.

7   Give five cycles of CPR.*
Check rhythm.
Shockable rhythm?   No

               Shockable

8
Continue CPR while defibrillator is charging.   ● Consider antiarrhythmics; give during
Give one shock.   CPR (before or after the shock).
● Manual biphasic: device-specific (same as   – amiodarone (300 mg I.V./I.O. once, then
  first shock or higher dose).   consider additional 150 mg I.V./I.O. once)
● AED: device-specific   – lidocaine (1 to 1.5 mg/kg first dose, then
● Monophasic: 360 joules   0.5 to 0.75 mg/kg I.V./I.O.; maximum 3 dos-
Resume CPR immediately after the shock.   es or 3 mg/kg).
                                                   ● Consider magnesium, loading dose 1 to
                                                     2 g I.V./I.O. for torsades de pointes.
                                                   ● After five cycles of CPR,* go to Box 5.

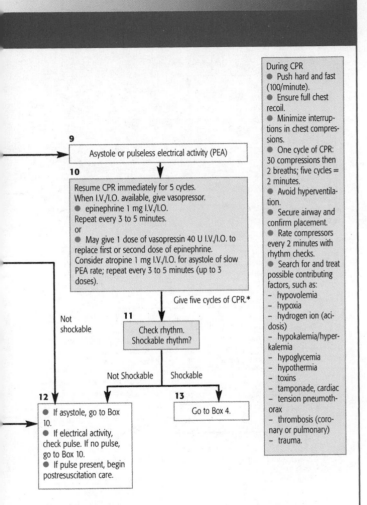

During CPR
- Push hard and fast (100/minute).
- Ensure full chest recoil.
- Minimize interruptions in chest compressions.
- One cycle of CPR: 30 compressions then 2 breaths; five cycles = 2 minutes.
- Avoid hyperventilation.
- Secure airway and confirm placement.
- Rate compressors every 2 minutes with rhythm checks.
- Search for and treat possible contributing factors, such as:
  – hypovolemia
  – hypoxia
  – hydrogen ion (acidosis)
  – hypokalemia/hyperkalemia
  – hypoglycemia
  – hypothermia
  – toxins
  – tamponade, cardiac
  – tension pneumothorax
  – thrombosis (coronary or pulmonary)
  – trauma.

9
Asystole or pulseless electrical activity (PEA)

10
Resume CPR immediately for 5 cycles. When I.V./I.O. available, give vasopressor.
- epinephrine 1 mg I.V./I.O. Repeat every 3 to 5 minutes.
or
- May give 1 dose of vasopressin 40 U I.V./I.O. to replace first or second dose of epinephrine. Consider atropine 1 mg I.V./I.O. for asystole of slow PEA rate; repeat every 3 to 5 minutes (up to 3 doses).

Give five cycles of CPR.*

11
Check rhythm. Shockable rhythm?

Not Shockable   Shockable

Not shockable

12
- If asystole, go to Box 10.
- If electrical activity, check pulse. If no pulse, go to Box 10.
- If pulse present, begin postresuscitation care.

13
Go to Box 4.

* After an advanced airway is placed, rescuers no longer deliver "cycles" of CPR. Give continuous chest compressions without pauses for breaths. Give 8 to 10 breaths/minute. Check rhythm every 2 minutes.

TACHYCARDIA

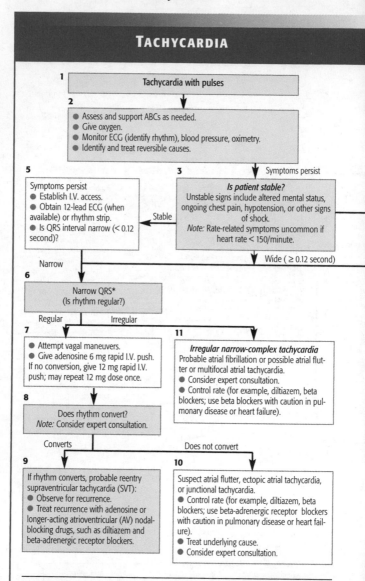

1

Tachycardia with pulses

2

- Assess and support ABCs as needed.
- Give oxygen.
- Monitor ECG (identify rhythm), blood pressure, oximetry.
- Identify and treat reversible causes.

Symptoms persist

5

Symptoms persist
- Establish I.V. access.
- Obtain 12-lead ECG (when available) or rhythm strip.
- Is QRS interval narrow (< 0.12 second)?

3

Is patient stable?
Unstable signs include altered mental status, ongoing chest pain, hypotension, or other signs of shock.
Note: Rate-related symptoms uncommon if heart rate < 150/minute.

Stable

Narrow

Wide (≥ 0.12 second)

6

Narrow QRS*
(Is rhythm regular?)

Regular   Irregular

7

- Attempt vagal maneuvers.
- Give adenosine 6 mg rapid I.V. push. If no conversion, give 12 mg rapid I.V. push; may repeat 12 mg dose once.

11

Irregular narrow-complex tachycardia
Probable atrial fibrillation or possible atrial flutter or multifocal atrial tachycardia.
- Consider expert consultation.
- Control rate (for example, diltiazem, beta blockers; use beta blockers with caution in pulmonary disease or heart failure).

8

Does rhythm convert?
Note: Consider expert consultation.

Converts

Does not convert

9

If rhythm converts, probable reentry supraventricular tachycardia (SVT):
- Observe for recurrence.
- Treat recurrence with adenosine or longer-acting atrioventricular (AV) nodal-blocking drugs, such as diltiazem and beta-adrenergic receptor blockers.

10

Suspect atrial flutter, ectopic atrial tachycardia, or junctional tachycardia.
- Control rate (for example, diltiazem, beta blockers; use beta-adrenergic receptor blockers with caution in pulmonary disease or heart failure).
- Treat underlying cause.
- Consider expert consultation.

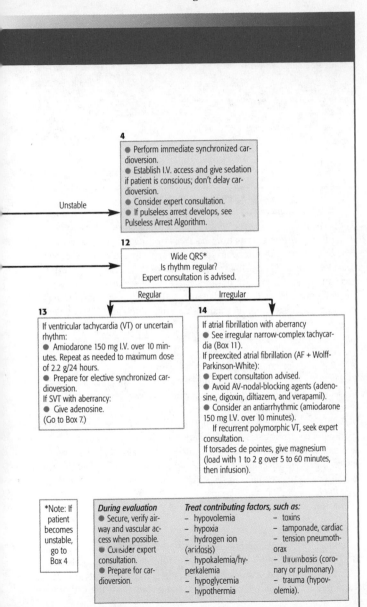

4
- Perform immediate synchronized cardioversion.
- Establish I.V. access and give sedation if patient is conscious; don't delay cardioversion.
- Consider expert consultation.
- If pulseless arrest develops, see Pulseless Arrest Algorithm.

Unstable →

12
Wide QRS*
Is rhythm regular?
Expert consultation is advised.

Regular — Irregular

13
If ventricular tachycardia (VT) or uncertain rhythm:
- Amiodarone 150 mg I.V. over 10 minutes. Repeat as needed to maximum dose of 2.2 g/24 hours.
- Prepare for elective synchronized cardioversion.
If SVT with aberrancy:
- Give adenosine.
(Go to Box 7.)

14
If atrial fibrillation with aberrancy
- See irregular narrow-complex tachycardia (Box 11).
If preexcited atrial fibrillation (AF + Wolff-Parkinson-White):
- Expert consultation advised.
- Avoid AV-nodal-blocking agents (adenosine, digoxin, diltiazem, and verapamil).
- Consider an antiarrhythmic (amiodarone 150 mg I.V. over 10 minutes).
  If recurrent polymorphic VT, seek expert consultation.
If torsades de pointes, give magnesium (load with 1 to 2 g over 5 to 60 minutes, then infusion).

*Note: If patient becomes unstable, go to Box 4

During evaluation
- Secure, verify airway and vascular access when possible.
- Consider expert consultation.
- Prepare for cardioversion.

Treat contributing factors, such as:
- hypovolemia
- hypoxia
- hydrogen ion (acidosis)
- hypokalemia/hyperkalemia
- hypoglycemia
- hypothermia

- toxins
- tamponade, cardiac
- tension pneumothorax
- thrombosis (coronary or pulmonary)
- trauma (hypovolemia).

Inflammatory disorders

ENDOCARDITIS

Endocarditis is an infection of the endocardium, heart valves, or cardiac prosthesis that results from bacterial or fungal invasion.

In patients with infective endocarditis, fibrin and platelets cluster on valve tissue and engulf circulating bacteria or fungi. This produces vegetation, which, in turn, may cover the valve surfaces, causing deformities and destruction of valvular tissue. It may also extend to the chordae tendineae, causing them to rupture, which leads to valvular insufficiency.

Sometimes vegetation forms on the endocardium, usually in areas altered by rheumatic, congenital, or syphilitic heart disease. It may also form on normal surfaces. Vegetative growth on the heart valves, endocardial lining of a heart chamber, or the endothelium of a blood vessel may embolize to the spleen, kidneys, central nervous system, and lungs.

Endocarditis can be classified as native valve endocarditis, endocarditis in I.V. drug users, or prosthetic valve endocarditis. It can be acute or subacute. Untreated, endocarditis is usually fatal. With proper treatment, however, about 70% of patients recover. The prognosis is worse when endocarditis causes severe valvular damage—leading to insufficiency and left-sided heart failure—or when it involves a prosthetic valve.

Pathophysiology

In endocarditis, bacteremia—even transient bacteremia after dental or urogenital procedures—introduces the pathogen into the bloodstream. This infection causes fibrin and platelets to aggregate on the valve tissue and engulf circulating bacteria or fungi that flourish and

DEGENERATIVE CHANGES IN ENDOCARDITIS

This illustration shows typical growths on the endocardium produced by fibrin and platelet deposits on infection sites.

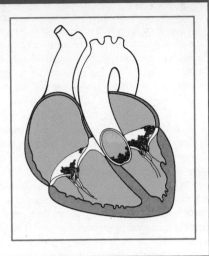

form on fragile, wartlike vegetative growths on the heart valves, the endocardial lining of a heart chamber, or the epithelium of a blood vessel. (See *Degenerative changes in endocarditis*.) Such growths may cover the valve surfaces, causing ulceration and necrosis. They may also extend to the chordae tendineae, leading to rupture and subsequent valvular insufficiency. Ultimately, they may embolize to the spleen, kidneys, central nervous system, and lungs.

Most cases of endocarditis occur in patients who:
- are I.V. drug abusers
- have mitral valve prolapse (especially with a systolic murmur)
- have prosthetic heart valves
- have rheumatic heart disease.

Other predisposing conditions include:
- coarctation of the aorta
- tetralogy of Fallot
- subaortic and valvular aortic stenosis
- ventricular septal defects
- pulmonary stenosis
- Marfan's syndrome

- degenerative heart disease, especially calcific aortic stenosis
- rarely, a syphilitic aortic valve.

However, some patients with endocarditis have no underlying heart disease.

Infecting organisms differ among these groups. In patients with native valve endocarditis who aren't I.V. drug abusers, causative organisms usually include (in order of frequency) streptococci, especially *Streptococcus viridans,* staphylococci, or enterococci. Although other bacteria occasionally cause the disorder, fungal causes are rare in this group. The mitral valve is the most common valve involved, followed by the aortic valve.

In patients who are I.V. drug abusers, *Staphylococcus aureus* is the most common infecting organism. Less common causes of the disorder are streptococci, enterococci, gram-negative bacilli, or fungi. The tricuspid valve is the most common valve involved, followed by the aortic valve and then the mitral valve.

In patients with prosthetic valve endocarditis, early cases (those that develop within 60 days of valve insertion) are usually caused by staphylococcal infection. However, gram-negative aerobic organisms, fungi, streptococci, enterococci, or diphtheroids may also cause the disorder. The course is usually sudden and severe and is associated with a high mortality rate. Late cases (occurring after 60 days) show signs and symptoms similar to native valve endocarditis.

Complications
- Heart failure
- Death
- Aortic root abscess
- Myocardial abscesses
- Pericarditis
- Cardiac arrhythmia
- Meningitis
- Cerebral emboli
- Brain abscesses
- Septic pulmonary infarcts
- Arthritis
- Glomerulonephritis
- Acute renal failure

Assessment findings
- The patient may report a predisposing condition and complain of nonspecific signs and symptoms, such as weakness, fatigue, weight

loss, anorexia, arthralgia, night sweats, and an intermittent fever that may recur for weeks.
- Inspection may reveal petechiae of the skin (especially common on the upper anterior trunk) and the buccal, pharyngeal, or conjunctival mucosa, and splinter hemorrhages under the nails.
- Rarely, you may see Osler's nodes (tender, raised, subcutaneous lesions on the fingers or toes), Roth's spots (hemorrhagic areas with white centers on the retina), and Janeway lesions (purplish macules on the palms or soles).
- Clubbing of the fingers may be present in patients with long-standing disease.
- Auscultation may reveal a murmur in most patients, except those with early acute endocarditis and I.V. drug abusers with tricuspid valve infection. The murmur is usually loud and regurgitant, which is typical of the underlying rheumatic or congenital heart disease. A murmur that changes suddenly or a new murmur that develops in the presence of fever is a classic sign of endocarditis.
- Percussion and palpation may reveal splenomegaly in long-standing disease. In patients who have developed left-sided heart failure, your assessment may reveal dyspnea, tachycardia, and bibasilar crackles.
- In 12% to 35% of patients with subacute endocarditis, embolization from vegetating lesions or diseased valve tissue may produce typical characteristics of splenic, renal, cerebral, or pulmonary infarction, or peripheral vascular occlusion:
  - Splenic infarction causes pain in the left upper quadrant, radiating to the left shoulder, and abdominal rigidity.
  - Renal infarction causes hematuria, pyuria, flank pain, and decreased urine output.
  - Cerebral infarction causes hemiparesis, aphasia, and other neurologic deficits.
  - Pulmonary infarction causes cough, pleuritic pain, pleural friction rub, dyspnea, and hemoptysis. These signs and symptoms are most common in patients with right-sided endocarditis, which typically occurs among I.V. drug abusers and after cardiac surgery.
  - Peripheral vascular occlusion causes numbness and tingling in an arm, leg, finger, or toe, or signs of impending peripheral gangrene.

Diagnostic test results
- Three or more blood cultures during a 24- to 48-hour period identify the causative organism in up to 90% of patients. The remaining

10% may have negative blood cultures, possibly suggesting fungal or difficult-to-diagnose infections such as *Haemophilus parainfluenzae*.

- Other abnormal but nonspecific laboratory results include:
  - normal or elevated white blood cell count and differential
  - abnormal histiocytes (macrophages)
  - normocytic, normochromic anemia (in patients with subacute infective endocarditis)
  - elevated erythrocyte sedimentation rate and serum creatinine level
  - positive serum rheumatoid factor in about half of patients with endocarditis after the disease is present for 6 weeks
  - proteinuria and microscopic hematuria.
- Echocardiography may identify valvular damage in most patients with native valve disease.
- An electrocardiogram reading may show atrial fibrillation and other arrhythmias that accompany valvular disease.

Treatment

The goal of treatment is to eradicate all infecting organisms from the vegetation. Therapy should start promptly and continue over 4 to 6 weeks. Selection of an anti-infective drug is based on the infecting organism and sensitivity studies. Although blood cultures are negative in 10% to 20% of the subacute cases, the practitioner may want to determine the probable infecting organism.

Supportive treatment includes bed rest, aspirin for fever and aches, and sufficient fluid intake. Severe valvular damage, especially aortic insufficiency or infection of a cardiac prosthesis, may require corrective surgery if refractory heart failure develops or if an infected prosthetic valve must be replaced.

Nursing interventions

- Stress the importance of bed rest. Assist the patient with bathing if necessary. Provide a bedside commode because using a commode puts less stress on the heart than using a bedpan. Offer the patient diversionary, physically undemanding activities.
- To reduce anxiety, allow the patient to express his concerns about the effects of activity restrictions on his responsibilities and routines. Reassure him that the restrictions are temporary.
- Before giving an antibiotic, obtain a patient history of allergies. Administer the prescribed antibiotic on time to maintain a consistent drug level in the blood.

TEACHING THE PATIENT WITH ENDOCARDITIS

● Teach the patient about the anti-infective medication that he'll continue to take. Stress the importance of taking the medication and restricting activity for as long as recommended.

● Tell the patient to watch for and report signs of embolization and to watch closely for fever, anorexia, and other signs of relapse that could occur about 2 weeks after treatment stops.

● Discuss the importance of completing the full course of antibiotics, even if he's feeling better. Make sure susceptible patients understand the need for prophylactic antibiotics before, during, and after dental work, childbirth, and genitourinary, GI, or gynecologic procedures.

● Teach the patient to brush his teeth with a soft toothbrush and rinse his mouth thoroughly. Tell him to avoid flossing his teeth and using irrigation devices.

● Teach the patient how to recognize symptoms of endocarditis. Tell him to notify the practitioner immediately if such symptoms occur.

■ Observe the venipuncture site for signs of infiltration or inflammation, a complication of long-term I.V. administration. To reduce the risk of this complication, rotate venous access sites.

■ Assess cardiovascular status frequently, and watch for signs and symptoms of left-sided heart failure, such as dyspnea, hypotension, tachycardia, tachypnea, crackles, and weight gain. Check for changes in cardiac rhythm or conduction.

■ Administer oxygen and evaluate arterial blood gas levels, as needed, to ensure adequate oxygenation.

RED FLAG Watch for signs and symptoms of embolization (hematuria, pleuritic chest pain, left upper quadrant pain, or paresis), a common occurrence during the first 3 months of treatment. Tell the patient to watch for and report these signs and symptoms, which may indicate impending peripheral vascular occlusion or splenic, renal, cerebral, or pulmonary infarction.

■ Monitor the patient's renal status (including blood urea nitrogen levels, creatinine clearance, and urine output) to check for signs of renal emboli and drug toxicity.

■ Make sure the susceptible patient understands the need for a prophylactic antibiotic before, during, and after dental work, childbirth, and genitourinary, GI, or gynecologic procedures. (See *Teaching the patient with endocarditis*.)

MYOCARDITIS

Myocarditis—a focal or diffuse inflammation of the myocardium—is typically uncomplicated and self-limiting. It may be acute or chronic and can occur at any age. In many patients, myocarditis fails to produce specific cardiovascular symptoms or electrocardiogram (ECG) abnormalities. Recovery usually is spontaneous and without residual defects.

Occasionally, myocarditis becomes serious and induces myofibril degeneration, right- and left-sided heart failure with cardiomegaly, and arrhythmias.

Pathophysiology

Damage to the myocardium occurs when an infectious organism triggers an autoimmune, cellular, and humoral reaction. The resulting inflammation may lead to hypertrophy, fibrosis, and inflammatory changes of the myocardium and conduction system. The heart muscle weakens and contractility is reduced. The heart muscle becomes flabby and dilated, and pinpoint hemorrhages may develop.

Causes of myocarditis include:

- bacterial infections, such as diphtheria, tuberculosis, typhoid fever, tetanus, and staphylococcal, pneumococcal, and gonococcal infections
- fungal infections, including candidiasis and aspergillosis
- helminthic infections such as trichinosis
- hypersensitive immune reactions, including acute rheumatic fever and postcardiotomy syndrome
- parasitic infections, especially South American trypanosomiasis (Chagas' disease) in infants and immunosuppressed adults; also toxoplasmosis
- radiation therapy; large doses of radiation to the chest in treating lung or breast cancer
- toxins, such as lead, chemicals, and cocaine, and alcoholism
- viral infections (most common cause in the United States and western Europe), such as coxsackievirus A and B strains and, possibly, poliomyelitis, influenza, Epstein-Barr virus, human immunodeficiency virus, cytomegalovirus, measles, mumps, rubeola, rubella, and adenoviruses and echoviruses.

Complications

- Recurrence of myocarditis
- Chronic valvulitis (when it results from rheumatic fever)

- Dilated cardiomyopathy
- Arrhythmias and sudden death
- Heart failure
- Pericarditis
- Ruptured myocardial aneurysm
- Thromboembolism

Assessment findings

- The history commonly reveals a recent upper respiratory tract infection with fever, viral pharyngitis, or tonsillitis.
- The patient may complain of nonspecific signs and symptoms, such as fatigue, dyspnea, palpitations, persistent tachycardia, and persistent fever, all of which reflect the accompanying systemic infection.
- Occasionally, the patient may complain of a mild, continuous pressure or soreness in the chest. This pain is unlike the recurring, stress-related pain of angina pectoris.
- Auscultation usually reveals S_3 and S_4 gallops, a muffled S_1, possibly a murmur of mitral insufficiency (from papillary muscle dysfunction) and, if the patient has pericarditis, a pericardial friction rub.
- If the patient has left-sided heart failure, you may notice pulmonary congestion, dyspnea, and resting or exertional tachycardia disproportionate to the degree of fever.
- If myofibril degeneration occurs, it may lead to right-sided and left-sided heart failure, with cardiomegaly, jugular vein distention, dyspnea, edema, pulmonary congestions, persistent fever with resting or exertional tachycardia disproportionate to the degree of fever, and supraventricular and ventricular arrhythmias.

Diagnostic test results

- Endomyocardial biopsy can be used to confirm a myocarditis diagnosis.
- Cardiac enzyme levels, including creatine kinase (CK), CK-MB, serum aspartate aminotransferase, and lactate dehydrogenase, are elevated.
- White blood cell count and erythrocyte sedimentation rate are elevated.
- Antibody titers, such as antistreptolysin-O titer, are elevated in patients with rheumatic fever.
- ECG typically shows diffuse ST-segment and T-wave abnormalities, as in patients with pericarditis, conduction defects (prolonged PR

interval), or other ventricular and supraventricular ectopic arrhythmias.

- Cultures of stool, throat, pharyngeal washings, blood, or other body fluids may identify the causative bacteria or virus.
- Echocardiography may show a weak heart muscle, an enlarged heart, or fluid surrounding the heart.

Treatment

An antibiotic is prescribed to treat the bacterial infections. An antipyretic is used to reduce fever and help decrease the stress on the heart. The patient will be placed on bed rest to reduce oxygen demands and to reduce the heart's workload. Activity restrictions will help minimize myocardial oxygen consumption. The patient will be given supplemental oxygen therapy. His sodium intake will be restricted, and he'll be given a diuretic to decrease fluid retention. An angiotensin-converting enzyme inhibitor will also be prescribed. For patients with heart failure, digoxin (Lanoxin) will be used to increase myocardial contractility. (Administer digoxin carefully because some patients may show a paradoxical sensitivity to even small doses.)

An antiarrhythmic, such as quinidine (Quinaglute) or procainamide (Pronestyl), is used to treat arrhythmias. Use these drugs cautiously because they may depress myocardial contractility. A temporary pacemaker may be inserted if complete atrioventricular block occurs.

Anticoagulation is used to prevent thromboembolism. A corticosteroid and an immunosuppressant, while controversial, are sometimes used to combat life-threatening complications, such as intractable heart failure.

Nonsteroidal anti-inflammatory drugs are contraindicated during the acute phase (first 2 weeks) because they increase myocardial damage. Cardiac assist devices or transplantation may be used as a last resort in severe cases that resist treatment.

Nursing interventions

- Stress the importance of bed rest. Assist the patient with bathing if necessary. Provide a bedside commode because using a commode puts less stress on the heart than using a bedpan. Offer the patient diversionary, physically undemanding activities.
- To reduce anxiety, allow the patient to express his concerns about the effects of activity restrictions on his responsibilities and routines. Reassure him that the restrictions are temporary.
- Assess cardiovascular status frequently, watching for signs and symptoms of left-sided heart failure (such as dyspnea, hypotension,

TEACHING THE PATIENT WITH MYOCARDITIS

● Teach the patient about anti-infectives. Stress the importance of taking the prescribed drug and restricting activities for as long as the practitioner orders.
● Teach the patient to check his pulse for 1 full minute before taking a cardiac glycoside at home. Direct him to withhold the dose and notify the practitioner if his heart rate falls below the predetermined rate (usually 60 beats/minute).
● During recovery, recommend that the patient resume normal activities slowly and avoid competitive sports.

and tachycardia). Check for changes in cardiac rhythm or conduction.
■ Administer oxygen and evaluate arterial blood gas levels, as needed, to ensure adequate oxygenation.
■ Observe the patient for signs and symptoms of digoxin toxicity (such as anorexia, nausea, vomiting, blurred vision, and cardiac arrhythmias) and for complicating factors that may potentiate toxicity, such as electrolyte imbalance and hypoxia.
■ Administer a parenteral anti-infective as indicated. (See *Teaching the patient with myocarditis*.)

PERICARDITIS

The pericardium is the fibroserous sac that envelops, supports, and protects the heart. Inflammation of this sac is called pericarditis. This condition occurs in acute and chronic forms. The acute form can be fibrinous or effusive, with serous, purulent, or hemorrhagic exudate. The chronic form (called constrictive pericarditis) is characterized by dense fibrous pericardial thickening. (See *Understanding pericarditis*, pages 344 and 345.)

The prognosis depends on the underlying cause, but typically the prognosis is good in patients with acute pericarditis, unless constriction occurs.

Pathophysiology
Pericardial tissue damaged by bacteria or other substances results in the release of chemical mediators in inflammation (prostaglandins,

(Text continues on page 346.)

UNDERSTANDING PERICARDITIS

Pericarditis occurs when a pathogen or other substance attacks the pericardium, leading to the following events.

Inflammation

Pericardial tissue damaged by bacteria or other substances releases chemical mediators of inflammation (such as prostaglandins, histamines, bradykinins, and serotonins) into the surrounding tissue, starting the inflammatory process. Friction occurs as the inflamed pericardial layers rub against each other.

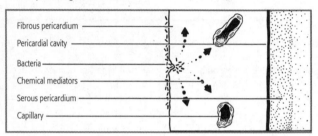

Vasodilation and clotting

Histamines and other chemical mediators cause vasodilation and increased vessel permeability. Local blood flow (hyperemia) increases. Vessel walls leak fluids and proteins (including fibrinogen) into tissues, causing extracellular edema. Clots of fibrinogen and tissue fluid form a wall, blocking tissue spaces and lymph vessels in the injured area. This wall prevents the spread of bacteria and toxins to adjoining healthy tissues.

Initial phagocytosis

Macrophages already present in the tissues begin to phagocytize the invading bacteria but usually fail to stop the infection.

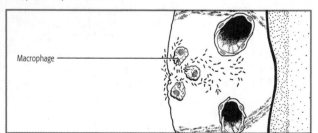

Enhanced phagocytosis

Substances released by the injured tissue stimulate neutrophil production in the bone marrow. Neutrophils then travel to the injury site through the bloodstream and join macrophages in destroying pathogens. Meanwhile, additional macrophages and monocytes migrate to the injured area and continue phagocytosis.

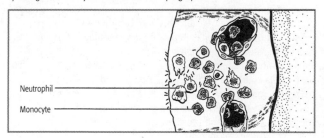

Exudation

After several days, the infected area fills with an exudate composed of necrotic tissue and dead and dying bacteria, neutrophils, and macrophages. This exudate, which is thinner than pus, forms until all infection ceases, creating a cavity that remains until tissue destruction stops. The contents of the cavity autolyze and are gradually reabsorbed into healthy tissue.

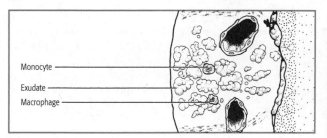

Fibrosis and scarring

As the end products of the infection slowly disappear, fibrosis and scar tissue may form. Scarring, which can be extensive, can ultimately cause heart failure if it restricts movement.

histamines, bradykinins, and serotonins) into the surrounding tissue, thereby initiating the inflammatory process. Friction occurs as the inflamed pericardial layers rub against each other. Histamines and other chemical mediators dilate vessels and increase vessel permeability. Vessel walls then leak fluids and protein (including fibrinogen) into tissues, causing extracellular edema. Macrophages already present in the tissue begin to phagocytize the invading bacteria and are joined by neutrophils and monocytes. After several days, the area fills with an exudate composed of necrotic tissue and dead and dying bacteria, neutrophils, and macrophages. Eventually, the contents of the cavity autolyze and are gradually reabsorbed into healthy tissue.

A pericardial effusion develops if fluid accumulates in the pericardial cavity. Cardiac tamponade results when fluid accumulates rapidly in the pericardial space, compressing the heart, preventing it from filling during diastole, and resulting in a drop in cardiac output.

Chronic constrictive pericarditis develops if the pericardium becomes thick and stiff from chronic or recurrent pericarditis, encasing the heart in a stiff shell and preventing it from properly filling during diastole. This causes an increase in left- and right-sided filling pressures, leading to a drop in stroke volume and cardiac output.

Common causes of pericarditis include:
- aortic aneurysm with pericardial leakage (less common)
- bacterial, fungal, or viral infection (infectious pericarditis)
- drugs, such as hydralazine (Apresoline) or procainamide (Procan SR)
- high dose radiation to the chest
- hypersensitivity or autoimmune disease, such as acute rheumatic fever (most common cause of pericarditis in children), systemic lupus erythematosus, and rheumatoid arthritis
- idiopathic factors (most common in acute pericarditis)
- myxedema with cholesterol deposits in the pericardium (less common)
- neoplasms (primary or metastases from lungs, breasts, or other organs)
- previous cardiac injury, such as a myocardial infarction (MI; Dressler's syndrome), trauma, or surgery (postcardiotomy syndrome), that leaves the pericardium intact but causes blood to leak into the pericardial cavity
- uremia.

Complications
- Pericardial effusion (major complication of acute pericarditis)
- Cardiac tamponade

Assessment findings

- The patient's history may include an event or disease that can cause pericarditis, such as a chest trauma, an MI, or a recent bacterial infection.
- The patient with acute pericarditis typically reports sharp, sudden pain, usually starting over the sternum and radiating to the neck, shoulders, back, and arms. The pain is usually pleuritic, increasing with deep inspiration and decreasing when the patient sits up and leans forward. This decrease occurs because leaning forward pulls the heart away from the diaphragmatic pleurae of the lungs.

  Pericarditis can mimic the pain of an MI. However, the patient may have no pain if he has slowly developing tuberculous pericarditis or postirradiation, neoplastic, or uremic pericarditis.
- The patient may also report dyspnea.
- Auscultation almost always reveals a pericardial friction rub, which is a grating sound heard as the heart moves. You can hear it best during forced expiration, while the patient leans forward or is on his hands and knees in bed. The rub may have up to three components that correspond to atrial systole, ventricular systole, and the rapid-filling phase of ventricular diastole.
- Occasionally, the friction rub is heard only briefly or not at all. If acute pericarditis has caused very large pericardial effusions, heart sounds may be distant.
- Palpation may reveal a diminished or an absent apical impulse.
- Chronic constrictive pericarditis causes the membrane to calcify and become rigid. It also causes a gradual increase in systemic venous pressure and symptoms similar to those of chronic right-sided heart failure (such as fluid retention, ascites, and hepatomegaly).
- Tachycardia, an ill-defined substernal chest pain, and a feeling of fullness in the chest may indicate pericardial effusion.

RED FLAG Pallor, clammy skin, hypotension, paradoxical pulse (a drop in systolic blood pressure of 15 mm Hg or greater during slow inspiration), jugular vein distention, and dyspnea indicate cardiac tamponade.

Diagnostic test results

Laboratory results indicate inflammation and may identify the disorder's cause. They include:

- normal or elevated white blood cell count, especially in patients with infectious pericarditis
- elevated erythrocyte sedimentation rate
- slightly elevated CK-MB level with associated myocarditis

- culture of pericardial fluid obtained by open surgical drainage or pericardiocentesis (which sometimes identifies a causative organism in patients with bacterial or fungal pericarditis).
- Other pertinent laboratory data include a blood urea nitrogen level to check for uremia, an antistreptolysin-O titer to detect rheumatic fever, and a purified protein derivative skin test to check for tuberculosis.
- Electrocardiography shows characteristic changes in patients with acute pericarditis. Such changes include elevated ST segments in the limb leads and most precordial leads. Downsloping PR segments and upright T waves are present in most leads. The QRS complexes may be diminished when pericardial effusion is present. Rhythm changes may also occur, including atrial ectopic rhythms (such as atrial fibrillation) or sinus arrhythmias. In chronic constrictive pericarditis, there may be low-voltage QRS complexes, T-wave inversion or flattening, and P mitral (wide P waves) in leads I, II, and V_6.
- Echocardiography indicates pericardial effusion when it shows an echo-free space between the ventricular wall and the pericardium.
- Chest X-rays may be normal with acute pericarditis. The cardiac silhouette may be enlarged with a water bottle shape caused by fluid accumulation if pleural effusion is present.

Treatment

Appropriate treatment aims to relieve symptoms, manage underlying systemic disease, and prevent or treat pericardial effusion and cardiac tamponade.

In patients with idiopathic pericarditis, postmyocardial infarction pericarditis, or postthoracotomy pericarditis, treatment consists of bed rest as long as fever and pain persist and administration of a nonsteroidal drug, such as aspirin or indomethacin (Indocin), to relieve pain and reduce inflammation. If symptoms continue, the practitioner may prescribe a corticosteroid. Although corticosteroids provide rapid, effective relief, they must be used cautiously because the disorder may recur when drug therapy stops. If an infectious cause is suspected, the patient may be started on antibacterial, antifungal, or antiviral therapy.

When infectious pericarditis results from disease of the left pleural space, mediastinal abscesses, or septicemia, the patient requires an antibiotic, surgical drainage, or both. If cardiac tamponade develops, the practitioner may perform emergency pericardiocentesis and may inject an antibiotic directly into the pericardial sac.

TEACHING THE PATIENT WITH PERICARDITIS

- Explain all tests and treatments to the patient.
- If surgery is necessary, teach the patient how to perform deep-breathing and coughing exercises before he undergoes the procedure.
- Tell the patient to resume his daily activities slowly and to schedule rest periods into his daily routine as instructed by the practitioner.

Recurrent pericarditis may require partial pericardectomy, which creates a window that allows fluid to drain into the pleural space. In patients with constrictive pericarditis, total pericardectomy may be necessary to permit the heart to fill and contract adequately. Treatment must also include management of rheumatic fever, uremia, tuberculosis, and other underlying disorders.

Nursing interventions

- Stress the importance of bed rest. Assist the patient with bathing if necessary. Provide a bedside commode because using a commode puts less stress on the heart than using a bedpan. Offer the patient diversionary, physically undemanding activities.
- Place the patient in an upright position to relieve dyspnea and chest pain.
- Provide an analgesic to relieve pain and oxygen to prevent tissue hypoxia.
- Because cardiac tamponade requires immediate treatment, keep a pericardiocentesis set handy if you suspect pericardial effusion.
- Assess cardiovascular status frequently, watching for signs of cardiac tamponade.
- To reduce anxiety, allow the patient to express his concerns about the effects of activity restrictions on his responsibilities and routines. Reassure him that the restrictions are temporary.
- Before giving an antibiotic, obtain a patient history of allergies. Administer the prescribed antibiotic on time to maintain a consistent level in the blood.
- Observe the venipuncture site for signs of infiltration or inflammation, a possible complication of long-term I.V. administration. To reduce the risk of this complication, rotate venous access sites.
- Provide appropriate postoperative care, similar to that given after cardiothoracic surgery. (See *Teaching the patient with pericarditis*.)

RHEUMATIC FEVER AND RHEUMATIC HEART DISEASE

A systemic inflammatory disease of childhood, acute rheumatic fever develops after infection of the upper respiratory tract with group A beta-hemolytic streptococci.

Rheumatic fever principally involves the heart, joints, central nervous system, skin, and subcutaneous tissues. It commonly recurs.

The term rheumatic heart disease refers to the cardiac involvement of rheumatic fever—its most destructive effect. Cardiac involvement develops in up to 50% of patients and may affect the endocardium, myocardium, or pericardium during the early acute phase. It may later affect the heart valves, causing chronic valvular disease.

Long-term antibiotic therapy can minimize the recurrence of rheumatic fever, reducing the risks of permanent cardiac damage and valvular deformity.

Although rheumatic fever tends to be familial, this tendency may reflect contributing environmental factors. For example, in lower socioeconomic groups, incidence is highest in children ages 5 to 15, probably resulting from malnutrition and crowded living conditions. Rheumatic fever usually strikes during cool, damp weather in winter and early spring. In the United States, it's most common in the northern states.

Pathophysiology

Rheumatic fever appears to be a hypersensitivity reaction to group A beta-hemolytic streptococcal infection. Because few patients with streptococcal infections contract rheumatic fever, altered host resistance must be involved in its development or recurrence. The antigens of group A streptococci bind to receptors in the heart, muscle, brain, and synovial joints, causing an autoimmune response. Because of a similarity between the antigens of the streptococcus bacteria and the antigens of the body's own cells, antibodies may attack healthy body cells by mistake.

Carditis may affect the endocardium, myocardium, or pericardium during the early acute phase. Later, the heart valves may be damaged, causing chronic valvular disease.

The extent of damage to the heart depends on where the disorder strikes. Pericarditis causes a pericardial friction rub and, occasionally, pain and effusion. Myocarditis produces characteristic lesions called Aschoff bodies in the acute stages as well as cellular swelling and fragmentation of interstitial collagen, leading to formation of a progressively fibrotic nodule and interstitial scars. Endocarditis causes valve leaflet swelling, erosion along the lines of leaflet closure, and blood, platelet, and fibrin deposits, which form beadlike vegetation. It usually affects the mitral valve in females and the aortic valve in males; in both, it affects the tricuspid valves occasionally and the pulmonic valve rarely.

Complications
- Destruction of the mitral and aortic valves
- Pancarditis (pericarditis, myocarditis, and endocarditis)
- Heart failure

Assessment findings
- Nearly all affected patients report having a streptococcal infection a few days to 6 weeks earlier.
- They usually have a recent history of low-grade fever that spikes to at least 100.4° F (38° C) late in the afternoon, unexplained epistaxis, and abdominal pain.
- Most patients complain of migratory joint pain (polyarthritis). Swelling, redness, and signs of effusion typically accompany such pain, which usually affects the knees, ankles, elbows, and hips.
- If the patient has pericarditis, he may complain of sharp, sudden pain that usually starts over the sternum and radiates to the neck, shoulders, back, and arms. The pain is usually pleuritic, increases with deep inspiration, and decreases when the patient sits up and leans forward. (This position pulls the heart away from the diaphragmatic pleurae of the lungs.) The pain may mimic that of a myocardial infarction.
- A patient with heart failure caused by severe rheumatic carditis may complain of dyspnea, right upper quadrant pain, and a hacking, nonproductive cough.

  Inspection may reveal skin lesions such as erythema marginatum, a nonpruritic, macular, transient rash. The lesions are red with blanched centers and well-demarcated borders. Lesions typically appear on the trunk and extremities.
- Near tendons or the bony prominences of joints, you may notice subcutaneous nodules that are firm, movable, nontender, and about ⅛″ to ¾″ (0.3 to 2 cm) in diameter. They occur around the elbows, knuckles, wrists, and knees, and less commonly on the scalp and backs of the hands. These nodules persist for a few days to several weeks and, like erythema marginatum, commonly accompany carditis.

- You may notice edema and tachypnea if the patient has left-sided heart failure.
- Up to 6 months after the original streptococcal infection, you may notice transient chorea. Mild chorea may produce hyperirritability, deterioration in handwriting, or inability to concentrate. Severe chorea causes purposeless, nonrepetitive, involuntary muscle spasms and speech disturbances; poor muscle coordination; and weakness. Chorea resolves with rest and causes no residual neurologic damage.
- Palpation may reveal a rapid pulse rate, and auscultation may reveal a pericardial friction rub (a grating sound heard as the heart moves) if the patient has pericarditis. You can hear it best during forced expiration, with the patient leaning forward or on his hands and knees.
- Murmurs and gallops may also occur. With left-sided heart failure, you may hear bibasilar crackles and a ventricular or an atrial gallop. The most common murmurs include:
  – a systolic murmur of mitral insufficiency (a high-pitched, blowing, holosystolic murmur, loudest at apex, possibly radiating to the anterior axillary line)
  – a midsystolic murmur caused by stiffening and swelling of the mitral leaflet
  – occasionally a diastolic murmur of aortic insufficiency (a low-pitched, rumbling, almost inaudible murmur).
- Valvular disease may eventually cause chronic valvular stenosis and insufficiency, including mitral stenosis and insufficiency and aortic insufficiency. In children, mitral insufficiency remains the major effect of rheumatic heart disease.

Diagnostic test results

No specific laboratory tests help determine the presence of rheumatic fever, but the following test results support the diagnosis:

- Jones criteria revealing either two major criteria or one major criterion and two minor criteria, plus evidence of a previous group A streptococcal infection, are necessary for diagnosis. (See *Jones criteria for diagnosing rheumatic fever.*)
- White blood cell count and erythrocyte sedimentation rate may be elevated (during the acute phase); blood studies show slight anemia caused by suppressed erythropoiesis during inflammation.
- C-reactive protein is positive (especially during the acute phase).
- Cardiac enzyme levels may be increased in patients with severe carditis.

JONES CRITERIA FOR DIAGNOSING RHEUMATIC FEVER

The Jones criteria are used to standardize the diagnosis of rheumatic fever. Diagnosis requires that the patient have either two major criteria *or* one major criterion and two minor criteria, plus evidence of a previous streptococcal infection.

Major criteria
- Carditis
- Migratory polyarthritis
- Sydenham's chorea
- Subcutaneous nodules
- Erythema marginatum

Minor criteria
- Fever
- Arthralgia
- Elevated acute phase reactants
- Prolonged PR interval

- Antistreptolysin-O titer is elevated in almost all patients within 2 months of onset. (Rising anti-DNase B test results can also detect recurrent streptococcal infection.)
- Throat cultures may continue to show the presence of group A streptococci; however, they usually occur in small numbers. Isolating them is difficult.
- Electrocardiography reveals no diagnostic changes, but some patients show a prolonged PR interval.
- Chest X-rays show normal heart size, except in patients with myocarditis, heart failure, and pericardial effusion.
- Echocardiography helps evaluate valvular damage, chamber size, ventricular function, and the presence of a pericardial effusion.
- Cardiac catheterization is used to help evaluate valvular damage and left ventricular function in patients with severe cardiac dysfunction.

Treatment

Effective management eradicates the streptococcal infection, relieves symptoms, and prevents recurrence, thus reducing the risk of permanent cardiac damage. During the acute phase, treatment includes penicillin or erythromycin (E-Mycin) (for patients with penicillin hypersensitivity). Salicylates, such as aspirin, relieve fever and minimize joint swelling and pain. If the patient has carditis or if salicylates fail to relieve pain and inflammation, the practitioner may prescribe a corticosteroid.

Supportive treatment requires strict bed rest for about 5 weeks during the acute phase for patients with active carditis, followed by a progressive increase in physical activity. The increase depends on clinical and laboratory findings and the patient's response to treatment.

After the acute phase subsides, a monthly I.M. injection of penicillin G benzathine (Bicillin) or daily doses of oral sulfadiazine (Sulfasalazine) or penicillin G may be used to prevent recurrence. Such preventive treatment usually continues for 5 to 10 years.

Heart failure requires continued bed rest, sodium restriction, digoxin (Lanoxin), an angiotensin-converting enzyme inhibitor, and a diuretic. Severe mitral or aortic valvular dysfunction that causes persistent heart failure requires corrective surgery, such as commissurotomy, valvuloplasty, or valve replacement. Corrective valvular surgery seldom is necessary before late adolescence.

Nursing interventions

- Before giving penicillin, ask the patient (or, if the patient is a child, his parents) if he has ever had a hypersensitivity reaction to it. Even if he hasn't, warn him that such a reaction is possible.
- Administer the prescribed antibiotic on time to maintain a consistent drug level in the blood.
- Stress the importance of bed rest. Assist with bathing as necessary. Provide a bedside commode because using a commode puts less stress on the heart than using a bedpan. Offer the patient diversionary, physically undemanding activities.
- Place the patient in an upright position to relieve dyspnea and chest pain if needed.
- Provide an analgesic to relieve pain and oxygen to prevent tissue hypoxia as needed.
- To reduce anxiety, allow the patient to express his concerns about the effects of activity restrictions on his responsibilities and routines. Reassure him that the restrictions are temporary.
- If the patient's status is unstable because of chorea, clear his environment of objects that could make him fall.
- After the acute phase, encourage the patient's family and friends to spend as much time as possible with the patient to minimize his boredom. Advise parents to secure a tutor to help their child keep up with schoolwork during the long convalescence.
- Help the parents overcome any guilt feelings they may have about their child's illness. Failure to seek treatment for streptococcal infection is common because the illness may seem no worse than a cold.

TEACHING THE PATIENT WITH RHEUMATIC FEVER AND RHEUMATIC HEART DISEASE

● Explain all tests and treatments to the patient.

● Tell the patient to resume activities of daily living slowly and to schedule rest periods in his routine, as instructed by the practitioner.

● Tell the parents or patient to stop penicillin therapy and call the physician immediately if the patient develops a rash, fever, chills, or other signs or symptoms of an allergic reaction.

● Instruct the patient and family to watch for and report early signs and symptoms of left-sided heart failure, such as dyspnea and a hacking, nonproductive cough.

● Teach the patient and family about this disease and its treatment. Warn the parents to watch for and immediately report signs and symptoms of recurrent streptococcal infection: sudden sore throat, diffuse throat redness and oropharyngeal exudate, swollen and tender cervical lymph glands, pain on swallowing, temperature of 101° to 104° F (38.3° to 40° C), headache, and nausea. Urge them to keep the child away from people with respiratory tract infections.

● Help the patient's family understand the frustrations associated with chorea (such as nervousness, restlessness, poor coordination, weakness, and inattentiveness). Emphasize that these effects are transient.

● Make sure the patient and his family understand the need to comply with prolonged antibiotic therapy and follow-up care. Arrange for a visiting nurse to oversee home care if necessary.

● Explain that an antibiotic must be given prophylactically before any dental work or other invasive procedure.

■ Encourage the parents and the child to vent their frustrations during the long, tedious recovery. If the child has severe carditis, help them prepare for permanent changes in the child's lifestyle. (See *Teaching the patient with rheumatic fever and rheumatic heart disease.*)

Valvular disorders

AORTIC INSUFFICIENCY

Aortic insufficiency by itself occurs most commonly in men. When associated with mitral valve disease, however, it's more common in women. This disorder may also be associated with Marfan syndrome, ankylosing spondylitis, syphilis, essential hypertension, and a ventricular septal defect, even after surgical closure.

Pathophysiology

In patients with aortic insufficiency (also called *aortic regurgitation*), blood flows back into the left ventricle during diastole. The ventricle becomes overloaded, dilated, and eventually hypertrophies. The excess fluid volume also overloads the left atrium and, eventually, the pulmonary system.

Aortic insufficiency results from rheumatic fever, syphilis, hypertension, endocarditis, or trauma. In some patients, it may be idiopathic.

Complications
- Left-sided heart failure
- Fatal pulmonary edema resulting from fever, infection, or cardiac arrhythmia
- Myocardial ischemia (left ventricular dilation and elevated left ventricular systolic pressure alter myocardial oxygen requirements)

Assessment findings
- A patient with chronic severe aortic insufficiency may report that he has an uncomfortable awareness of his heartbeat, especially when lying down on his left side.
- He may report palpitations along with a pounding head.

IDENTIFYING THE MURMUR OF AORTIC INSUFFICIENCY

A high-pitched, blowing decrescendo murmur that radiates from the aortic valve area to the left sternal border characterizes aortic insufficiency.

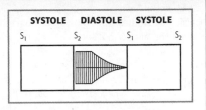

- The patient may experience exertional dyspnea and paroxysmal nocturnal dyspnea with diaphoresis, orthopnea, and cough.
- He may become fatigued and syncopal with exertion or emotion.
- He may also have a history of angina unrelieved by sublingual nitroglycerin.
- On inspection, you may note that each heartbeat seems to jar the patient's entire body and that his head bobs with each systole.
- Inspection of arterial pulsations shows a rapidly rising pulse that collapses suddenly as arterial pressure falls late in systole.
- The patient's nail beds may appear to be pulsating. If you apply pressure at the nail tip, the root will alternately flush and pale.
- Inspection of the chest may reveal a visible apical pulse.
- If the patient has left-sided heart failure, he may have ankle edema and ascites.
- When palpating the peripheral pulses, you may note rapidly rising and collapsing pulses (called *pulsus biferiens*). If the patient has cardiac arrhythmias, pulses may be irregular. You'll be able to feel the apical impulse. (The apex is displaced laterally and inferiorly.) A diastolic thrill probably is palpable along the left sternal border, and you may be able to feel a prominent systolic thrill in the jugular notch and along the carotid arteries.
- Auscultation may reveal an S_3, occasionally an S_4, and a loud systolic ejection sound. A high-pitched, blowing, decrescendo diastolic murmur is best heard at the left sternal border, at the third intercostal space. Use the diaphragm of the stethoscope to hear it, and have the patient sit up, lean forward, and hold his breath in forced expiration. (See *Identifying the murmur of aortic insufficiency*.)

- You may also hear a grade 5 or 6 midsystolic ejection murmur at the base of the heart, typically higher pitched, shorter, and less rasping than the murmur heard in aortic stenosis.
- Another murmur that may occur is a soft, low-pitched, rumbling, middiastolic or presystolic bruit; this murmur is best heard at the base of the heart.
- Place the stethoscope lightly over the femoral artery to hear a booming, pistol-shot sound and a to-and-fro murmur.
- Arterial pulse pressure is widened.
- Auscultating blood pressure may be difficult because you can hear the patient's pulse after you inflate the cuff. To determine systolic pressure, note when Korotkoff sounds begin to muffle.

Diagnostic test results

- Cardiac catheterization shows reduced arterial diastolic pressures, aortic insufficiency, other valvular abnormalities, and increased left ventricular end-diastolic pressure.
- Chest X-rays display left ventricular enlargement and pulmonary vein congestion.
- Echocardiography reveals left ventricular enlargement, dilation of the aortic annulus and left atrium, and thickening of the aortic valve. It also reveals a rapid, high-frequency fluttering of the anterior mitral leaflet that results from the impact of aortic insufficiency.
- Electrocardiography shows sinus tachycardia, left ventricular hypertrophy, and left atrial hypertrophy in patients with severe disease. ST-segment depressions and T-wave inversions appear in leads I, aV_L, V_5, and V_6 and indicate left ventricular strain.

Treatment

Valve replacement is the treatment of choice and should be performed before significant ventricular dysfunction occurs. This may be impossible, however, because signs and symptoms seldom occur until after myocardial dysfunction develops.

A cardiac glycoside, a low-sodium diet, a diuretic, a vasodilator and, especially, an angiotensin-converting enzyme inhibitor are used to treat patients with left-sided heart failure. For acute episodes, supplemental oxygen may be necessary.

Nursing interventions

- If the patient needs bed rest, stress its importance. Assist with bathing if necessary. Provide a bedside commode because using a

DISCHARGE TEACHING

TEACHING THE PATIENT WITH AORTIC INSUFFICIENCY

- Advise the patient to plan for periodic rest in his daily routine to prevent undue fatigue.
- Teach the patient about diet restrictions, drugs, signs and symptoms that should be reported, and the importance of consistent follow-up care.
- Tell the patient to elevate his legs whenever he sits.

commode puts less stress on the heart than using a bedpan. Offer the patient diversionary, physically undemanding activities.

- Alternate periods of activity with periods of rest to prevent extreme fatigue and dyspnea.
- To reduce anxiety, allow the patient to express his concerns about the effects of activity restrictions on his responsibilities and routines. Reassure him that the restrictions are temporary.
- Keep the patient's legs elevated while he sits in a chair to improve venous return to the heart.
- Place the patient in an upright position to relieve dyspnea, if necessary, and administer oxygen to prevent tissue hypoxia.
- Keep the patient on a low-sodium diet. Consult a dietitian to ensure that the patient receives foods that he likes while adhering to diet restrictions. (See *Teaching the patient with aortic insufficiency*.)
- Monitor the patient for signs of heart failure, pulmonary edema, and adverse reactions to drug therapy.

 RED FLAG If the patient undergoes surgery, watch for hypotension, arrhythmias, and thrombus formation.

- Monitor his vital signs, arterial blood gas level, intake and output, daily weight, blood chemistry results, chest X-ray, and pulmonary artery catheter readings.

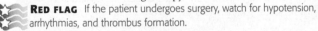

AORTIC STENOSIS

Aortic stenosis is hardening of the aortic valve or of the aorta itself. About 80% of patients with aortic stenosis are male.

AGE AWARE Signs and symptoms of aortic stenosis may not appear until the patient reaches ages 50 to 70, even though the lesion has been present since childhood. Incidence increases with age. Aortic stenosis is the most significant valvular lesion seen among elderly people.

Pathophysiology

In aortic stenosis, the opening of the aortic valve narrows, and the left ventricle exerts increased pressure to drive blood through the opening. The added workload increases the demand for oxygen, and diminished cardiac output reduces coronary artery perfusion, causes ischemia of the left ventricle, and leads to heart failure.

Aortic stenosis may result from congenital aortic bicuspid valve (from coarctation of the aorta), congenital stenosis of pulmonic valve cusps, rheumatic fever or, in elderly patients, atherosclerosis.

Complications

- Left-sided heart failure, usually after age 70, within 4 years after the onset of signs and symptoms; fatal in up to two-thirds of patients
- Sudden death, usually around age 60, in 20% of patients, possibly caused by an arrhythmia

Assessment findings

- Even with severe aortic stenosis (narrowing to about one-third of the normal opening), the patient may be asymptomatic.
- The patient may complain of exertional dyspnea, fatigue, exertional syncope, angina, and palpitations.
- If left-sided heart failure develops, the patient may complain of orthopnea and paroxysmal nocturnal dyspnea.
- Inspection may reveal peripheral edema if the patient has left-sided heart failure.
- Palpation may detect diminished carotid pulses and alternating pulses. If the patient has left-sided heart failure, the apex of the heart may be displaced inferiorly and laterally. If the patient has pulmonary hypertension, you may be able to palpate a systolic thrill at the base of the heart, at the jugular notch, and along the carotid arteries. Occasionally, it may be palpable only during expiration and when the patient leans forward.
- Auscultation may uncover an early systolic ejection murmur in children and adolescents who have noncalcified valves. The murmur begins shortly after S_1 and increases in intensity to reach a peak toward the middle of the ejection period. It diminishes just before the aortic valve closes. (See *Identifying the murmur of aortic stenosis.*)

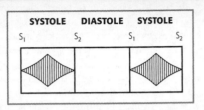

IDENTIFYING THE MURMUR OF AORTIC STENOSIS

A low-pitched, harsh crescendo-decrescendo murmur that radiates from the aortic valve area to the carotid artery characterizes aortic stenosis.

- The murmur is low-pitched, rough, and rasping and is loudest at the base at the second intercostal space. In patients with stenosis, the murmur is at least grade 3 or 4. It disappears when the valve calcifies. A split S_2 develops as aortic stenosis becomes more severe. An S_4 reflects left ventricular hypertrophy and may be heard at the apex in patients with severe aortic stenosis.

Diagnostic test results

- Cardiac catheterization reveals the pressure gradient across the valve (indicating the severity of the obstruction), increased left ventricular end-diastolic pressures (indicating left ventricular function), and the location of the left ventricular outflow obstruction.
- Chest X-rays show valvular calcification, left ventricular enlargement, pulmonary vein congestion and, in later stages, left atrial, pulmonary arterial, right atrial, and right ventricular enlargement.
- Echocardiography demonstrates a thickened aortic valve and left ventricular wall and, possibly, coexistent mitral valve stenosis.
- Electrocardiography reveals left ventricular hypertrophy. In advanced stages, the patient exhibits ST-segment depression and T-wave inversion in standard leads I and aV_L and in the left precordial leads. Up to 10% of patients have atrioventricular and intraventricular conduction defects.

Treatment

A cardiac glycoside, a low-sodium diet, a diuretic and, for acute cases, oxygen are used to treat patients with heart failure. Nitroglycerin helps to relieve angina.

AGE AWARE For children who don't have calcified valves, simple commissurotomy under direct visualization is usually effective.

Adults with calcified valves need valve replacement when they become symptomatic or are at risk for developing left-sided heart failure.

Percutaneous balloon aortic valvuloplasty is useful in a child or young adult with congenital aortic stenosis and in an elderly patient with severe calcifications. This procedure may improve left ventricular function so the patient can tolerate valve replacement surgery.

A Ross procedure is usually performed in patients younger than age 55. During this procedure, the pulmonic valve is used to replace the aortic valve, and the pulmonic valve of a cadaver is inserted. This allows longer valve life and makes anticoagulant therapy unnecessary.

Nursing interventions

- If the patient needs bed rest, stress its importance. Assist the patient with bathing if necessary; provide a bedside commode because using a commode puts less stress on the heart than using a bedpan. Offer the patient diversionary, physically undemanding activities.
- Alternate periods of activity with periods of rest to prevent extreme fatigue and dyspnea.
- To reduce anxiety, allow the patient to express his concerns about the effects of activity restrictions on his responsibilities and routines. Reassure him that the restrictions are temporary.
- Keep the patient's legs elevated while he sits in a chair to improve venous return to the heart.
- Place the patient in an upright position to relieve dyspnea, if needed. Administer oxygen to prevent tissue hypoxia, as needed.
- Keep the patient on a low-sodium diet. Consult with a dietitian to ensure that the patient receives foods that he likes while adhering to diet restrictions. (See *Teaching the patient with aortic stenosis*.)
- Monitor the patient for signs of heart failure, pulmonary edema, and adverse reactions to drug therapy.
- Allow the patient to express his fears and concerns about the disorder, its impact on his life, and any upcoming surgery. Reassure him as needed.
- After cardiac catheterization, apply firm pressure to the catheter insertion site, usually in the groin. Monitor the site every 15 minutes for at least 6 hours for signs of bleeding. If the site bleeds, remove the pressure dressing and apply firm pressure.

- Notify the practitioner of any changes in peripheral pulses distal to the insertion site, changes in cardiac rhythm and vital signs, and complaints of chest pain.

  RED FLAG If the patient has surgery, watch for hypotension, arrhythmias, and thrombus formation.

- Monitor vital signs, arterial blood gas levels, intake and output, daily weight, blood chemistry results, chest X-rays, and pulmonary artery catheter readings.

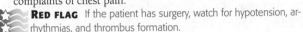

MITRAL INSUFFICIENCY

Mitral insufficiency—also known as *mitral regurgitation*—occurs when a damaged mitral valve allows blood from the left ventricle to flow back into the left atrium during systole.

Pathophysiology

In mitral insufficiency, blood from the left ventricle flows back into the left atrium during systole. As a result, the atrium enlarges to accommodate the backflow. The left ventricle also dilates to accommodate the increased volume of blood from the atrium and to compensate for diminishing cardiac output.

Mitral insufficiency tends to be progressive because left ventricular dilation increases the insufficiency, which further enlarges the left atrium and ventricle, which further increases the insufficiency.

Damage to the mitral valve can result from rheumatic fever, hypertrophic cardiomyopathy, mitral valve prolapse, a myocardial infarction, severe left-sided heart failure, or ruptured chordae tendineae.

In older patients, mitral insufficiency may occur because the mitral annulus has become calcified. The cause is unknown, but it may

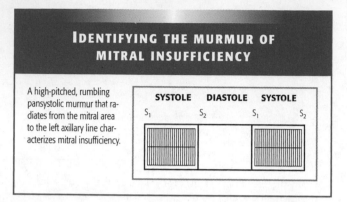

IDENTIFYING THE MURMUR OF MITRAL INSUFFICIENCY

A high-pitched, rumbling pansystolic murmur that radiates from the mitral area to the left axillary line characterizes mitral insufficiency.

be linked to a degenerative process. Mitral insufficiency is sometimes associated with congenital anomalies such as transposition of the great arteries.

Complications

- Left- and right-sided heart failure with pulmonary edema and cardiovascular collapse, resulting from ventricular hypertrophy and increased end-diastolic pressure

Assessment findings

- Depending on the severity of the disorder, the patient may be asymptomatic or complain of orthopnea, exertional dyspnea, fatigue, weakness, weight loss, chest pain, and palpitations.
- Inspection may reveal jugular vein distention with an abnormally prominent *a* wave. You may also note peripheral edema.
- Auscultation may detect a soft S_1 that may be buried in the systolic murmur. A grade 3 to 6 or louder holosystolic murmur, most characteristic of mitral insufficiency, is best heard at the apex.
- You also hear a split S_2 and a low-pitched S_3. The S_3 may be followed by a short, rumbling diastolic murmur. An S_4 may be evident in patients who have experienced a recent onset of severe mitral insufficiency and who are in normal sinus rhythm. (See *Identifying the murmur of mitral insufficiency*.)
- Auscultation of the lungs may reveal crackles if the patient has pulmonary edema.
- Palpation of the chest may disclose a regular pulse rate with a sharp upstroke. You can probably palpate a systolic thrill at the apex. In

patients with marked pulmonary hypertension, you may be able to palpate a right ventricular tap and the shock of the pulmonic valve closing. When the left atrium is markedly enlarged, it may be palpable along the sternal border late during ventricular systole. It resembles a right ventricular lift.

■ Abdominal palpation may reveal hepatomegaly if the patient has right-sided heart failure.

Diagnostic test results

■ Cardiac catheterization is used to detect mitral insufficiency with increased left ventricular end-diastolic volume and pressure, increased left atrial and pulmonary artery wedge pressures, and decreased cardiac output.

■ Chest X-rays demonstrate left atrial and ventricular enlargement, pulmonary vein congestion, and calcification of the mitral leaflets in patients with long-standing mitral insufficiency and stenosis.

■ Echocardiography reveals abnormal motion of the valve leaflets, left atrial enlargement, and a hyperdynamic left ventricle.

■ Electrocardiography may show left atrial and ventricular hypertrophy, sinus tachycardia, and atrial fibrillation.

Treatment

The nature and severity of associated symptoms determine treatment for a patient with valvular heart disease. For example, he may need to restrict activities to avoid extreme fatigue and dyspnea.

Heart failure requires digoxin (Lanoxin), a diuretic, a sodium-restricted diet and, for acute cases, oxygen. Other appropriate measures include anticoagulant therapy to prevent thrombus formation around diseased or replaced valves and a prophylactic antibiotic before and after surgery or dental care.

If the patient has severe signs and symptoms that can't be managed medically, he may need open-heart surgery with cardiopulmonary bypass for valve replacement.

 AGE AWARE Valvuloplasty may be used for elderly patients who have end-stage disease and can't tolerate general anesthesia.

Nursing interventions

■ Provide rest periods between periods of activity to prevent excessive fatigue.

■ To reduce anxiety, allow the patient to express his concerns about the effects of activity restrictions on his responsibilities and routines. Reassure him that the restrictions are temporary.

TEACHING THE PATIENT WITH MITRAL INSUFFICIENCY

- Teach the patient about diet restrictions, drugs, signs and symptoms that should be reported, and the importance of consistent follow-up care.
- Explain all tests and treatments.
- Make sure the patient and his family understand the need to comply with prolonged antibiotic therapy and follow-up care, and the need for an additional antibiotic during dental procedures.
- Tell the parents or patient to stop the drug and call the practitioner immediately if the patient develops a rash, fever, chills, or other signs or symptoms of allergy at any time during penicillin therapy.
- Instruct the patient and his family to watch for and report early signs and symptoms of heart failure, such as dyspnea and a hacking, unproductive cough.

- Keep the patient on a low-sodium diet; consult with the dietitian to ensure that the patient receives as many favorite foods as possible during diet restrictions. (See *Teaching the patient with mitral insufficiency*.)
- Monitor the patient for left-sided heart failure, pulmonary edema, and adverse reactions to drug therapy. Provide oxygen to prevent tissue hypoxia, as needed.
- If the patient has surgery, monitor him postoperatively for hypotension, arrhythmias, and thrombus formation.
- Monitor the patient's vital signs, arterial blood gas level, intake and output, daily weight, blood chemistry results, chest X-ray, and pulmonary artery catheter readings.

RED FLAG Before giving penicillin, ask the patient or his parents if he has ever had a hypersensitivity reaction to it. Even if he hasn't, warn that such a reaction is possible. Give the ordered antibiotic on time to maintain a consistent drug level in the blood.

MITRAL STENOSIS

Mitral stenosis is the hardening of the mitral valve. Two-thirds of all patients with mitral stenosis are women.

Pathophysiology

In patients with mitral stenosis, valve leaflets become diffusely thickened by fibrosis and calcification. The mitral commissures fuse, the chordae tendineae fuse and shorten, the valvular cusps become rigid, and the apex of the valve becomes narrowed, obstructing blood flow from the left atrium to the left ventricle.

As a result of these changes, left atrial volume and pressure increase and the atrial chamber dilates. The increased resistance to blood flow causes pulmonary hypertension, right ventricular hypertrophy and, eventually, right-sided heart failure. Also, inadequate filling of the left ventricle reduces cardiac output.

Mitral stenosis most commonly results from rheumatic fever. It may also be associated with congenital anomalies.

Complications

- Rupture of pulmonary-bronchial venous connections, causing hemorrhage
- Fibrosis in the alveoli and pulmonary capillaries resulting from increased transudation of fluid from pulmonary capillaries and reduced vital capacity, total lung capacity, maximal breathing capacity, and oxygen uptake per unit of ventilation
- Thrombi in the left atrium, embolizing and traveling to the brain, kidneys, spleen, and extremities, possibly causing infarction; most common in patients with arrhythmias

Assessment findings

- Patients with mild mitral stenosis may have no symptoms.
- Those with moderate to severe mitral stenosis may have a history of exertional dyspnea, paroxysmal nocturnal dyspnea, orthopnea, weakness, fatigue, and palpitations.
- A dry cough and dysphagia may occur because of an enlarged left atrium or bronchus.
- Hemoptysis suggests rupture of pulmonary-bronchial venous connections.
- Inspection may reveal peripheral and facial cyanosis, particularly in severe cases. The patient's face may appear pinched and blue, and she may have a malar rash. You may note jugular vein distention and ascites in the patient with severe pulmonary hypertension or associated tricuspid stenosis.
- Palpation may reveal peripheral edema, hepatomegaly, and a diastolic thrill at the cardiac apex.

IDENTIFYING THE MURMUR OF MITRAL STENOSIS

A low, rumbling crescendo-decrescendo murmur in the mitral valve area characterizes mitral stenosis.

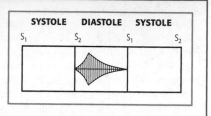

- Auscultation may reveal a loud S_1 or opening snap and a diastolic murmur at the apex, along the left sternal border or at the base of the heart. (See *Identifying the murmur of mitral stenosis*.)
- In patients with pulmonary hypertension, the S_2 is commonly accentuated, and the two components of the S_2 are closely split. A pulmonary systolic ejection click may be heard in patients with severe pulmonary hypertension. Crackles may be heard when the lungs are auscultated.
- Because mitral insufficiency is a form of heart disease, the practitioner may need to differentiate it from other forms of valvular heart disease.

Diagnostic test results

- Cardiac catheterization shows a diastolic pressure gradient across the valve. It also shows elevated pulmonary artery wedge pressure (greater than 15 mm Hg) and pulmonary artery pressure in the left atrium with severe pulmonary hypertension. It detects elevated right ventricular pressure, decreased cardiac output, and abnormal contraction of the left ventricle. However, this test may not be indicated for patients who have isolated mitral stenosis with mild symptoms.
- Chest X-rays show left atrial and ventricular enlargement (in patients with severe mitral stenosis), straightening of the left border of the cardiac silhouette, enlarged pulmonary arteries, dilation of the upper lobe pulmonary veins, and mitral valve calcification.
- Echocardiography discloses thickened mitral valve leaflets and left atrial enlargement.

- Electrocardiography reveals left atrial enlargement, right ventricular hypertrophy, right axis deviation and, in about half of cases, atrial fibrillation.

Treatment

Treatment for patients with valvular heart disease depends on the nature and severity of associated symptoms. In a young patient with asymptomatic mitral stenosis, penicillin is an important prophylactic.

If the patient is symptomatic, treatment varies. Heart failure requires bed rest, digoxin (Lanoxin), a diuretic, a sodium-restricted diet and, for acute cases, oxygen. Small doses of a beta-adrenergic receptor blocker may also be used to slow the ventricular rate when digoxin fails to control atrial fibrillation or flutter. Synchronized cardioversion may be used to correct atrial fibrillation in a patient whose status is unstable.

If hemoptysis develops, the patient requires bed rest, a sodium-restricted diet, and a diuretic to decrease pulmonary venous pressure. Embolization mandates an anticoagulant along with symptomatic treatments.

A patient with severe, medically uncontrollable symptoms may need open-heart surgery with cardiopulmonary bypass for commissurotomy or valve replacement.

Percutaneous balloon valvuloplasty may be used in young patients who have no calcification or subvalvular deformity, in symptomatic pregnant women, and in elderly patients with end-stage disease who can't tolerate general anesthesia. This procedure is performed in the cardiac catheterization laboratory.

Nursing interventions

- Before giving penicillin, ask the patient if she has ever had a hypersensitivity reaction to it. Even if she hasn't, warn her that such a reaction is possible.
- If the patient needs bed rest, stress its importance. Assist with bathing as necessary. Provide a bedside commode because using a commode puts less stress on the heart than using a bedpan. Offer the patient diversionary, physically undemanding activities.
- To reduce anxiety, allow the patient to express concerns over her inability to meet her responsibilities because of activity restrictions. Give reassurance that activity limitations are temporary.
- Watch closely for signs of heart failure, pulmonary edema, and adverse reactions to drug therapy.

DISCHARGE TEACHING

TEACHING THE PATIENT WITH MITRAL STENOSIS

- Explain all tests and treatments to the patient.
- Advise the patient to plan for periodic rest in her daily routine to prevent undue fatigue.
- Teach the patient about diet restrictions, medications, signs and symptoms that should be reported, and the importance of consistent follow-up care.
- Make sure the patient and her family understand the need to comply with prolonged antibiotic therapy and follow-up care, and the need for an additional antibiotic during dental or other surgical procedures.

■ Place the patient in an upright position to relieve dyspnea, if needed. Administer oxygen to prevent tissue hypoxia as needed.

■ If the patient has had surgery, watch for hypotension, arrhythmias, and thrombus formation. Monitor her vital signs, arterial blood gas level, intake and output, daily weight, blood chemistry results, chest X-ray, and pulmonary artery catheter readings.

■ Keep the patient on a low-sodium diet; provide as many favorite foods as possible. (See *Teaching the patient with mitral stenosis*.)

PULMONIC INSUFFICIENCY

Pulmonic insufficiency is the leaking of the pulmonic valve, which lets blood flow back into the right ventricle.

Pathophysiology

In patients with pulmonic insufficiency, blood ejected into the pulmonary artery during systole flows back into the right ventricle during diastole, causing fluid overload in the ventricle, ventricular hypertrophy, and eventual right-sided heart failure.

Pulmonic insufficiency may be congenital or may result from pulmonary hypertension. The most common acquired cause is dilation of the pulmonic valve ring from severe pulmonary hypertension.

Rarely, pulmonic insufficiency may result from prolonged use of a pressure-monitoring catheter in the pulmonary artery.

Complications

■ Right-sided heart failure possible with pulmonary hypertension

IDENTIFYING THE MURMUR OF PULMONIC INSUFFICIENCY

A high-pitched, blowing decrescendo murmur at Erb's point characterizes pulmonic insufficiency.

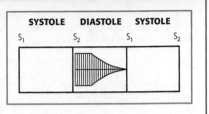

Assessment findings

- The patient may complain of exertional dyspnea, fatigue, chest pain, and syncope.
- Peripheral edema may cause him discomfort.
- A patient with severe insufficiency that progresses to right-sided heart failure may appear jaundiced with severe peripheral edema and ascites. He may also appear malnourished.
- Auscultation may reveal a high-pitched, decrescendo, diastolic blowing murmur along the left sternal border. This murmur may be difficult to distinguish from the murmur of aortic insufficiency. (See *Identifying the murmur of pulmonic insufficiency*.)
- Palpation may disclose hepatomegaly if the patient has right-sided heart failure.

Diagnostic test results

- Cardiac catheterization shows pulmonic insufficiency, increased right ventricular pressure, and associated cardiac defects.
- Chest X-rays show right ventricular and pulmonary arterial enlargement.
- Echocardiography can be used to visualize the pulmonic valve abnormality.
- Electrocardiography findings may be normal in mild cases or reveal right ventricular hypertrophy.

Treatment

Treatment is based on the patient's symptoms. A low-sodium diet and a diuretic helps to reduce hepatic congestion before surgery. Valvulotomy or valve replacement may be required in severe cases.

DISCHARGE TEACHING

TEACHING THE PATIENT WITH PULMONIC INSUFFICIENCY

- Teach the patient about diet restrictions, drugs, signs and symptoms that should be reported, and the importance of consistent follow up care.
- Tell the patient to elevate his legs whenever he sits.

Nursing interventions

- Alternate periods of activity and rest to prevent extreme fatigue and dyspnea.
- Keep the patient's legs elevated while he sits in a chair to improve venous return to the heart.
- Elevate the head of the bed to improve ventilation.
- Keep the patient on a low-sodium diet. Consult with a dietitian to ensure that the patient receives foods that he likes while adhering to diet restrictions. (See *Teaching the patient with pulmonic insufficiency*.)
- Monitor the patient for signs of heart failure, pulmonary edema, and adverse reactions to drug therapy.
- To reduce anxiety, allow the patient to express his concerns about the effects of activity restrictions on his responsibilities and routines. Reassure him that the restrictions are temporary.
- If the patient has surgery, watch for hypotension, arrhythmias, and thrombus formation. Monitor his vital signs, arterial blood gas level, intake and output, daily weight, blood chemistry results, chest X-ray, and pulmonary artery catheter readings.

PULMONIC STENOSIS

Pulmonic stenosis is a hardening or narrowing of the opening between the pulmonary artery and right ventricle. A congenital defect, pulmonic stenosis is associated with other congenital heart defects such as tetralogy of Fallot. It's rare among elderly patients.

IDENTIFYING THE MURMUR OF PULMONIC STENOSIS

A medium-pitched, harsh crescendo-decrescendo murmur in the area of the pulmonic valve characterizes pulmonic stenosis.

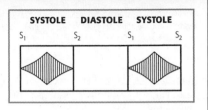

Pathophysiology

In patients with pulmonic stenosis, obstructed right ventricular outflow causes right ventricular hypertrophy as the right ventricle attempts to overcome resistance to the narrow valvular opening.

Pulmonic stenosis results from congenital stenosis of the pulmonic valve cusp or, infrequently, from rheumatic heart disease or cancer.

Complications

- Right-sided heart failure resulting from untreated pulmonic stenosis

Assessment findings

- Depending on the severity of the obstruction, the patient with mild stenosis may be asymptomatic.
- A patient with moderate to severe stenosis may complain of exertional dyspnea, fatigue, chest pain, and syncope. Accompanying peripheral edema may cause him discomfort.
- Inspection may reveal a prominent *a* wave in the jugular venous pulse.
- If severe stenosis has progressed to right-sided heart failure, the patient may appear jaundiced with severe peripheral edema and ascites. He may also appear malnourished.
- Auscultation may reveal an S_4, a thrill at the upper left sternal border, a harsh systolic ejection murmur, and a holosystolic decrescendo murmur of tricuspid insufficiency, particularly if the patient has heart failure. (See *Identifying the murmur of pulmonic stenosis*.)

DISCHARGE TEACHING

TEACHING THE PATIENT WITH PULMONIC STENOSIS

● Teach the patient about diet restrictions, drugs, signs and symptoms that should be reported, and the importance of consistent follow-up care.
● Teach the patient to elevate his legs when sitting.

■ Palpation may detect hepatomegaly if the patient has right-sided heart failure, presystolic pulsations of the liver, and a right parasternal lift.

Diagnostic test results

■ Chest X-rays usually show normal heart size and lung vascularity, although the pulmonary arteries may be evident. With severe obstruction and right-sided heart failure, the right atrium and ventricle typically appear enlarged.
■ Echocardiography can be used to visualize the pulmonic valve abnormality.
■ Electrocardiography results may be normal in mild cases, or they may show right-axis deviation and right ventricular hypertrophy. High-amplitude P waves in leads II and VI indicate right atrial enlargement.

Treatment

A low-sodium diet and a diuretic help reduce hepatic congestion before surgery. Also, cardiac catheter balloon valvuloplasty is usually effective, even with moderate to severe obstruction.

Nursing interventions

■ Alternate periods of activity with periods of rest to prevent extreme fatigue and dyspnea.
■ Keep the patient's legs elevated while he sits in a chair to improve venous return to the heart.
■ Elevate the head of the bed to improve ventilation.
■ Keep the patient on a low-sodium diet. Consult with a dietitian to ensure that the patient receives foods that he likes while adhering to diet restrictions. (See *Teaching the patient with pulmonic stenosis.*)
■ Monitor the patient for signs of heart failure, pulmonary edema, and adverse reactions to drug therapy.

- To reduce anxiety, allow the patient to express his concerns about the effects of activity restrictions on his responsibilities and routines. Reassure him that the restrictions are temporary.
- After cardiac catheterization, apply firm pressure to the catheter insertion site, usually in the groin. Monitor the site for signs of bleeding every 15 minutes for at least 6 hours. If the site bleeds, remove the pressure dressing and manually apply firm pressure to the site.
- Notify the practitioner of changes in peripheral pulses distal to the insertion site, changes in cardiac rhythm and vital signs, and complaints of chest pain.

TRICUSPID INSUFFICIENCY

Tricuspid insufficiency occurs when the tricuspid valve doesn't close completely, allowing blood to flow back into the right atrium.

Pathophysiology

In patients with tricuspid insufficiency (also known as *tricuspid regurgitation*), an incompetent tricuspid valve allows blood to flow back into the right atrium during systole, decreasing blood flow to the lungs and left side of the heart. Cardiac output also decreases.

Tricuspid insufficiency results from marked dilation of the right ventricle and tricuspid valve ring. It most commonly occurs in the late stages of heart failure because of rheumatic or congenital heart disease.

Less commonly, it results from congenitally deformed tricuspid valves, atrioventricular canal defects, or Ebstein's malformation of the tricuspid valve. Other causes include infarction of the right ventricular papillary muscles, tricuspid valve prolapse, carcinoid heart disease, endomyocardial fibrosis, infective endocarditis, and trauma.

Complications

- Right-sided heart failure possible if fluid overload in right side of heart

Assessment findings

- The patient may have a history of a disorder that can cause tricuspid insufficiency.
- The patient may complain of dyspnea, fatigue, weakness, and syncope.
- Peripheral edema may cause him discomfort.

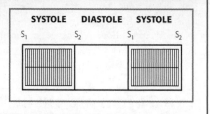

IDENTIFYING THE MURMUR OF TRICUSPID INSUFFICIENCY

A high-pitched, blowing holosystolic murmur in the tricuspid area characterizes tricuspid insufficiency.

- Inspection may reveal jugular vein distention with prominent *v* waves in a patient with normal sinus rhythm.
- A patient with severe tricuspid insufficiency that has progressed to right-sided heart failure may appear jaundiced, with severe peripheral edema and ascites.
- Auscultation may disclose a blowing holosystolic murmur at the lower left sternal border that increases with inspiration and decreases with expiration and Valsalva's maneuver. (See *Identifying the murmur of tricuspid insufficiency.*)
- Palpation may reveal hepatomegaly when the patient has right-sided heart failure, systolic pulsations of the liver, and a positive hepatojugular reflex. You may also feel a prominent right ventricular pulsation along the left parasternal region.

Diagnostic test results
- Cardiac catheterization demonstrates markedly decreased cardiac output. The right atrial pressure pulse may exhibit no *x* descent during early systole, but instead a prominent *c-v* wave with a rapid *y* descent. The mean right atrial and right ventricular end-diastolic pressures typically are elevated.
- Chest X-rays show right atrial and ventricular enlargement.
- Echocardiography reveals right ventricular dilation and prolapse or flailing of the tricuspid leaflets.
- Electrocardiography discloses right atrial hypertrophy, right or left ventricular hypertrophy, atrial fibrillation, and incomplete right bundle-branch block.

Treatment

A sodium-restricted diet and a diuretic help reduce hepatic congestion before surgery. When rheumatic fever has deformed the tricuspid valve, resulting in severe insufficiency, the patient usually needs open-heart surgery for tricuspid annuloplasty or tricuspid valve replacement.

Nursing interventions

- Alternate periods of activity with rest periods to prevent extreme fatigue and dyspnea.
- Keep the patient's legs elevated while he's sitting to improve venous return to the heart.
- Elevate the head of the bed to improve ventilation.
- Maintain a low-sodium diet. Consult with a dietitian to ensure that the patient receives foods that he likes while adhering to diet restrictions. (See *Teaching the patient with tricuspid insufficiency*.)
- Monitor the patient for signs of heart failure, pulmonary edema, and adverse reactions to drug therapy.
- To reduce anxiety, allow the patient to express his concerns about the effects of activity restrictions on his responsibilities and routines. Reassure him that the restrictions are temporary.
- If the patient has surgery, watch for hypotension, arrhythmias, and thrombus formation. Monitor his vital signs, arterial blood gas level, intake and output, daily weight, blood chemistry results, chest X-ray, and pulmonary artery catheter readings.

TRICUSPID STENOSIS

Tricuspid stenosis is a relatively uncommon disorder in which the tricuspid valve is hardened, resulting in increased blood in the right atrium.

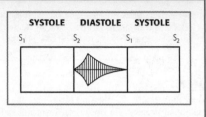

IDENTIFYING THE MURMUR OF TRICUSPID STENOSIS

A low, rumbling crescendo-decrescendo murmur in the tricuspid area characterizes tricuspid stenosis.

SYSTOLE	DIASTOLE	SYSTOLE	
S_1	S_2	S_1	S_2

Tricuspid stenosis seldom occurs alone and is usually associated with mitral stenosis. It's most common in women.

Pathophysiology

In tricuspid stenosis, blood flow is obstructed from the right atrium to the right ventricle, causing the right atrium to dilate and hypertrophy. Eventually, this leads to right-sided heart failure and increases pressure in the vena cava.

Although tricuspid stenosis is usually caused by rheumatic fever, it may also be congenital.

Complications

■ Right-sided heart failure possible with untreated tricuspid stenosis

Assessment findings

■ The patient with tricuspid stenosis may report dyspnea, fatigue, weakness, and syncope. Peripheral edema may cause her discomfort.

■ Inspection may reveal jugular vein distention with giant *a* waves in a patient who has normal sinus rhythm.

■ A patient with severe tricuspid stenosis that has progressed to right-sided heart failure may appear jaundiced, with severe peripheral edema and ascites; she may also appear malnourished.

■ Auscultation may reveal a diastolic murmur at the lower left sternal border and over the xiphoid process. It's most prominent during presystole in sinus rhythm. The murmur increases with inspiration and decreases with expiration and during Valsalva's maneuver. (See *Identifying the murmur of tricuspid stenosis*.)

■ Palpation may reveal hepatomegaly when the patient has right-sided heart failure.

Diagnostic test results

■ Cardiac catheterization shows an increased pressure gradient across the valve, increased right atrial pressure, and decreased cardiac output.

■ Chest X-rays demonstrate right atrial and superior vena cava enlargement.

■ Echocardiography indicates a thick tricuspid valve and right atrial enlargement.

■ Electrocardiography reveals right atrial hypertrophy, right or left ventricular hypertrophy, and atrial fibrillation. Tall, peaked P waves appear in lead II; prominent, upright P waves appear in lead V_1.

Treatment

Treatment for tricuspid stenosis is based on the patient's symptoms. A sodium-restricted diet and a diuretic can help to reduce hepatic congestion before surgery.

A patient with moderate to severe stenosis probably requires open-heart surgery for valvulotomy or valve replacement.

 AGE AWARE Valvuloplasty may be performed on elderly patients with end-stage disease in the cardiac catheterization laboratory.

Nursing interventions

■ Alternate periods of activity and rest to prevent extreme fatigue and dyspnea.

■ When the patient sits in a chair, elevate her legs to improve venous return to the heart.

■ Elevate the head of the bed to improve ventilation.

■ Keep the patient on a low-sodium diet. Consult with a dietitian to ensure that the patient receives foods that she likes while adhering to diet restrictions. (See *Teaching the patient with tricuspid stenosis,* page 380.)

■ Monitor the patient for signs of heart failure, pulmonary edema, and adverse reactions to drug therapy.

■ Allow the patient to express her fears and concerns about the disorder, its impact on her life, and upcoming surgery. Reassure her as needed.

■ If the patient has surgery, watch for hypotension, arrhythmias, and thrombus formation. Monitor her vital signs, arterial blood gas level, intake and output, daily weight, blood chemistry results, chest X-ray, and pulmonary artery catheter readings.

8

Degenerative disorders

ACUTE CORONARY SYNDROMES

Acute myocardial infarction (MI), including ST-segment elevation MI (STEMI) and non-ST-segment elevation MI (NSTEMI), and unstable angina are now recognized as part of a group of clinical diseases called acute coronary syndromes (ACS).

Rupture or erosion of plaque—an unstable and lipid-rich substance—initiates all coronary syndromes. The rupture and erosion result in platelet adhesions, fibrin clot formation, and activation of thrombin.

In cardiovascular disease—the leading cause of death in the United States and Western Europe—death usually results from cardiac damage after an MI. Each year, about 1 million people in the United States experience an MI. The incidence is higher in men younger than age 70. (Women have the protective effects of estrogen until menopause.) Mortality is high when treatment is delayed, and almost one-half of sudden deaths caused by an MI occur before hospitalization or within 1 hour of the onset of symptoms. The prognosis improves if vigorous treatment begins immediately.

Pathophysiology

ACS most commonly results when a thrombus progresses and occludes blood flow. The degree of blockage and the time that the affected vessel remains occluded determine the type of infarct that occurs. The underlying effect is an imbalance in myocardial oxygen supply and demand. (See *Stages of myocardial ischemia, injury, and infarct,* pages 382 and 383.)

For the patient with unstable angina, a thrombus full of platelets partially occludes a coronary vessel. The partially occluded vessel may

STAGES OF MYOCARDIAL ISCHEMIA, INJURY, AND INFARCT

Ischemia

Ischemia is the first stage and indicates that blood flow and oxygen demand are out of balance. It can be resolved by improving flow or reducing oxygen needs. Electrocardiogram (ECG) changes reveal ST-segment depression or T-wave changes.

Injury

The second stage, injury, occurs when ischemia is prolonged enough to damage the area of the heart. ECG changes usually reveal ST-segment elevation (usually in two or more leads).

Infarct

Infarct is the third stage and occurs with actual death of myocardial cells. Scar tissue eventually replaces the dead tissue, and the damage caused is irreversible.

In the earliest stage of a myocardial infarction (MI), hyperacute or very tall and narrow T waves may be seen on the ECG. Within hours, the T waves become inverted and ST-segment elevation occurs in the leads facing the area of damage. The last change to occur in the evolution of an MI is the development of the pathologic Q wave, which is the only permanent ECG evidence of myocardial necrosis. Q waves are considered pathologic when they appear greater than or equal to 0.04 second wide and their height is greater than 25% of the R-wave height in that lead. Pathologic Q waves develop in over 90% of patients with ST-segment elevation MI. About 25% of patients with a non–ST-segment elevation MI develop pathologic Q waves, and the remaining patients have a non–Q-wave MI.

have distal microthrombi that cause necrosis in some myocytes. The smaller vessels infarct, thus placing the patient at higher risk for NSTEMI. If a thrombus fully occludes the vessel for a prolonged time, a STEMI usually develops. (See *What happens during an MI,* pages 384 and 385.) This type of MI involves a greater concentration of thrombin and fibrin. (See *How ACS affects the body,* pages 386 and 387.)

The location of the area of damage depends on the blood vessels involved.

■ Anterior-wall MI occurs when the left anterior descending artery becomes occluded.

■ Septal-wall MI typically accompanies an anterior wall MI because the ventricular septum is supplied by the left anterior descending artery as well.

■ Lateral-wall MI is caused by a blockage in the left circumflex artery, and usually accompanies an anterior- or inferior-wall MI.

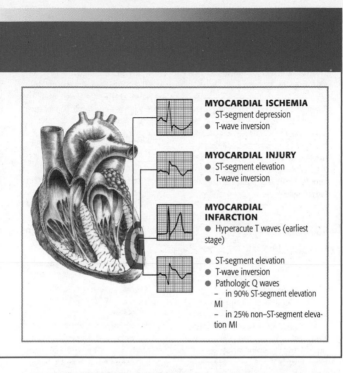

MYOCARDIAL ISCHEMIA
- ST-segment depression
- T-wave inversion

MYOCARDIAL INJURY
- ST-segment elevation
- T-wave inversion

MYOCARDIAL INFARCTION
- Hyperacute T waves (earliest stage)

- ST-segment elevation
- T-wave inversion
- Pathologic Q waves
  – in 90% ST-segment elevation MI
  – in 25% non–ST-segment elevation MI

- Inferior-wall MI is caused by occlusion of the right coronary artery; it usually occurs alone or with a lateral-wall or right-ventricular MI.
- Posterior-wall MI is caused by occlusion of the right coronary artery or the left circumflex arteries.
- Right-ventricular MI follows occlusion of the right coronary artery; this type of an MI rarely occurs alone. (In 40% of patients, a right-ventricular MI accompanies an inferior-wall MI.)

  Predisposing factors for ACS include:
- aging
- diabetes mellitus
- elevated triglyceride, low-density lipoprotein, and cholesterol levels, and decreased high-density lipoprotein levels
- excessive intake of saturated fats, carbohydrates, or salt
- hypertension
- obesity
- positive family history of coronary artery disease (CAD)

What happens during an MI

When blood supply to the myocardium is interrupted, the following events occur:

1. Injury to the endothelial lining of the coronary arteries causes platelets, white blood cells, fibrin, and lipids to converge at the injured site. Foam cells, or resident macrophages, congregate under the damaged lining and absorb oxidized cholesterol, forming a fatty streak that narrows the arterial lumen.

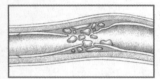

2. Because the arterial lumen narrows gradually, collateral circulation develops and helps maintain myocardial perfusion distal to the obstruction. During this stage, the patient may have chest pain when myocardial oxygen demand increases.

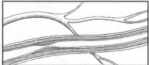

3. When myocardial demand for oxygen is more than the collateral circulation can supply, myocardial metabolism shifts from

aerobic to anaerobic, producing lactic acid (A), which stimulates pain nerve endings. The patient experiences worsening angina that requires rest and medication for relief.

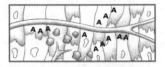

4. Lacking oxygen, the myocardial cells die. This decreases contractility, stroke volume, and blood pressure. The patient experiences tachycardia, hypotension, diminished heart sounds, cyanosis, tachypnea, and poor perfusion to vital organs.

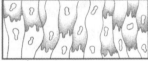

5. Hypoperfusion stimulates baroreceptors, which in turn stimulate the adrenal glands to release epinephrine and norepinephrine. These catecholamines (C) increase heart rate and cause peripheral vasoconstriction, further increasing myocardial oxygen demand. The patient may experience tachyarrhythmias, changes in pulses, decreased level of consciousness, and cold, clammy skin.

- sedentary lifestyle
- smoking
- stress or a type A personality (aggressive, competitive attitude, addiction to work, chronic impatience).

In addition, use of such drugs as amphetamines or cocaine can cause an MI.

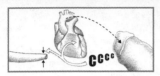

6. Damaged cell membranes in the infarcted area allow intracellular contents into the vascular circulation. Ventricular arrhythmias then develop with elevated serum levels of potassium (■), creatine kinase (CK) and CK-MB (▲), and troponin (●).

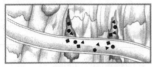

7. All myocardial cells are capable of spontaneous depolarization and repolarization, so the electrical conduction system may be affected by infarct, injury, and ischemia. The patient may have a fever, leukocytosis, tachycardia, and electrocardiogram signs of tissue ischemia (altered T waves), injured tissue (altered ST segment), and infarcted tissue (deep Q waves).

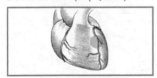

8. Extensive damage to the left ventricle may impair its ability to pump, allowing blood to back up into the left atrium and, eventually, into the pulmonary veins and capillaries. When this occurs, the patient may be dyspneic, orthopneic, tachypneic, and cyanotic. Crackles may be heard in the lungs on auscultation. Pulmonary artery pressure and pulmonary artery wedge pressure are increased.

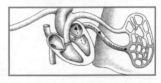

9. As back pressure increases, fluid crosses the alveolar-capillary membrane, impeding diffusion of oxygen (O_2) and carbon dioxide (CO_2). The patient experiences increasing respiratory distress, and arterial blood gas results may show decreased partial pressure of oxygen and arterial pH and increased partial pressure of carbon dioxide.

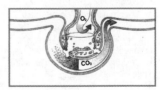

Men are more susceptible to MIs than premenopausal women, although incidence is rising among women who smoke and take a hormonal contraceptive. The incidence in postmenopausal women resembles that in men.

Complications
- Arrhythmias
- Heart failure causing pulmonary edema

How ACS affects the body

Acute coronary syndromes (ACS) can have far-reaching effects and requires a multidisciplinary approach to care. Here's what happens in ACS:

Cardiovascular system

● An area of viable ischemic tissue surrounds the zone of injury.

● When the heart muscle is damaged, the integrity of the cell membrane is impaired.

● Intracellular contents, including cardiac enzymes (such as creatine kinase and aspartate aminotransferase) and proteins (such as troponin T, troponin I, and myoglobin) are released.

● Within 24 hours, the infarcted area becomes edematous and cyanotic.

● During the next several days, leukocytes infiltrate the necrotic area and begin to remove necrotic cells, thinning the ventricular wall.

● Scar formation begins by the 3rd week after a myocardial infarction (MI); by the 6th week, scar tissue is well established.

● The scar tissue that forms on the necrotic area inhibits contractility.

● Compensatory mechanisms (vascular constriction, increased heart rate, and renal retention of sodium and water) try to maintain cardiac output.

● Ventricular dilation may also occur in a process called *remodeling*.

● Functionally, an MI may cause reduced contractility with abnormal wall motion, altered left ventricular compliance, reduced stroke volume, reduced ejection fraction, and elevated left ventricular end-diastolic pressure.

● Cardiogenic shock is caused by failure of the heart to perform as an effective pump and can result in low cardiac output, diminished peripheral perfusion, pulmonary congestion, and elevated systemic vascular resistance and pulmonary vascular pressures.

● Ineffective contractility of the heart leads to accumulation of blood in the venous circulation distal to the failing ventricle.

● Arrhythmias can occur in the patient with an acute MI as a result of autonomic nervous system imbalance, electrolyte disturbances, ischemia, and slowed conduction in zones of ischemic myocardium.

Neurologic system

● Hypoperfusion of the brain results in altered mental status, involving changes in the level of consciousness, restlessness, irritability, confusion, or disorientation.

● Stupor or coma may result if the decrease in cerebral perfusion continues.

Renal system

● Shock and hypoperfusion from an MI cause the kidney to respond by conserving salt and water.

● Poor perfusion results in diminished renal blood flow, and increased afferent arteriolar resistance occurs, causing a decreased glomerular filtration rate.

● Increased amounts of antidiuretic hormone and aldosterone are released to help maintain perfusion. Urine formation, however, is reduced.

● Depletion of renal adenosine triphosphate stores results from prolonged renal hypoperfusion, causing impaired renal function.

HOW ACS AFFECTS THE BODY *(continued)*

Respiratory system

● Cardiogenic shock with left-sided heart failure results in increased fluid in the lungs. This process can overwhelm the capacity of the pulmonary lymphatics, resulting in interstitial and alveolar edema.

● Lung edema occurs when pulmonary capillary pressure exceeds 18 mm Hg.

● Pulmonary alveolar edema develops when pressures exceed 24 mm Hg, impairing oxygen diffusion.

● Increased interstitial and intra-alveolar fluid causes progressive reduction in lung compliance, increasing the work of ventilation and increasing perfusion of poorly ventilated alveoli.

Collaborative management

A cardiologist is consulted for initial assessment and treatment. A cardiothoracic surgeon may also be consulted if the patient requires invasive therapy. Other specialists may be required after initial therapy and treatment, such as a physical therapist for cardiac rehabilitation and a nutritionist for dietary and lifestyle changes.

■ Cardiogenic shock
■ Rupture of the atrial or ventricular septum, ventricular wall, or valves
■ Pericarditis
■ Ventricular aneurysms
■ Mural thrombi causing cerebral or pulmonary emboli
■ Dressler's syndrome (post-MI pericarditis) occurring days to weeks after an MI and causing residual pain, malaise, and fever (see *Complications of an MI,* pages 388 to 390)

 AGE AWARE An elderly patient is more prone to complications and death. Psychological problems can also occur, either from the patient's fear of another MI or from an organic brain disorder caused by tissue hypoxia. Occasionally, a patient may have a personality change.

Assessment findings

■ Typically, the patient reports the cardinal symptom of an MI: persistent, crushing substernal pain that may radiate to the left arm, jaw, neck, and shoulder blades. He commonly describes the pain as heavy, squeezing, or crushing, and it may persist for 12 or more hours.

(Text continues on page 390.)

COMPLICATIONS OF AN MI

COMPLICATION	ASSESSMENT	TREATMENT
Arrhythmias	● Electrocardiogram (ECG) shows premature ventricular contractions, ventricular tachycardia, or ventricular fibrillation; in an inferior myocardial infarction (MI), bradycardia and junctional rhythms or atrioventricular (AV) block; in an anterior MI, tachycardia or heart block.	● Antiarrhythmic, atropine, cardioversion, defibrillation, and pacemaker
Heart failure	● In left-sided heart failure, chest X-rays show venous congestion and cardiomegaly. ● Catheterization shows increases in pulmonary artery systolic and diastolic pressures, pulmonary artery wedge pressure (PAWP), central venous pressure, and systemic vascular resistance (SVR).	● Diuretic, angiotensin-converting enzyme inhibitor, beta-adrenergic receptor blocker, vasodilator, inotropic, and cardiac glycoside
Cardiogenic shock	● Catheterization shows decreased cardiac output, increased pulmonary artery systolic and diastolic pressures, decreased cardiac index, increased SVR, and increased PAWP. ● Signs are hypotension, tachycardia, decreased level of consciousness, decreased urine output, jugular vein distention, S_3 and S_4, and cool, pale skin.	● I.V. fluids, vasodilator, diuretic, cardiac glycoside, intra-aortic balloon pump (IABP), vasopressor, and beta-adrenergic receptor stimulant
Mitral insufficiency	● Auscultation reveals apical holosystolic murmur. ● Dyspnea is prominent. ● Catheterization shows increased pulmonary artery pressure (PAP) and PAWP.	● Nitroglycerin (Nitrostat), nitroprusside (Nitropress), IABP, and surgical replacement of the mitral valve; possible myocardial revascularization with significant coronary artery disease

COMPLICATIONS OF AN MI *(continued)*

COMPLICATION	ASSESSMENT	TREATMENT
Ventricular septal rupture	● Echocardiogram shows valve dysfunction. ● In left-to-right shunt, auscultation reveals a harsh holosystolic murmur and thrill. ● Catheterization shows increased PAP and PAWP. ● Increased oxygen saturation of right ventricle and pulmonary artery confirms the diagnosis. ● Color-flow and Doppler echocardiography demonstrate left-to-right blood flow across the septum.	● Surgical correction (may be postponed, but more patients have surgery immediately or up to 7 days after septal rupture), IABP, nitroglycerin, nitroprusside, low-dose inotropic (dopamine [Inocor]), and cardiac pacing when high-grade AV blocks occur
Pericarditis or Dressler's syndrome	● Auscultation reveals a pericardial friction rub. ● Chest pain is relieved in sitting position. ● Sharp pain is unlike previously experienced angina.	● Anti-inflammatory agent, such as aspirin (Ecotrin) or other nonsteroidal anti-inflammatory drug or corticosteroid
Ventricular aneurysm	● Chest X-rays may show cardiomegaly. ● ECG may show arrhythmias and persistent ST-segment elevation. ● Left ventriculography shows altered or paradoxical left ventricular motion.	● Cardiopulmonary resuscitation (CPR), cardioversion, defibrillation (if ventricular tachycardia or fibrillation occurs), antiarrhythmic, vasodilator, anticoagulant, cardiac glycoside, diuretic and, possibly, surgery
Cerebral or pulmonary embolism	● Dyspnea and chest pain or neurologic changes occur. ● Nuclear scan shows ventilation-perfusion mismatch in pulmonary embolism. ● Angiography shows arterial blockage.	● Oxygen and heparin ● CPR, epinephrine, or cardiac pacing

(continued)

COMPLICATIONS OF AN MI *(continued)*

COMPLICATION	ASSESSMENT	TREATMENT
Ventricular rupture	● Cardiac tamponade occurs. ● Arrhythmias, such as ventricular tachycardia and ventricular fibrillation, occur or sudden death results.	● Resuscitation as per Advanced Cardiac Life Support protocol ● Possible emergency surgical repair if CPR successful

■ In some patients—particularly elderly patients or those with diabetes—pain may not occur; in others, it may be mild and confused with indigestion.

■ Patients with CAD may report increasing anginal frequency, severity, or duration (especially when not precipitated by exertion, a heavy meal, or cold and wind).

■ The patient may also report a feeling of impending doom, fatigue, nausea, vomiting, and shortness of breath. Sudden death, however, may be the first and only indication of an MI.

■ Women may experience atypical signs and symptoms of an MI, which may go unnoticed. These include:
  – burning sensation or discomfort in the upper abdomen
  – difficulty breathing
  – nausea and vomiting
  – weakness or fatigue
  – profuse sweating
  – light-headedness and fainting.

  Practitioners may also not recognize these signs and symptoms as cardiac related and may delay prompt diagnosis and treatment.

■ Inspection may reveal an extremely anxious and restless patient with dyspnea and diaphoresis.

■ If right-sided heart failure is present, you may note jugular vein distention.

■ Within the first hour after an anterior MI, about 25% of patients exhibit sympathetic nervous system hyperactivity, such as tachycardia and hypertension.

■ Up to 50% of patients with an inferior MI exhibit parasympathetic nervous system hyperactivity, such as bradycardia and hypotension.

- In patients who develop ventricular dysfunction, auscultation may disclose an S_4, an S_3, paradoxical splitting of S_2, and decreased heart sounds. A systolic murmur of mitral insufficiency may be heard with papillary muscle dysfunction secondary to infarction. A pericardial friction rub may also be heard, especially in patients who have a transmural MI or have developed pericarditis.
- Fever is unusual at the onset of an MI, but a low-grade fever may develop during the next few days.

Diagnostic test results

- Serial 12-lead electrocardiogram (ECG) readings may be normal or inconclusive during the first few hours after an MI. Characteristic abnormalities include serial ST-segment depression in patients with a subendocardial MI, and ST-segment elevation and Q waves, representing scarring and necrosis, in those with a transmural MI. (See *ECG characteristics in ACS*, page 392.)
- The creatine kinase (CK) level is elevated, especially the CK-MB isoenzyme, the cardiac muscle fraction of CK.
- White blood cell count usually appears elevated on the 2nd day and lasts 1 week.
- Myoglobin (the hemoprotein found in cardiac and skeletal muscle) is released with muscle damage and may be detected as soon as 2 hours after an MI.
- Troponin I, a structural protein found in cardiac muscle, is elevated only in patients with cardiac muscle damage. It's more specific than the CK-MB level. Troponin levels increase within 4 to 6 hours of myocardial injury and may remain elevated for 5 to 11 days.
- Echocardiography shows ventricular-wall dyskinesia with a transmural MI and helps evaluate the ejection fraction.
- Nuclear ventriculography (multiple gated acquisition scanning or radionuclide ventriculography) can identify acutely damaged muscle by picking up accumulations of radioactive nucleotide, which appears as a hot spot on the film. Myocardial perfusion imaging with thallium-201 or Cardiolite reveals a "cold spot" in most patients during the first few hours after a transmural MI.
- Elevated homocysteine and C-reactive protein levels have been found incidentally in patients with an MI and may indicate a newer risk factor. Folic acid supplementation is used to treat elevated homocysteine levels.

Treatment

The goals of treatment for patients with ACS include reducing the amount of myocardial necrosis in those with ongoing infarction, de-

ECG CHARACTERISTICS IN ACS

The first step in assessing a patient complaining of chest pain is to obtain an electrocardiogram (ECG). This should be done within 10 minutes of being seen by a practitioner. It's crucial in determining the presence of myocardial ischemia, and the findings will direct the treatment plan.

Angina

Most patients with angina show ischemic changes on an ECG only during the attack. Because these changes may be fleeting, always obtain an order for and perform a 12-lead ECG as soon as the patient reports chest pain.

Myocardial infarction (MI)

According to the American Heart Association, patients should be classified as having ST-segment elevation or new left bundle-branch block (LBBB), ST-segment depression or dynamic T-wave inversion, or nondiagnostic or normal ECG.

ST-segment elevation or new LBBB

● Patients with an ST-segment elevation greater than 1 mm in two or more contiguous leads or with new LBBB need to be treated for an acute MI.
● More than 90% of patients with this presentation will develop new Q waves and have positive serum cardiac markers.

● Repeating the ECG may be helpful for patients who present with hyperacute T waves.

ST-segment depression or dynamic T-wave inversion

● Patients with ST-segment depression indicating a posterior MI benefit most when an acute MI is diagnosed.
● Ischemia should be suspected with findings of ST-segment depression greater than or equal to 0.5 mm, marked symmetrical T-wave inversion in multiple precordial leads, and dynamic ST-T changes with pain.
● Patients who display persistent symptoms and recurrent ischemia, diffuse or widespread ECG abnormalities, heart failure, and positive serum markers are considered high risk.

Nondiagnostic or normal ECG

● A normal ECG won't show ST-segment changes or arrhythmias.
● If the ECG is nondiagnostic, it may show an ST-segment depression of less than 0.5 mm or a T-wave inversion or flattening in leads with dominant R waves.
● Continue assessment of myocardial changes through use of serial ECGs, ST-segment monitoring, and serum cardiac markers.
● If further assessment is warranted, perform perfusion radionuclide imaging and stress echocardiography.

creasing cardiac workload and increasing oxygen supply to the myocardium, preventing major adverse cardiac events, and providing for cardiopulmonary resuscitation and defibrillation when ventricular fibrillation or pulseless ventricular tachycardia (VT) is present. (See *Treating an MI*, pages 394 and 395.)

Initial treatment for the patient with ACS includes the following:
- Obtain a 12-lead ECG and cardiac markers to help confirm the diagnosis of an acute MI. Cardiac markers (especially troponin I and CK-MB) are used to distinguish unstable angina and NSTEMI.
- Use the memory aid "MONA," which stands for morphine, oxygen, nitroglycerin, and aspirin, to treat any patient experiencing ischemic chest pain or suspected ACS. Administer:
  - morphine to relieve pain
  - oxygen to increase oxygenation of the blood
  - nitroglycerin sublingually to relieve chest pain (unless systolic blood pressure is less than 90 mm Hg or heart rate is less than 50 beats/minute or greater than 100 beats/minute)
  - aspirin to inhibit platelet aggregation.

For the patient with unstable angina and NSTEMI, treatment includes the above initial measures, and:
- a beta-adrenergic receptor blocker to reduce the heart's workload and oxygen demands
- heparin and a glycoprotein IIb/IIIa inhibitor to minimize platelet aggregation and the danger of coronary occlusion with high-risk patients (patients with planned cardiac catheterization and positive troponin)
- nitroglycerin I.V. to dilate coronary arteries and relieve chest pain (unless systolic blood pressure is less than 90 mm Hg or heart rate is less than 50 beats/minute or greater than 100 beats/minute)
- an antiarrhythmic, transcutaneous pacing (or transvenous pacemaker), or defibrillation if the patient has ventricular fibrillation or pulseless VT
- percutaneous transluminal coronary angioplasty (PTCA) or coronary artery bypass graft (CABG) surgery for obstructive lesions
- an antilipemic to reduce elevated cholesterol or triglyceride levels.

For the patient with STEMI, treatment includes the above initial measures and these additional measures:
- thrombolytic therapy (unless contraindicated) within 12 hours of onset of symptoms to restore vessel patency and minimize necrosis in STEMI
- I.V. heparin to promote patency in the affected coronary artery
- a beta-adrenergic receptor blocker to reduce myocardial workload
- an antiarrhythmic, transcutaneous pacing (or transvenous pacemaker), or defibrillation if the patient has ventricular fibrillation or pulseless VT

(Text continues on page 396.)

TREATING AN MI

This flowchart shows how treatments can be applied to a myocardial infarction (MI) at various stages of its development.

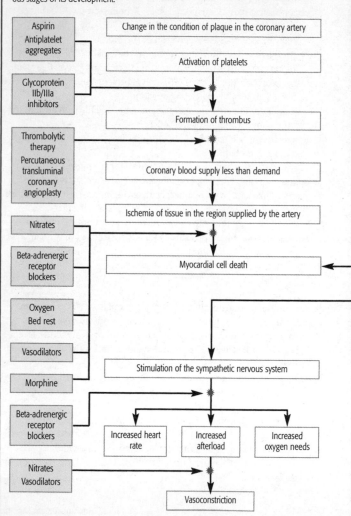

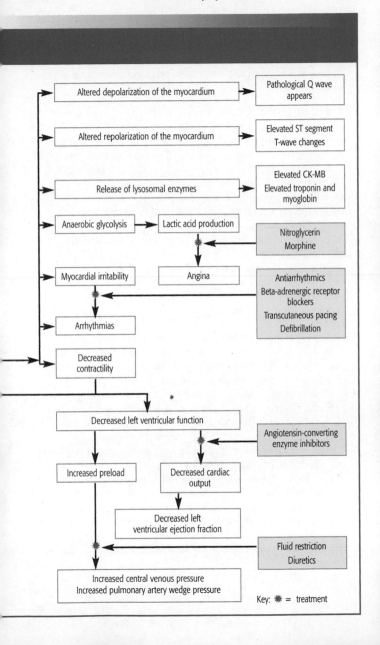

- an angiotensin-converting enzyme inhibitor to reduce afterload and preload and prevent remodeling (begin in STEMI 6 hours after admission or when the patient's condition is stable)
- interventional procedures (such as PTCA, stent placement, or surgical procedures such as CABG) may open blocked or narrowed arteries.

Nursing interventions

- Care for patients who have suffered an MI is directed toward detecting complications, preventing further myocardial damage, and promoting comfort, rest, and emotional well-being. Most patients receive treatment in the coronary care unit (CCU), where they're under constant observation for complications.
- On admission to the CCU, monitor and record the patient's ECG readings, blood pressure, temperature, and heart and breath sounds.
- Assess pain and give an analgesic. Record the severity, location, type, and duration of pain. Don't give I.M. injections because absorption from the muscle is unpredictable, the CK level may be falsely elevated, and I.V. administration gives more rapid relief of signs and symptoms.
- Check the patient's blood pressure after giving nitroglycerin, especially the first dose.
- Frequently monitor the ECG to detect rate changes and arrhythmias. Analyze rhythm strips. Place a representative strip in the patient's chart if any new arrhythmias are documented, if chest pain occurs, at every shift change, or according to facility protocol.
- During episodes of chest pain, obtain a 12-lead ECG (before and after nitroglycerin therapy as well). Also obtain blood pressure and pulmonary artery catheter measurements, if applicable, to determine changes.
- Watch for crackles, cough, tachypnea, and edema, which may indicate impending left-sided heart failure. Carefully monitor daily weight, intake and output, respiratory rate, enzyme levels, ECG readings, and blood pressure. Auscultate for adventitious breath sounds periodically (patients on bed rest frequently have atelectatic crackles, which may disappear after coughing) and for S_3 or S_4 gallops.
- Organize patient care and activities to maximize periods of uninterrupted rest.

DISCHARGE TEACHING

TEACHING THE PATIENT WITH ACS

● To promote compliance with the prescribed medication regimen and other treatment measures, thoroughly explain dosages and therapy. Inform the patient of the drug's adverse reactions, and advise him to watch for and report signs and symptoms of toxicity (for example, anorexia, nausea, vomiting, mental depression, vertigo, blurred vision, and yellow vision, if the patient is receiving a cardiac glycoside).

● Review dietary restrictions with the patient. If he must follow a low-sodium, low-fat, or low-cholesterol diet, provide a list of foods to avoid. Ask the dietitian to speak to the patient and his family.

● Encourage the patient to participate in a cardiac rehabilitation exercise program. The practitioner and the exercise physiologist should determine the level of exercise and then discuss it with the patient and secure his agreement to a stepped-care program.

● Counsel the patient to resume sexual activity progressively. He may need to take nitroglycerin before sexual intercourse to prevent chest pain from the increased activity.

● Advise the patient about appropriate responses to new or recurrent symptoms.

● Advise the patient to report typical or atypical chest pain. Post-myocardial infarction (MI) syndrome may develop, producing chest pain that must be differentiated from a recurrent MI, pulmonary infarction, and heart failure.

● Stress the need to stop smoking. If necessary, refer the patient to a support group.

● If the patient has a Holter monitor in place, explain its purpose and use.

● Review follow-up procedures, such as office visits and treadmill testing, with the patient.

- Ask the dietary department to provide a clear liquid diet until nausea subsides. A low-cholesterol, low-sodium diet, without caffeine, may be ordered. (See *Teaching the patient with ACS*.)
- Provide a stool softener to prevent straining during defecation, which causes vagal stimulation and may slow heart rate.
- Allow the patient to use a bedside commode, and provide as much privacy as possible.
- Assist with range-of-motion exercises. If the patient is immobilized by a severe MI, turn him often. Antiembolism stockings help prevent venostasis and thrombophlebitis.
- Initiate a cardiac rehabilitation program, which typically includes education regarding heart disease, exercise, and emotional support for the patient and his family.
- Provide emotional support, and help reduce stress and anxiety; administer a tranquilizer if needed.

- If the patient has undergone PTCA, sheath care is necessary. Keep the sheath line open with a heparin drip. Observe the patient for generalized and site bleeding. Keep the leg with the sheath insertion site immobile. Maintain strict bed rest. Check peripheral pulses in the affected leg frequently. Provide an analgesic for back pain, if needed.

- After thrombolytic therapy, administer continuous heparin. Monitor the partial thromboplastin time every 6 hours, and monitor the patient for evidence of bleeding.

- Monitor ECG rhythm strips for reperfusion arrhythmias, and treat them according to facility protocol. If the artery reoccludes, the patient experiences the same symptoms as before. If this occurs, prepare the patient for return to the cardiac catheterization laboratory.

CORONARY ARTERY DISEASE

Coronary artery disease (CAD) results from the narrowing of the coronary arteries over time resulting from atherosclerosis. The foremost effect of CAD is the loss of oxygen and nutrients to myocardial tissue because of diminished coronary blood flow. As the population ages, the prevalence of CAD is increasing. About 13 million Americans have CAD, and it's more common in men, whites, and middle-aged and elderly people. With proper care, the prognosis for CAD is favorable.

Pathophysiology

Fatty, fibrous plaque progressively narrow the coronary artery lumina, reducing the volume of blood that can flow through them and leading to myocardial ischemia.

As atherosclerosis progresses, luminal narrowing is accompanied by vascular changes that impair the ability of the diseased vessel to dilate. This causes a precarious balance between myocardial oxygen supply and demand, threatening the myocardium beyond the lesion. When oxygen demand exceeds what the diseased vessel can supply, localized myocardial ischemia results.

Myocardial cells become ischemic within 10 seconds of a coronary artery occlusion. Transient ischemia causes reversible changes at the cellular and tissue levels, depressing myocardial function. Untreated, this can lead to tissue injury or necrosis. Within several minutes, oxygen deprivation forces the myocardium to shift from aerobic to anaerobic metabolism, leading to accumulation of lactic acid and reduction of cellular pH.

EXPLORING THE GENETIC LINK TO CAD

Researchers have identified more than 250 genes that may play a role in coronary artery disease (CAD). It commonly results from the combined effects of multiple genes, making it difficult to determine the impact of specific genes that can influence a person's risk of contracting the disease.

Some of the best understood genes linked to CAD include:

● low-density lipoprotein (LDL) receptor—a protein that removes LDL from the bloodstream; a mutation in this gene is responsible for familial hypercholesterolemia

● apolipoprotein E—mutations in this gene, commonly called *apo E,* also affects blood levels of LDL

● apolipoprotein B-100—commonly called *apo B-11*, it's a component of LDL; mutations of the gene cause LDL to stay in the blood longer than normal, leading to high LDL levels

● apolipoprotein A—a glycoprotein that combines with LDL to form a particle called *Lp(a);* it appears as a part of plaque on blood vessels

● MTHFR—an enzyme that clears homocysteine from the blood; mutations in MTHFR genes may cause high homocysteine levels

● cystathione B-synthase—also known as *CBS,* it's another enzyme involved in homocysteine metabolism; CBS mutations cause a condition known as *homocystinuria* (homocysteine levels are so high that homocysteine can be detected in urine).

The combination of hypoxia, reduced energy availability, and acidosis rapidly impairs left ventricular function. The strength of the contractions in the affected myocardial region is reduced as the fibers shorten inadequately, resulting in less force and velocity. Moreover, wall motion is abnormal in the ischemic area, resulting in less blood being ejected from the heart with each contraction. Restoring blood flow through the coronary arteries restores aerobic metabolism and contractility; however, if blood flow isn't restored, myocardial infarction (MI) results.

Atherosclerosis, the most common cause of CAD, has been linked to many risk factors. Some risk factors can't be controlled:

■ age—Atherosclerosis usually occurs after age 40.

■ sex—Men are eight times more susceptible than premenopausal women.

■ heredity—A positive family history of CAD increases the risk. (See *Exploring the genetic link to CAD.*)

■ race—White men are more susceptible than nonwhite men, and nonwhite women are more susceptible than white women.

The patient can modify the following risk factors with good medical care and appropriate lifestyle changes:

- high blood pressure—Systolic blood pressure that's higher than 160 mm Hg or diastolic blood pressure that's higher than 95 mm Hg increases the risk.
- high cholesterol levels—Increased low-density lipoprotein and decreased high-density lipoprotein levels substantially heighten the risk.
- smoking—Cigarette smokers are twice as likely to have an MI and four times as likely to experience sudden death. The risk dramatically drops within 1 year after smoking ceases.
- obesity—Added weight increases the risk of diabetes mellitus, hypertension, and elevated cholesterol levels.
- physical inactivity—Regular exercise reduces the risk.
- stress—Added stress or a type A personality increases the risk.
- diabetes mellitus—This disorder raises the risk, especially in women.
- other modifiable factors—Increased fibrinogen and uric acid levels, elevated hematocrit, reduced vital capacity; high resting heart rate, thyrotoxicosis, and use of a hormonal contraceptive heightens the risk.

Uncommon causes of reduced coronary artery blood flow include dissecting aneurysms, infectious vasculitis, syphilis, and congenital defects in the coronary vascular system. Coronary artery spasms may also impede blood flow. (See *Understanding coronary artery spasm*.)

Complications
- Arrhythmias
- Ischemic cardiomyopathy
- MI

Assessment findings
- The classic symptom of CAD is angina, the direct result of inadequate oxygen flow to the myocardium. The patient usually describes it as a burning, squeezing, or crushing tightness in the substernal or precordial chest that may radiate to the left arm, neck, jaw, or shoulder blade. Typically, the patient clenches his fist over his chest or rubs his left arm when describing the pain. Nausea, vomiting, fainting, sweating, and cool extremities may accompany the tightness.

    Angina commonly occurs after physical exertion but may also follow emotional excitement, exposure to cold, or a large meal. Angina

UNDERSTANDING CORONARY ARTERY SPASM

In patients with coronary artery spasm, a spontaneous, sustained contraction of one or more coronary arteries causes ischemia and dysfunction of the heart muscle. This disorder may also cause Prinzmetal's angina and even a myocardial infarction (MI) in patients with nonoccluded coronary arteries.

Causes

The direct cause of coronary artery spasm is unknown, but possible contributing factors include:
- altered influx of calcium across the cell membrane
- intimal hemorrhage into the medial layer of the blood vessel
- hyperventilation
- an elevated catecholamine level
- fatty buildup in the lumen.

Signs and symptoms

The major symptom of coronary artery spasm is angina. Unlike classic angina, this pain commonly occurs spontaneously and may be unrelated to physical exertion or emotional stress; it may, however, follow cocaine use. It's usually more severe than classic angina, lasts longer, and may be cyclic—recurring every day at the same time. Ischemic episodes may cause arrhythmias, altered heart rate, lower blood pressure and, occasionally, fainting caused by decreased cardiac output. Spasm in the left coronary artery may result in mitral valve prolapse, producing a loud systolic murmur and, possibly, pulmonary edema, with dyspnea, crackles,

and hemoptysis. An MI and sudden death may occur.

Treatment

After diagnosis by coronary angiography and 12-lead electrocardiography, the patient may receive a calcium channel blocker (such as verapamil [Calan], nifedipine [Procardia], or diltiazem [Cardizem]) to reduce coronary artery spasm and to decrease vascular resistance, and a nitrate (such as nitroglycerin [Nitro-Bid] or isosorbide dinitrate [Isordil]) to relieve chest pain. During cardiac catheterization, the patient with clean arteries may receive ergotamine to induce the spasm and aid in the diagnosis.

Nursing interventions

When caring for a patient with coronary artery spasm, explain all necessary procedures and teach him how to take his drugs safely. For calcium antagonist therapy, monitor the patient's blood pressure, pulse rate, and cardiac rhythm strips to detect arrhythmias.

For nifedipine and verapamil therapy, monitor the digoxin (Lanoxin) level, and check for signs of digoxin toxicity. Because nifedipine may cause peripheral and periorbital edema, watch for fluid retention.

Because coronary artery spasm is sometimes associated with atherosclerotic disease, advise the patient to stop smoking, avoid overeating, minimize alcohol intake, and maintain a balance between exercise and rest.

Types of Angina

There are four types of angina:

● Stable angina–pain is predictable in frequency and duration and is relieved by rest and nitroglycerin.

● Unstable angina–pain increases in frequency and duration and is more easily induced; it indicates a worsening of coronary artery disease that may progress to a myocardial infarction.

● Prinzmetal's, or variant, angina–pain is caused by spasm of the coronary arteries; it may occur spontaneously and may be unrelated to physical exercise or emotional stress.

● Microvascular angina–impairment of vasodilator reserve causes angina-like chest pain in a person with normal coronary arteries.

may also develop during sleep from which symptoms awaken the patient. (See *Types of angina*.)

- Inspection may reveal evidence of atherosclerotic disease, such as xanthelasma and xanthoma.
- Ophthalmoscopic inspection may show increased light reflexes and arteriovenous nicking, suggesting hypertension, an important risk factor of CAD.
- Palpation can uncover thickened or absent peripheral arteries, signs of cardiac enlargement, and abnormal contraction of the cardiac impulse, such as left ventricular akinesia or dyskinesia.
- Auscultation may detect bruits, an S_3, an S_4, or a late systolic murmur (if mitral insufficiency is present).

AGE AWARE In the older adult, CAD may be asymptomatic because of a decrease in sympathetic response. Dyspnea and fatigue are two key signals of ischemia in an active, older adult.

Diagnostic test results

- An electrocardiogram (ECG) during angina shows ischemia as demonstrated by T-wave inversion or ST-segment depression and possibly arrhythmias, such as premature ventricular contractions. ECG results may be normal during pain-free periods. Arrhythmias may occur without infarction, secondary to ischemia. A Holter monitor may be used to obtain continuous graphic tracing of the ECG as the patient performs daily activities.
- Treadmill or bicycle exercise testing may provoke chest pain and ECG signs of myocardial ischemia in response to physical exertion.

Monitoring electrical rhythm may demonstrate T-wave inversion or ST-segment depression in the ischemic areas.

- Coronary angiography reveals coronary artery stenosis or obstruction, collateral circulation, and the arteries' condition beyond the narrowing.
- Myocardial perfusion imaging with thallium-201, Cardiolite, or Myoview during treadmill exercise helps detect ischemic areas of the myocardium, visualized as "cold spots."
- In pharmacologic myocardial perfusion imaging, a patent coronary artery vasodilator, such as adenosine (Adenocard) or dipyridamole (Persantine), is given and response is tested. This can be done along with stress testing. In normal arteries, coronary blood flow is increased to three to four times baseline. In arteries with stenosis, the decrease in blood flow is proportional to the percentage of occlusion.
- Multiple-gated acquisition scanning demonstrates cardiac wall motion and reflects injury to cardiac tissue.
- Stress echocardiography may show wall motion abnormalities.
- Electron-beam computed tomography identifies calcium within arterial plaque; the more calcium seen, the higher the likelihood of CAD.

Treatment

The goal of treatment in patients with angina is to reduce myocardial oxygen demand or increase the oxygen supply and reduce pain. Activity restrictions may be required to prevent onset of pain. Rather than eliminating activities, performing them more slowly can help avert pain. Stress-reduction techniques are also essential, especially if known stressors precipitate pain.

Pharmacologic therapy consists primarily of a nitrate, such as nitroglycerin, isosorbide dinitrate, or a beta-adrenergic receptor blocker or calcium channel blocker. A nitrate, such as nitroglycerin (Nitrostat) may be given to help reduce myocardial oxygen consumption. A beta-adrenergic receptor blocker is given to reduce the heart's workload and oxygen demands by reducing heart rate and peripheral resistance to blood flow. A calcium channel blocker is used to prevent coronary artery spasm. An antiplatelet drug helps to minimize platelet aggregation and the risk of coronary occlusion. A glycoprotein IIb/IIIa inhibitor, such as abciximab (ReoPro), eptifibatide (Integrilin), or tirofiban (Aggrastat), helps reduce the risk of blood clots. An antilipemic is given to reduce serum cholesterol or triglyceride levels. An antihypertensive is used to help control hypertension.

Obstructive lesions may necessitate atherectomy or coronary artery bypass graft (CABG) surgery, using vein grafts. A surgical technique available as an alternative to traditional CABG surgery is minimally invasive coronary artery bypass surgery, also known as *keyhole surgery*. This procedure requires a shorter recovery period and has fewer postoperative complications. Instead of sawing open the patient's sternum and spreading the ribs apart, several small incisions are made in the torso through which small surgical instruments and fiber-optic cameras are inserted. This procedure was initially designed to correct blockages in just one or two easily reached arteries; it may be unsuitable for more complicated cases.

Percutaneous transluminal coronary angioplasty (PTCA) may be performed during cardiac catheterization to compress fatty deposits and relieve occlusion. In patients with calcification, PTCA may reduce the obstruction by fracturing the plaque. (See *Relieving occlusions with angioplasty*.)

RED FLAG PTCA carries certain risks but causes fewer complications than surgery. Complications after PTCA can include circulatory insufficiency, death (rarely), an MI, restenosis of the vessels, retroperitoneal bleeding, sudden coronary occlusions, or vasovagal response and arrhythmias.

PTCA is a viable alternative to grafting in elderly patients or in those who otherwise can't tolerate cardiac surgery. However, patients with a left main coronary artery occlusion, lesions in extremely tortuous vessels, or occlusions older than 3 months aren't candidates for PTCA.

PTCA may be done along with coronary stenting, or stents may be placed alone. Stents provide a framework to hold an artery open by securing flaps of tunica media against an artery wall. Intravascular coronary stenting is done to reduce the incidence of restenosis. Prosthetic intravascular cylindrical stents made of stainless steel coil are positioned at the site of the occlusion. To be eligible for this procedure, the patient must be able to tolerate anticoagulant therapy and the vessel to be stented must be at least ⅛" (0.3 cm) in diameter. Some stents have a drug already placed in them that's released over time to help minimize the risk of in-stent restenosis. Coronary brachytherapy, which involves delivering beta or gamma radiation into the coronary arteries, may be used in patients who have undergone stent implantation in a coronary artery but then developed such problems as diffuse in-stent restenosis. Brachytherapy is a promising technique, but its use is restricted to the treatment of stent-related problems because of complications and the unknown long-term effects of

RELIEVING OCCLUSIONS WITH ANGIOPLASTY

For a patient with an occluded coronary artery, percutaneous transluminal coronary angioplasty can open the artery without opening the chest—an important advantage over bypass surgery.

First, coronary angioplasty must confirm the presence and location of the arterial occlusion. Then, a guide catheter is threaded through the patient's femoral artery into the coronary artery under fluoroscopic guidance.

When angiography shows the guide catheter positioned at the occlusion site, a smaller double-lumen balloon catheter is carefully inserted through the guide catheter and the balloon is directed through the occlusion (near right). A marked pressure gradient is obvious.

The balloon is alternately inflated and deflated until an angiogram verifies successful arterial dilation (far right) and that the pressure gradient has decreased.

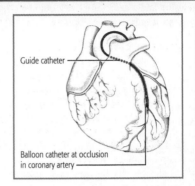

Guide catheter

Balloon catheter at occlusion in coronary artery

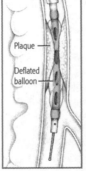

Plaque

Deflated balloon

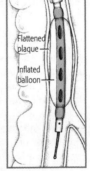

Flattened plaque

Inflated balloon

the radiation. However, in some facilities, brachytherapy is being studied as a first-line treatment for coronary disease.

Laser angioplasty corrects occlusion by vaporizing fatty deposits with the excimer or hot-tip laser device. Percutaneous myocardial revascularization (PMR) is a procedure that uses a laser to create channels in the heart muscle to improve perfusion to the myocardium. A carbon dioxide laser is used to create transmural channels from the epicardial layer to the myocardium, extending into the left ventricle. This technique is also known as *transmyocardial revascularization* and appears to be up to 90% effective in treating severe symptoms.

Rotational ablation (or rotational atherectomy) removes atheromatous plaque with a high-speed, rotating burr covered with diamond crystals. Another method recently approved is an AngioJet system septa to remove clots in symptomatic coronary arteries and CABGs. It's an alternative to thrombolytic therapy and involves a jet stream of saline solution and a catheter to seek out clots. After the clot is removed, the patient can undergo angioplasty.

Nursing interventions

- During anginal episodes, monitor blood pressure and heart rate. Take a 12-lead ECG before administering nitroglycerin or other nitrates. Record the duration of pain, the amount of medication required to relieve it, and accompanying symptoms.
- Ask the patient to grade the severity of his pain on a scale of 0 to 10. This allows him to give his individual assessment of pain as well as of the effectiveness of pain-relieving medications.
- Keep nitroglycerin available for immediate use. Instruct the patient to call immediately whenever he feels chest, arm, or neck pain and before taking nitroglycerin.
- Before cardiac catheterization, explain the procedure to the patient. Make sure he knows why it's necessary, understands the risks, and realizes that it may indicate a need for surgery.
- During catheterization, monitor the patient for dye reactions. If symptoms, such as falling blood pressure, bradycardia, diaphoresis, and light-headedness appear, increase parenteral fluids as ordered, administer nasal oxygen, place the patient in the Trendelenburg position, and administer I.V. atropine if necessary.
- After catheterization, review the expected course of treatment with the patient and his family. Monitor the catheter site for bleeding. Also, check for distal pulses. To counter the diuretic effect of the dye, increase I.V. fluids and make sure the patient drinks plenty of fluids. Assess potassium levels, and add potassium to the I.V. fluid if necessary.
- After PTCA and intravascular stenting, maintain heparinization, observe the patient for bleeding systemically at the site, and keep the affected leg immobile. If the patient undergoes PMR, he must also remain immobile because the stents are left in the patient until his clotting time is less than 180 seconds. Precordial blood must be taken every 8 hours for 24 hours for cardiac enzyme levels. Complete blood count and electrolyte levels are monitored.
- After rotational ablation, monitor the patient for chest pain, hypotension, coronary artery spasm, and bleeding from the catheter

TEACHING THE PATIENT WITH CAD

● Help the patient determine which activities precipitate episodes of pain. Help him identify and select more effective coping mechanisms to deal with stress. Occupational change may be needed to prevent symptoms, but many patients reject this alternative.

● Stress the need to follow the ordered drug regimen.

● Encourage the patient to maintain the ordered low-sodium diet and start a low-calorie diet as well.

● Explain that recurrent angina symptoms after percutaneous transluminal coronary angioplasty or rotational ablation may signal reobstruction.

● Encourage regular, moderate exercise. Refer the patient to a cardiac reha-

bilitation center or cardiovascular fitness program near his home or workplace. The staff can set up a program of exercise that best meets the patient's needs and limitations. Encourage other family members or a friend to join in the physical activity to encourage the patient's commitment to the exercise program.

● Reassure the patient that he will be able to resume sexual activity and that modifications can allow for sexual fulfillment without fear of overexertion, pain, or reocclusion.

● Refer the patient to a program to stop smoking. Acknowledge that this will be difficult but that he should make every attempt to stop smoking immediately and never restart.

site. Provide heparin and antibiotic therapy for 24 to 48 hours, as ordered.

■ If the patient is scheduled for surgery, explain the procedure, provide a tour of the intensive care unit, introduce him to the staff, and discuss postoperative care.

■ After bypass surgery, provide care for the I.V. set, pulmonary artery catheter, and endotracheal tube. Monitor blood pressure, intake and output, breath sounds, chest tube drainage, and cardiac rhythm, watching for signs of ischemia and arrhythmias. I.V. epinephrine, nitroprusside (Nitropress), dopamine (Inocor), albumin, potassium, and blood products may be necessary. The patient may also need temporary epicardial pacing, especially if the surgery included replacement of the aortic valve.

■ Intra-aortic balloon pump insertion may be necessary until the patient's condition stabilizes. Also, watch for and treat chest pain. Perform vigorous chest physiotherapy, and guide the patient in pulmonary self-care.

■ Before discharge, stress the need to follow the prescribed drug regimen, exercise program, and diet. (See *Teaching the patient with CAD*.)

DILATED CARDIOMYOPATHY

Dilated cardiomyopathy—also called *congestive cardiomyopathy*—results from extensively damaged myocardial muscle fibers. It interferes with myocardial metabolism and grossly dilates every heart chamber, giving the heart a globular shape. When hypertrophy coexists with dilated cardiomyopathy, the heart ejects blood less efficiently than normal and a large volume of blood remains in the left ventricle after systole, causing signs of heart failure.

Dilated cardiomyopathy most commonly affects middle-aged men but can occur in any age-group. Because it isn't usually diagnosed until the advanced stages, the prognosis is generally poor. Most patients, especially those older than age 55, die within 2 years of symptom onset.

Pathophysiology

Dilated cardiomyopathy primarily affects systolic function. It results from extensively damaged myocardial muscle fibers. Consequently, contractility in the left ventricle decreases.

As systolic function declines, stroke volume, ejection fraction, and cardiac output decrease. As end-diastolic volumes increase, pulmonary congestion may occur. The elevated end-diastolic volume is a compensatory response to preserve stroke volume despite a reduced ejection fraction.

The sympathetic nervous system is also stimulated to increase heart rate and contractility. The kidneys are stimulated to retain sodium and water to maintain cardiac output, and vasoconstriction also occurs as the renin-angiotensin system is stimulated. When these compensatory mechanisms can no longer maintain cardiac output, the heart begins to fail. Left ventricular dilation occurs as venous return and systemic vascular resistance increase. Eventually, the atria also dilate, as more work is required to pump blood into the full ventricles. Blood pooling in the ventricles increases the risk of emboli.

The cause of most cardiomyopathies is unknown. Dilated cardiomyopathy can result from myocardial destruction by a toxic, infectious, or metabolic agent; an endocrine or electrolyte disorder; a nutritional deficiency; a muscle disorder (such as myasthenia gravis, muscular dystrophy, or myotonic dystrophy); an infiltrative disorder (such as hemochromatosis or amyloidosis); or sarcoidosis.

Cardiomyopathy may be associated with alcoholism, viral myocarditis (especially after infection with coxsackievirus B, poliovirus, or influenza virus), or acquired immunodeficiency syndrome.

Metabolic cardiomyopathies are related to endocrine and electrolyte disorders and nutritional deficiencies. Dilated cardiomyopathy may develop in patients with hyperthyroidism, pheochromocytoma, beriberi, or kwashiorkor. Cardiomyopathy may also result from rheumatic fever, especially among children with myocarditis.

Cardiomyopathy may develop during the last trimester of pregnancy or within months after delivery. Its cause is unknown, but it's most common in multiparous women older than age 30, particularly those with malnutrition or preeclampsia. In these patients, cardiomegaly and heart failure may reverse with treatment, allowing a subsequent normal pregnancy. If cardiomegaly persists despite treatment, the prognosis is poor.

Dilated cardiomyopathy has been linked to the use of doxorubicin (Adriamycin), cyclophosphamide (Cytoxan), cocaine, and fluorouracil (Fluoroplex). Also, familial forms of this disorder may exist, possibly with an X-linked inheritance pattern.

Complications

- Intractable heart failure, arrhythmias, and emboli, resulting from dilated cardiomyopathy
- Syncope and sudden death, resulting from ventricular arrhythmias

Assessment findings

- The patient may have a history of a disorder that can cause cardiomyopathy. He commonly reports a gradual onset of shortness of breath, orthopnea, exertional dyspnea, paroxysmal nocturnal dyspnea, fatigue, dry cough at night, palpitations, and vague chest pain.
- Inspection may reveal peripheral edema, jugular vein distention, ascites, and peripheral cyanosis.
- Palpation of peripheral pulses may disclose tachycardia even at rest and alternating pulse in late stages. Palpation may also reveal hepatomegaly and splenomegaly.
- Percussion may detect hepatomegaly. Dullness is heard over lung areas that are fluid-filled.
- Blood pressure auscultation may show a narrow pulse pressure.
- Cardiac auscultation reveals irregular rhythms, diffuse apical impulses, pansystolic murmur (such as mitral and tricuspid insufficiency caused by cardiomegaly and weak papillary muscles), and

ASSESSMENT FINDINGS IN CARDIOMYOPATHIES

TYPE	ASSESSMENT FINDINGS
Dilated cardiomyopathy	<ul><li>Generalized weakness, fatigue</li><li>Chest pain, palpitations</li><li>Syncope</li><li>Tachycardia</li><li>Narrow pulse pressure</li><li>Pulmonary congestion, pleural effusions</li><li>Jugular vein distention, peripheral edema</li><li>Paroxysmal nocturnal dyspnea, orthopnea, dyspnea on exertion</li></ul>
Hypertrophic cardiomyopathy	<ul><li>Angina, palpitations</li><li>Syncope</li><li>Orthopnea, exertional dyspnea</li><li>Pulmonary congestion</li><li>Loud systolic murmur</li><li>Life-threatening arrhythmias</li><li>Sudden cardiac arrest</li></ul>
Restrictive cardiomyopathy	<ul><li>Generalized weakness, fatigue</li><li>Bradycardia</li><li>Dyspnea</li><li>Jugular vein distention, peripheral edema</li><li>Liver congestion, abdominal ascites</li></ul>

S_3 and S_4 gallop rhythms. Lung auscultation may reveal crackles and gurgles.

Dilated cardiomyopathy may need to be differentiated from other types of cardiomyopathy. (See *Assessment findings in cardiomyopathies*.)

Diagnostic test results

No single test confirms dilated cardiomyopathy. Diagnosis requires elimination of other possible causes of heart failure and arrhythmias.

■ An electrocardiogram (ECG) and angiography can help rule out ischemic heart disease. The ECG may also show biventricular hypertrophy, sinus tachycardia, atrial enlargement, ST-segment and T-wave abnormalities and, in 20% of patients, atrial fibrillation or left bundle branch block. QRS complexes are decreased in amplitude.

- Chest X-rays demonstrate moderate to marked cardiomegaly usually affecting all heart chambers, along with pulmonary congestion, pulmonary venous hypertension, and pleural effusion. Pericardial effusion may appear as a water-bottle shape.
- Echocardiography can help identify ventricular thrombi, global hypokinesis, and the degrees of left ventricular dilation and dysfunction.
- Cardiac catheterization can show left ventricular dilation and dysfunction, elevated left ventricular and (in some instances) right ventricular filling pressures, and diminished cardiac output.
- Gallium scans may identify patients with dilated cardiomyopathy and myocarditis.
- Transvenous endomyocardial biopsy may be useful in some patients to determine the underlying disorder, such as amyloidosis or myocarditis.

Treatment

In patients with dilated cardiomyopathy, the goal of treatment is to correct the underlying causes and to improve the heart's pumping ability with a cardiac glycoside, a diuretic, oxygen, an anticoagulant, a vasodilator, and a low-sodium diet supplemented by vitamin therapy. An antiarrhythmic may be used to treat arrhythmias. If cardiomyopathy results from alcoholism, alcohol consumption must be stopped. A woman of childbearing age should avoid pregnancy.

Therapy may also include prolonged bed rest and selective use of a corticosteroid, particularly when myocardial inflammation is present.

A vasodilator can help reduce preload and afterload, thereby decreasing congestion and increasing cardiac output. Acute heart failure necessitates vasodilation with I.V. nitroprusside (Nitropress), I.V. nesiritide (Natrecor), or I.V. nitroglycerin (Nitrostat). Long-term treatment may include prazosin (Minipress), hydralazine (Apresoline), isosorbide dinitrate (Isordil), an angiotensin-converting enzyme inhibitor and, if the patient is on prolonged bed rest, an anticoagulant. Dopamine (Inocor), dobutamine (Dobutrex), and milrinone (Primacor) may be useful during the acute stage.

When these treatments fail, therapy may require heart transplantation for carefully selected patients.

Cardiomyoplasty may be used for those who aren't candidates for transplants and who are symptomatic at rest. During cardiomyoplasty, the latissimus dorsi muscle is wrapped around the ventricle, helping the ventricle to effectively pump blood. A cardiomyostimulator delivers bursts of electrical impulses during systole to contract the muscle.

TEACHING THE PATIENT WITH DILATED CARDIOMYOPATHY

● Before discharge, teach the patient about the illness and its treatment.

● Emphasize the need to restrict sodium intake, watch for weight gain, and take a cardiac glycoside, as ordered, and watch for a toxic reaction to it (such as anorexia, nausea, and vomiting).

● Encourage family members to learn cardiopulmonary resuscitation because sudden cardiac arrest is possible.

Nursing interventions

■ Alternate periods of rest with required activities of daily living and treatments. Provide personal care as needed to prevent fatigue.

■ Provide active or passive range-of-motion exercises to prevent muscle atrophy while the patient is on bed rest.

■ Consult with the dietitian to provide a low-sodium diet that the patient can accept.

■ Monitor the patient for signs of progressive failure (decreased arterial pulses, increased jugular vein distention) and compromised renal perfusion (oliguria, increased blood urea nitrogen and serum creatinine levels, and electrolyte imbalances). Weigh the patient daily.

■ Administer oxygen as needed.

■ If the patient is receiving a vasodilator, check his blood pressure and heart rate frequently. If he becomes hypotensive, stop the infusion and place him in a supine position with his legs elevated to increase venous return and ensure cerebral blood flow.

■ If the patient is receiving a diuretic, monitor him for signs of resolving congestion (decreased crackles and dyspnea) or too-vigorous diuresis. Check his serum potassium level for hypokalemia, especially if therapy includes a cardiac glycoside.

■ Therapeutic restrictions and an uncertain prognosis usually cause profound anxiety and depression; offer support and let the patient express his feelings. Be flexible with visiting hours. If confinement to a facility is prolonged, try to obtain permission for the patient to spend occasional weekends at home. (See *Teaching the patient with dilated cardiomyopathy*.)

■ Allow the patient and his family to express their fears and concerns. As needed, help them identify effective coping strategies.

CLASSIFYING HEART FAILURE

Two sets of guidelines are available to classify heart failure. The New York Heart Association (NYHA) classification is based on functional capacity. The American College of Cardiology/American Heart Association (ACC/AHA) guidelines are based on objective assessment. These guidelines are compared side-by-side below.

NYHA CLASSIFICATION	ACC/AHA GUIDELINES
	Stage A. Patient at high risk for developing heart failure but without structural heart disease or signs and symptoms of heart failure
Class I. Ordinary physical activity doesn't cause undue fatigue, palpitations, dyspnea, or angina.	**Stage B.** Structural heart disease, but without signs and symptoms of heart failure
Class II. Slight limitation of physical activity but asymptomatic at rest. Ordinary physical activity causes fatigue, palpitations, dyspnea, or angina. **Class III.** Marked limitation of physical activity, but typically asymptomatic at rest. Less than ordinary physical activity causes fatigue, palpitations, dyspnea, or angina.	**Stage C.** Structural heart disease with prior or current signs and symptoms of heart failure
Class IV. Unable to perform any physical activity without discomfort; symptoms may be present at rest. Discomfort increases with physical activity.	**Stage D.** End-stage disease requiring specialized treatment strategies, such as mechanical circulatory support, continuous inotropic infusion, or heart transplant

HEART FAILURE

A syndrome rather than a disease, heart failure occurs when the heart can't pump enough blood to meet the body's metabolic needs. Heart failure results in intravascular and interstitial volume overload and poor tissue perfusion. An individual with heart failure experiences reduced exercise tolerance, a reduced quality of life, and a shortened life span. (See *Classifying heart failure*.)

Although the most common cause of heart failure is coronary artery disease, it also occurs in infants, children, and adults with congenital and acquired heart defects. The incidence of heart failure in-

WHAT HAPPENS DURING HEART FAILURE

These illustrations show, step-by-step, what happens when myocardial damage leads to heart failure.

Left-sided heart failure

Increased workload and end-diastolic volume enlarge the left ventricle. Because of the lack of oxygen, however, the ventricle enlarges with stretched tissue rather than functional tissue. The patient may experience increased heart rate, pale and cool tingling in the extremities, decreased cardiac output, and arrhythmias.

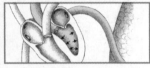

Diminished left ventricular function allows blood to pool in the ventricle and atrium and eventually back up into the pulmonary veins and capillaries. At this stage, the patient may experience exertional dyspnea, confusion, dizziness, orthostatic hypotension, decreased peripheral pulses and pulse pressure, cyanosis, and an S_3 gallop.

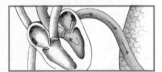

As the pulmonary circulation becomes engorged, rising capillary pressure pushes sodium (Na) and water (H_2O) into the interstitial space, causing pulmonary edema. Note coughing, subclavian retractions, crackles, tachypnea, elevated pulmonary artery pressure, diminished pulmonary compliance, and increased partial pressure of carbon dioxide.

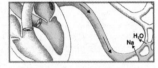

When the patient lies down, fluid in the extremities moves into the systemic circulation. Because the left ventricle can't handle the increased venous return, fluid pools in the pulmonary circulation, worsening pulmonary edema. You may note decreased breath sounds, dullness on percussion, crackles, and orthopnea.

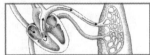

The right ventricle may now become stressed because it's pumping against greater pulmonary vascular resistance and left ventricular pressure. When this occurs, the patient's symptoms worsen.

creases with age. About 5 million people in the United States have heart failure. About 300,000 Americans die of heart failure each year. Mortality from heart failure is greater for males, blacks, and elderly people.

For many patients, the symptoms of heart failure restrict the ability to perform activities of daily living, severely affecting quality of life. Advances in diagnostic and therapeutic techniques have greatly im-

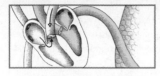

Right-sided heart failure

The stressed right ventricle hypertrophies with the formation of stretched tissue. Increasing conduction time and deviation of the heart from its normal axis can cause arrhythmias. If the patient doesn't already have left-sided heart failure, he may experience increased heart rate, cool skin, cyanosis, decreased cardiac output, palpitations, and dyspnea.

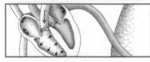

Blood pools in the right ventricle and right atrium. The backed-up blood causes pressure and congestion in the vena cava and systemic circulation. The patient has elevated central venous pressure, jugular vein distention, and hepatojugular reflux.

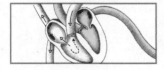

Backed-up blood also distends the visceral veins, especially the hepatic vein. As the liver and spleen become engorged, their function is impaired. The patient may develop anorexia, nausea, abdominal pain, palpable liver and spleen, weakness, and dyspnea secondary to abdominal distention.

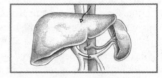

Increasing capillary pressure forces excess fluid from the capillaries into the interstitial space. This causes tissue edema, especially in the legs and abdomen. The patient may experience weight gain, pitting edema, and nocturia.

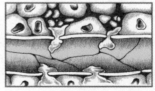

proved the outlook for these patients, but the prognosis still depends on the underlying cause and its response to treatment.

Pathophysiology

Heart failure may be classified according to the side of the heart it affects (left-sided or right-sided heart failure) or by the cardiac cycle involved (systolic or diastolic dysfunction). (See *What happens during heart failure.*)

LEFT-SIDED HEART FAILURE

Left-sided heart failure occurs as a result of ineffective left ventricular contractile function. As the pumping ability of the left ventricle fails, cardiac output falls. Blood is no longer effectively pumped out into the body; it backs up into the left atrium and then into the lungs, causing pulmonary congestion, dyspnea, and activity intolerance. If the condition persists, pulmonary edema and right-sided heart failure may result. Common causes include left ventricular infarctions, hypertension, and aortic and mitral valve stenosis.

RIGHT-SIDED HEART FAILURE

Right-sided heart failure results from ineffective right ventricular contractile function. Consequently, blood isn't pumped effectively through the right ventricle to the lungs, causing blood to back up into the right atrium and the peripheral circulation. The patient gains weight and develops peripheral edema and engorgement of the kidney and other organs. It may result from an acute right ventricular infarction, pulmonary hypertension, or a pulmonary embolus. However, the most common cause is profound backward blood flow due to left-sided heart failure.

SYSTOLIC DYSFUNCTION

Systolic dysfunction occurs when the left ventricle can't pump enough blood out to the systemic circulation during systole and the ejection fraction falls. Consequently, blood backs up into the pulmonary circulation and pressure increases in the pulmonary venous system. Cardiac output falls; weakness, fatigue, and shortness of breath may occur. Causes of systolic dysfunction include a myocardial infarction and dilated cardiomyopathy.

DIASTOLIC DYSFUNCTION

Diastolic dysfunction occurs when the ability of the left ventricle to relax and fill during diastole is reduced and the stroke volume falls. Therefore, higher volumes are needed in the ventricles to maintain cardiac output. Consequently, pulmonary congestion and peripheral edema develop. Diastolic dysfunction may occur as a result of left ventricular hypertrophy, hypertension, or restrictive cardiomyopathy. This type of heart failure is less common than systolic dysfunction, and its treatment isn't as clear.

All causes of heart failure eventually lead to reduced cardiac output, which triggers compensatory mechanisms, such as increased sympathetic activity, activation of the renin-angiotensin-aldosterone system, ventricular dilation, and hypertrophy. These mechanisms improve cardiac output at the expense of increased ventricular work.

Increased sympathetic activity—a response to decreased cardiac output and blood pressure—enhances peripheral vascular resistance, contractility, heart rate, and venous return. Signs of increased sympathetic activity, such as cool extremities and clamminess, may indicate impending heart failure.

Increased sympathetic activity also restricts blood flow to the kidneys, causing them to secrete renin, which in turn converts angiotensinogen to angiotensin I, which then becomes angiotensin II—a potent vasoconstrictor. Angiotensin causes the adrenal cortex to release aldosterone, leading to sodium and water retention and increased circulating blood volume. This renal mechanism is initially helpful; however, if it persists unchecked, it can aggravate heart failure as the heart struggles to pump against the increased volume.

In ventricular dilation, an increase in end-diastolic ventricular volume (preload) causes increased stroke work and stroke volume during contraction, stretching cardiac muscle fibers so that the ventricle can accept the intravascular volume. Eventually, the muscle becomes stretched beyond optimum limits and contractility declines.

In ventricular hypertrophy, an increase in ventricular muscle mass allows the heart to pump against increased resistance to the outflow of blood, improving cardiac output. However, this increased muscle mass also increases myocardial oxygen requirements. An increase in the ventricular diastolic pressure necessary to fill the enlarged ventricle may compromise diastolic coronary blood flow, limiting the oxygen supply to the ventricle and causing ischemia and impaired muscle contractility.

In heart failure, counterregulatory substances—prostaglandins and atrial natriuretic factor—are produced in an attempt to reduce the negative effects of volume overload and vasoconstriction caused by the compensatory mechanisms.

The kidneys release the prostaglandins, prostacyclin and prostaglandin E2, which are potent vasodilators. These vasodilators also act to reduce volume overload produced by the renin-angiotensin-aldosterone system by inhibiting sodium and water reabsorption by the kidneys.

Atrial natriuretic factor is a hormone secreted mainly by the atria in response to stimulation of the stretch receptors in the atria caused by excess fluid volume. B-type natriuretic factors work to counteract the negative effects of sympathetic nervous system stimulation and the

HOW HEART FAILURE AFFECTS THE BODY

This summary highlights how heart failure affects the major body systems and the multidisciplinary care required.

Cardiovascular system
● In left-sided heart failure, the pumping ability of the left ventricle fails and cardiac output falls. Blood backs up into the right atrium.
● In right-sided heart failure, the right ventricle becomes stressed and hypertrophies, leading to increased conduction time and arrhythmias.

Respiratory system
● As blood backs up into the right atrium (because the heart's pumping ability has failed), blood backs into the lungs, causing pulmonary congestion.

GI system
● Congestion of the peripheral tissues leads to GI tract congestion and anorexia, GI distress, and weight loss.
● Liver failure can occur as a result of blood backing up into the peripheral circulation and subsequent engorgement of organs.

Renal system
● With right-sided heart failure, blood backs up into the right atrium and the peripheral circulation. The patient gains weight and develops peripheral edema and engorgement of the kidney and other organs.

Collaborative management
Multidisciplinary care is needed to determine the underlying cause and precipitating factors of heart failure, and may include the expertise of a respiratory therapist, dietitian, and physical therapist. Surgery may be indicated if the patient has coronary artery disease or is experiencing severe limitations or recurrent hospitalizations despite maximal medical treatment. Social services may be necessary to help the patient's transition to his home setting after the acute situation is resolved.

renin-angiotensin-aldosterone system by producing vasodilation and diuresis. (See *How heart failure affects the body*.)

Complications

ACUTE
■ Acute renal failure
■ Arrhythmias
■ Pulmonary edema

CHRONIC
■ Activity intolerance
■ Cardiac cachexia
■ Metabolic impairment

- Renal impairment
- Thromboembolism

Assessment findings

- The patient's history reveals a disorder or condition that can precipitate heart failure. The patient frequently reports shortness of breath, which in early stages occurs during activity and in late stages also occurs at rest. He may report that dyspnea worsens at night when he lies down. He may use two or three pillows to elevate his head to sleep or have to sleep sitting up in a chair. He may state that his shortness of breath awakens him shortly after he falls asleep, causing him to sit up to catch his breath. He may remain dyspneic, coughing, and wheezing even when he sits up. This is referred to as paroxysmal nocturnal dyspnea.
- The patient may report that his shoes or rings have become too tight, a result of peripheral edema.
- He may also report increasing fatigue, weakness, insomnia, anorexia, nausea, and a sense of abdominal fullness (particularly if he has right-sided heart failure).
- Inspection may reveal a dyspneic, anxious patient in respiratory distress. In mild cases, dyspnea may occur while the patient is lying down or active; in severe cases, it's unrelated to position.
- The patient may have a cough that produces pink, frothy sputum. You may note cyanosis of the lips and nail beds, pale skin, diaphoresis, dependent peripheral and sacral edema, and jugular vein distention.
- Ascites may also be present, especially in patients with right-sided heart failure.
- If heart failure is chronic, the patient may appear cachectic.
- When palpating the pulse, you may note that the skin feels cool and clammy. The pulse rate is rapid, and an alternating pulse may be present. Hepatomegaly and, possibly, splenomegaly may also be present.
- Percussion reveals dullness over fluid-filled lung bases.
- Auscultation of the blood pressure may detect decreased pulse pressure, reflecting reduced stroke volume. Heart auscultation may disclose an S_3 and S_4. Lung auscultation reveals moist, bibasilar crackles. If pulmonary edema is present, you hear crackles throughout the lung, accompanied by rhonchi and expiratory wheezing.

Diagnostic test results

- Electrocardiography reflects heart strain or enlargement or ischemia. It may also reveal atrial enlargement, tachycardia, and extra systoles.
- Chest X-rays show increased pulmonary vascular markings, interstitial edema, or pleural effusion and cardiomegaly.
- Pulmonary artery pressure monitoring typically demonstrates elevated pulmonary artery and pulmonary artery wedge pressures, left ventricular end-diastolic pressure in patients with left-sided heart failure, and elevated right atrial or central venous pressure in those with right-sided heart failure.
- Echocardiography demonstrates left ventricular dysfunction with a reduced ejection fraction.
- Brain natriuretic peptide (BNP) assay helps to detect abnormal hormone levels produced by failing ventricles.
- Cardiopulmonary exercise testing determines oxygen consumption and severity of heart failure.

Treatment

The goal of therapy is to improve pump function by reversing the compensatory mechanisms producing the clinical effects. Heart failure can usually be controlled quickly with treatment consisting of a diuretic (such as furosemide [Lasix], hydrochlorothiazide [HydroDI-URIL], ethacrynic acid [Edecrin], bumetanide [Bumex], spironolactone [Aldactone], or triamterene [Dyrenium]) to reduce total blood volume and circulatory congestion; nesiritide (Natrecor), a recombinant form of human BNP, to increase diuresis and to decrease afterload; an angiotensin-converting enzyme (ACE) inhibitor to decrease peripheral vascular resistance; carvedilol (Coreg), a nonselective beta-adrenergic receptor blocker with alpha-receptor blockade to reduce mortality and improve quality of life; oxygen administration to increase oxygen delivery to the myocardium and other vital organ tissues; an inotropic drug, such as digoxin (Lanoxin), to strengthen myocardial contractility; a sympathomimetic, such as dopamine and dobutamine (Dobutrex), in acute situations; milrinone (Primacor), to increase contractility and cause arterial vasodilation; a vasodilator to increase cardiac output or an ACE inhibitor to decrease afterload; and antiembolism stockings to prevent venostasis and possible thromboembolism formation.

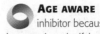 **AGE AWARE** An elderly patient may require lower doses of an ACE inhibitor because of impaired renal clearance. Monitor him for severe hypotension, signifying a toxic effect.

Acute pulmonary edema requires morphine; nitroglycerin or nitroprusside (Nitropress) as a vasodilator to diminish blood return to the heart; dobutamine, dopamine, or milrinone to increase myocardial contractility and cardiac output; a diuretic to reduce fluid volume; supplemental oxygen; and high Fowler's position.

After recovery, the patient usually must continue taking a cardiac glycoside, a diuretic, and a potassium supplement and must remain under medical supervision. If the patient with valve dysfunction has recurrent acute heart failure, surgical replacement may be necessary.

The patient may also require lifestyle modifications (to reduce symptoms of heart failure), such as weight loss, limited sodium (3 g/day) and alcohol intake, reduced fat intake, smoking cessation, stress reduction, and development of an exercise program.

A biventricular pacemaker may be used to control ventricular dyssynchrony. If heart failure is due to coronary artery disease, the patient may require coronary artery bypass graft surgery or angioplasty. The patient may also require valve surgery to reshape and support the mitral valve and improve cardiac functioning. If heart failure is severe enough that the patient requires a heart transplant, he may have a left ventricular assist device placed to improve the pumping ability of the heart until transplantation can be performed.

Nursing interventions

- Place the patient in Fowler's position and give him supplemental oxygen to help him breathe more easily. Organize all activity to provide maximum rest periods.
- Weigh the patient daily (the best index of fluid retention), and check for peripheral edema. Also, monitor I.V. intake and urine output (especially if the patient is receiving a diuretic).
- Assess vital signs (for increased respiratory and heart rates and for narrowing pulse pressure) and mental status. Auscultate the heart for abnormal sounds (S_3 gallop) and the lungs for crackles or rhonchi. Report any changes immediately.
- Frequently monitor blood urea nitrogen and serum creatinine, potassium, sodium, chloride, and magnesium levels.
- Provide continuous cardiac monitoring during acute and advanced stages to identify and treat arrhythmias promptly.

DISCHARGE TEACHING

TEACHING THE PATIENT WITH HEART FAILURE

● Advise the patient to follow a low-sodium diet, if ordered. Identify low-sodium food substitutes and foods to avoid, and show how to read labels to assess sodium content. To evaluate compliance, analyze the patient's 24-hour dietary intake.

● Show the patient how to take his own pulse by placing a finger on the radial artery and counting for 1 minute. Have him demonstrate the procedure.

● Tell the patient to take digoxin at the same time each day, to check his pulse rate and rhythm before taking it, and to call the practitioner if the rate is less than 60 beats/minute or if the rhythm is irregular.

● Teach the patient to report important signs and symptoms, such as dizziness, blurred vision, shortness of breath, persistent dry cough, palpitations, increased fatigue, paroxysmal nocturnal dyspnea, swollen ankles, and decreased urine output.

● Advise the patient to weigh himself at least three times per week and to report an increase of 3 to 5 lb (1.4 to 2.3 kg) in 1 week.

● Instruct the patient taking a potassium-wasting diuretic to eat high-potassium foods, such as bananas and orange juice.

● Instruct the patient to avoid fatigue by scheduling his activities to allow for rest periods.

■ To prevent deep vein thrombosis from vascular congestion, help the patient with range-of-motion exercises. Apply antiembolism stockings as needed. Check for calf pain and tenderness.

■ Allow adequate rest periods. (See *Teaching the patient with heart failure.*)

HYPERTENSION

Hypertension is an intermittent or sustained elevation of diastolic or systolic blood pressure. The two major types are essential (also called *primary* or *idiopathic*) hypertension—the most common (90% to 95% of cases)—and secondary hypertension, which results from renal disease or another identifiable cause. Malignant hypertension is a severe, fulminant form of hypertension that typically arises from both types. Hypertension is a major cause of stroke, cardiac disease, and renal failure.

Hypertension affects about 50 million adults in the United States. The risk of hypertension increases with age and is higher for blacks than for whites and in those with less education and lower income. Men have a higher incidence of hypertension in young and early middle adulthood; thereafter, women have a higher incidence.

Essential hypertension usually begins insidiously as a benign disease, slowly progressing to an accelerated or malignant state. If untreated, even mild hypertension can cause significant complications and a high mortality. In many cases, however, treatment with stepped care offers patients an improved prognosis.

Pathophysiology

Arterial blood pressure is a product of total peripheral resistance and cardiac output. Cardiac output is increased by conditions that increase heart rate, stroke volume, or both. Peripheral resistance is increased by factors that increase blood viscosity or reduce the lumen size of vessels, especially the arterioles.

Several theories help to explain the development of hypertension, including:

- changes in the arteriolar bed, causing increased peripheral vascular resistance
- abnormally increased tone in the sympathetic nervous system that originates in the vasomotor system centers, causing increased peripheral vascular resistance
- increased blood volume resulting from renal or hormonal dysfunction
- an increase in arteriolar thickening caused by genetic factors, leading to increased peripheral vascular resistance
- abnormal renin release, resulting in the formation of angiotensin II, which constricts the arteriole and increases blood volume. (See *How hypertension develops,* pages 424 and 425.)

Prolonged hypertension increases the heart's workload as resistance to left ventricular ejection increases. To increase contractile force, the left ventricle hypertrophies, raising the heart's oxygen demands and workload. Cardiac dilation and failure may occur when hypertrophy can no longer maintain sufficient cardiac output. Because hypertension promotes coronary atherosclerosis, the heart may be further compromised by reduced blood flow to the myocardium, resulting in angina or a myocardial infarction (MI). Hypertension also causes vascular damage, leading to accelerated atherosclerosis and target organ damage, such as retinal injury, renal failure, stroke, and aortic aneurysm and dissection.

The pathophysiology of secondary hypertension is related to the underlying disease. For example:

HOW HYPERTENSION DEVELOPS

Increased blood volume, cardiac rate, and stroke volume or arteriolar vasoconstriction that increases peripheral resistance causes blood pressure to rise. Hypertension may also result from the breakdown or inappropriate response of the following intrinsic regulatory mechanisms.

Renin-angiotensin system

Renal hypoperfusion causes the release of renin. Angiotensinogen, a liver enzyme, converts renin to angiotensin I, which increases preload and afterload. Angiotensin I then converts to angiotensin II in the lungs. A powerful vasoconstrictor, angiotensin II also helps increase preload and afterload by stimulating the adrenal cortex to secrete aldosterone. This serves to increase sodium reabsorption. Next comes hypertonic-stimulated release of antidiuretic hormone from the pituitary gland. This, in turn, increases water absorption, plasma volume, cardiac output, and blood pressure.

Autoregulation

Several intrinsic mechanisms work to change an artery's diameter to maintain tissue and organ perfusion, despite fluctuations in systemic blood pressure. Mechanisms include stress relaxation and capillary fluid shift. During stress relaxation, blood vessels gradually dilate when blood pressure rises to reduce peripheral resistance. During capillary fluid shift, plasma moves between vessels and extravascular spaces to maintain intravascular volume.

When blood pressure decreases, baroreceptors in the aortic arch and carotid sinuses decrease their inhibition of the medulla's vasomotor center. This action increases sympathetic stimulation of the heart by norepinephrine. This, in turn, increases cardiac output by strengthening the contractile force, increasing the heart rate, and augmenting peripheral resistance by vasoconstriction. Stress can also stimulate

- The most common cause of secondary hypertension is chronic renal disease. Insult to the kidney from chronic glomerulonephritis or renal artery stenosis interferes with sodium excretion, the renin-angiotensin-aldosterone system, or renal perfusion, causing blood pressure to increase.
- In Cushing's syndrome, increased cortisol levels raise blood pressure by increasing renal sodium retention, angiotensin II levels, and vascular response to norepinephrine.
- In primary aldosteronism, increased intravascular volume, altered sodium concentrations in vessel walls, or high aldosterone levels cause vasoconstriction and increased resistance.
- Pheochromocytoma is a chromaffin cell tumor of the adrenal medulla that secretes epinephrine and norepinephrine. Epineph-

the sympathetic nervous system to increase cardiac output and peripheral vascular resistance.

Blood vessel damage

Sustained hypertension damages blood vessels (as pictured below). Vascular injury begins with alternating areas of dilation and constriction in the arterioles. Increased intra-arterial pressure damages the endothelium (see illustration, below left). Independently, angiotensin induces endothelial wall contraction (see middle illustration below), allowing plasma to leak through interendothelial spaces. Eventually, plasma constituents deposited in the vessel wall cause medial necrosis (see illustration, below right).

VASCULAR DAMAGE

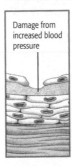

Damage from increased blood pressure

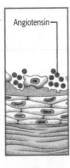

Angiotensin

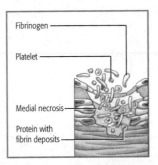

Fibrinogen

Platelet

Medial necrosis

Protein with fibrin deposits

rine increases cardiac contractility and rate, whereas norepinephrine increases peripheral vascular resistance.

The cause of essential hypertension is unknown. Family history, race, stress, obesity, a diet high in sodium or saturated fat, use of tobacco or hormonal contraceptives, excess alcohol intake, smoking, sedentary lifestyle, and aging have all been studied to determine their role in the development of hypertension. Other causes may include excessive renin production, mineral deficiencies (especially calcium, potassium, and magnesium), obesity, sleep apnea, and increased stress.

AGE AWARE Elderly people may have isolated systolic hypertension (ISH), in which just the systolic blood pressure is elevated, because atherosclerosis causes a loss of elasticity in large arteries. Previously, it was believed that ISH was a normal part of the aging process and shouldn't

be treated. Results of the Systolic Hypertension in the Elderly Program, however, found that treating ISH with an antihypertensive lowered the incidence
of stroke, coronary artery disease (CAD), and left-sided heart failure.

Secondary hypertension may result from renovascular disease; renal parenchymal disease; pheochromocytoma; primary hyperaldosteronism; Cushing's syndrome; diabetes mellitus; dysfunction of the
thyroid, pituitary, or parathyroid gland; coarctation of the aorta; pregnancy; or a neurologic disorder. Use of a hormonal contraceptive may
be the most common cause of secondary hypertension, probably because these drugs activate the renin-angiotensin-aldosterone system.
Other medications contributing to secondary hypertension include
glucocorticoids, mineralocorticoids, sympathomimetics, cyclosporine
(Sandimmune), cocaine, and epoetin alfa.

Complications

- Hypertensive crisis, peripheral arterial disease, dissecting aortic
  aneurysm, CAD, angina, MI, heart failure, arrhythmias, and sudden
  death (see *What happens in hypertensive crisis*)
- Transient ischemic attacks, stroke, retinopathy, and hypertensive
  encephalopathy
- Renal failure

Assessment findings

- In many cases, the hypertensive patient has no symptoms, and the
  disorder is revealed incidentally during evaluation for another disorder or during a routine blood pressure screening program. When
  symptoms do occur, they reflect the effect of hypertension on the
  organ systems.
- The patient may report awakening with a headache in the occipital
  region, which subsides spontaneously after a few hours. This
  symptom usually is associated with severe hypertension. He may
  also report dizziness, palpitations, fatigue, and impotence.
- With vascular involvement, the patient may complain of nose-
  bleeds, bloody urine, weakness, and blurred vision. Complaints of
  chest pain and dyspnea may indicate cardiac involvement.
- Inspection may reveal peripheral edema in late stages when heart
  failure is present.
- Ophthalmoscopic evaluation may reveal hemorrhages, exudates,
  and papilledema in late stages if hypertensive retinopathy is present.
- Palpation of the carotid artery may disclose stenosis or occlusion.

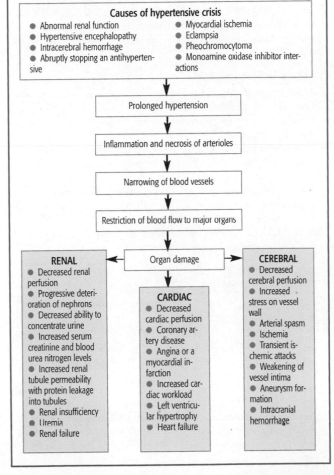

- Palpation of the abdomen may reveal a pulsating mass, suggesting an abdominal aneurysm.
- Enlarged kidneys may point to polycystic disease, a cause of secondary hypertension.
- Systolic or diastolic pressure, or both, may be elevated. An increase in diastolic blood pressure from a sitting to a standing position suggests essential hypertension, whereas a fall in blood pressure from the sitting to the standing position indicates secondary hypertension.
- Auscultation may reveal an abdominal bruit to the right or left of the umbilicus midline or in the flanks if renal artery stenosis is present. Bruits may also be heard over the abdominal aorta and the femoral or carotid arteries.

Diagnostic test results

The following tests may be used to find predisposing factors and help identify the cause of hypertension.

- Serial blood pressure measurements may be useful. (See *Classifying blood pressure readings*.)
- Urinalysis may show protein, red blood cells, or white blood cells, suggesting renal disease; glucose, suggesting diabetes mellitus; or presence of catecholamines associated with pheochromocytoma.
- Excretory urography may reveal renal atrophy, indicating chronic renal disease; one kidney that's more than ½" (1.3 cm) shorter than the other suggests unilateral renal disease.
- A serum potassium level less than 3.5 mEq/L may indicate adrenal dysfunction (primary hyperaldosteronism).
- A blood urea nitrogen level that's normal or elevated to more than 20 mg/dl and a serum creatinine level that's normal or elevated to more than 1.5 mg/dl suggest renal disease.

Other tests that help to detect cardiovascular damage and other complications include the following:

- Electrocardiography may show left ventricular hypertrophy or ischemia, and chest X-rays may show cardiomegaly.
- Ophthalmoscopy reveals arteriovenous nicking and, in patients with hypertensive encephalopathy, edema.
- An oral captopril (Capoten) challenge may be done to test for renovascular hypertension. This functional diagnostic test depends on the abrupt inhibition of circulatory angiotensin II by an angiotensin-converting enzyme (ACE) inhibitor, removing the major support for perfusion through a stenotic kidney. The acutely is-

CLASSIFYING BLOOD PRESSURE READINGS

In 2003, the National Institutes of Health issued The Seventh Report of the Joint National Committee on Prevention, Detection, Evaluation, and Treatment of High Blood Pressure (The JNC 7 Report). Updates since The JNC 6 report include a new category, prehypertension, and the combining of stages 2 and 3 hypertension. Categories now are normal, prehypertension, and stages 1 and 2 hypertension.

The revised categories are based on the average of two or more readings taken on separate visits after an initial screening. They apply to adults ages 18 and older. (If the systolic and diastolic pressures fall into different categories, use the higher of the two pressures to classify the reading. For example, a reading of 160/92 mm Hg should be classified as stage 2.)

Normal blood pressure with respect to cardiovascular risk is a systolic reading below 120 mm Hg and a diastolic reading below 80 mm Hg. Patients with prehypertension are at increased risk for developing hypertension and should follow health-promoting lifestyle modifications to prevent cardiovascular disease.

In addition to classifying stages of hypertension based on average blood pressure readings, practitioners should also take note of target organ disease and additional risk factors, such as a patient with diabetes, left ventricular hypertrophy, and chronic renal disease. This additional information is important to obtain a true picture of the patient's cardiovascular health.

CATEGORY	SYSTOLIC		DIASTOLIC
NORMAL	< 120 mm Hg	and	< 80 mm Hg
PREHYPERTENSION	120 to 139 mm Hg	or	80 to 89 mm Hg
HYPERTENSION Stage 1	140 to 159 mm Hg	or	90 to 99 mm Hg
Stage 2	≥ 160 mm Hg	or	≥ 100 mm Hg

chemic kidney immediately releases more renin and undergoes a marked decrease in glomerular filtration rate and renal blood flow.
■ Renal arteriography may show renal artery stenosis.

Treatment

The Seventh Report of the Joint National Committee on Prevention, Detection, Evaluation, and Treatment of High Blood Pressure of the National Institutes of Health, National Heart, Lung, and Blood Institute recommends:

■ Lifestyle modifications including weight reduction, use of a Dietary Approaches to Stop Hypertension (or DASH) diet (involves an increased intake of fruits, vegetables, and low-fat dairy products and a decreased intake of saturated and total fat), reduction of dietary sodium intake, physical activity (regular aerobic activity such as brisk walking), and moderation of alcohol intake.

- If the patient fails to achieve the desired blood pressure or make significant progress, continue lifestyle modifications and begin drug therapy.
- For stage 1 hypertension in the absence of compelling indications (heart failure, post-MI, high coronary disease risk, diabetes, chronic kidney disease, or recurrent stroke), give most patients a thiazide-type diuretic. Consider using an ACE inhibitor, an angiotensin receptor blocker, a beta-adrenergic receptor blocker, a calcium channel blocker, or a combination.
- For stage 2 hypertension in the absence of compelling indications, give most patients a two-drug combination (usually a thiazide-type diuretic and an ACE inhibitor, an angiotensin receptor blocker, a beta-adrenergic receptor blocker, or a calcium channel blocker).
- If the patient has one or more compelling indications, base drug treatment on benefits from outcome studies or existing clinical guidelines. Treatment may include the following, depending on indication:
  - heart failure—a diuretic, a beta-adrenergic receptor blocker, an ACE inhibitor, an angiotensin receptor blocker, or an aldosterone antagonist
  - post-MI—a beta-adrenergic receptor blocker, an ACE inhibitor, or an aldosterone antagonist
  - high CAD risk—a diuretic, a beta-adrenergic receptor blocker, an ACE inhibitor, or a calcium channel blocker
  - diabetes—a diuretic, a beta-adrenergic receptor blocker, an ACE inhibitor, an angiotensin receptor blocker, or a calcium channel blocker
  - chronic kidney disease—an ACE inhibitor or an angiotensin receptor blocker
  - recurrent stroke prevention—a diuretic or an ACE inhibitor
  - as needed—another antihypertensive.

Treatment for a patient with secondary hypertension includes correcting the underlying cause and controlling hypertensive effects.

Severely elevated blood pressure (hypertensive crisis) may be refractory to medications and may be fatal.

Hypertensive emergencies require parenteral administration of a vasodilator or an adrenergic inhibitor or oral administration of a se-

TEACHING THE PATIENT WITH HYPERTENSION

● Teach the patient to use a self-monitoring blood pressure cuff and to record the reading at least twice weekly in a journal for review by his practitioner at every office appointment. Tell the patient to take his blood pressure at the same hour each time with relatively the same type of activity preceding the measurement.

● Tell the patient and his family to keep a record of drugs used in the past, noting especially which ones are or aren't effective. Suggest recording this information on a card so the patient can show it to his practitioner.

● To encourage compliance with antihypertensive therapy, suggest establishing a daily routine for taking medication. Warn the patient that uncontrolled hypertension may cause stroke and heart attack. Tell him to report any adverse reactions to prescribed drugs. Advise him to avoid high-sodium antacids and over-the-counter cold and sinus medications containing harmful vasoconstrictors.

● Help the patient examine and modify his lifestyle. Suggest stress-reduction techniques, dietary changes, and an exercise program, particularly aerobic walking, to improve cardiac status and reduce obesity and serum cholesterol levels.

● Encourage a change in dietary habits. Help the obese patient plan a reducing diet. Tell him to avoid high-sodium foods (such as pickles, potato chips, canned soups, and cold cuts), table salt, and foods high in cholesterol and saturated fat.

lected drug (such as nifedipine [Procardia], captopril, clonidine [Catapres], or labetalol [Normodyne]), to rapidly reduce blood pressure.

The initial goal is to reduce mean arterial blood pressure by no more than 25% (within minutes to hours) and then to 160/110 within 2 hours while avoiding excessive falls in blood pressure that can precipitate renal, cerebral, or myocardial ischemia.

Examples of hypertensive emergencies include hypertensive encephalopathy, intracranial hemorrhage, acute left-sided heart failure with pulmonary edema, and dissecting aortic aneurysm. Hypertensive emergencies are also associated with eclampsia or severe gestational hypertension, unstable angina, and an acute MI.

Hypertension without accompanying symptoms or target-organ disease seldom requires emergency drug therapy.

Nursing interventions

■ If a patient is hospitalized with hypertension, find out if he was taking his prescribed antihypertensive. If he wasn't, ask why. If he can't afford the medication, refer him to the appropriate social service department. (See *Teaching the patient with hypertension*.)

■ When routine blood pressure screening reveals elevated pressure, make sure the sphygmomanometer cuff's size is appropriate for the patient's upper arm circumference. Take the pressure in both arms in lying, sitting, and standing positions. Ask the patient if he smoked, drank a beverage containing caffeine, or was emotionally upset before the test. Advise him to return for blood pressure testing at frequent and regular intervals.

■ To help identify hypertension and prevent untreated hypertension, participate in public education programs dealing with hypertension and ways to reduce risk factors. Encourage public participation in blood pressure screening programs. Routinely screen all patients, especially those at risk (blacks and those with family histories of hypertension, stroke, or heart attack).

HYPERTROPHIC CARDIOMYOPATHY

Hypertrophic cardiomyopathy—also known as *idiopathic hypertrophic subaortic stenosis, hypertrophic obstructive cardiomyopathy,* and *muscular aortic stenosis*—is a primary disease of cardiac muscle. It's characterized by left ventricular hypertrophy and disproportionate, asymmetrical thickening of the intraventricular septum and free wall of the left ventricle. In patients with hypertrophic cardiomyopathy, cardiac output may be low, normal, or high, depending on whether the stenosis is obstructive or nonobstructive. Eventually, left ventricular dysfunction—resulting from rigidity and decreased compliance—causes pump failure. If cardiac output is normal or high, stenosis may go undetected for years, but low cardiac output may lead to potentially fatal heart failure.

The course of this disorder varies. Some patients demonstrate progressive deterioration; others remain stable for several years.

Pathophysiology

The hypertrophied ventricle becomes stiff, noncompliant, and unable to relax during ventricular filling. Consequently, ventricular filling is reduced and left ventricular filling pressure rises, causing increases in left atrial and pulmonary venous pressures and leading to venous congestion and dyspnea.

Ventricular filling time is further reduced as a compensatory response to tachycardia. Reduced ventricular filling during diastole and obstruction of ventricular outflow lead to low cardiac output. If papillary muscles become hypertrophied and don't close completely during contraction, mitral insufficiency occurs. Moreover, intramural coronary arteries are abnormally small and may not be sufficient to supply the hypertrophied muscle with enough blood and oxygen to meet the increased needs to the hyperdynamic muscle.

About half of all cases of hypertrophic cardiomyopathy are transmitted as an autosomal dominant trait. Other causes aren't known.

Complications
- Pulmonary hypertension
- Heart failure
- Sudden death
- Ventricular arrhythmias, such as ventricular tachycardia and premature ventricular contractions

Assessment findings
- Generally, clinical features don't appear until the disease is well advanced. Then atrial dilation and, sometimes, atrial fibrillation abruptly reduce blood flow to the left ventricle.
- Most patients are asymptomatic but have a family history of hypertrophic cardiomyopathy.

  AGE AWARE In some cases, death occurs suddenly, particularly in children and young adults.
- Patients who have symptoms report exertional dyspnea (90% of patients) and orthopnea. They commonly have angina (75% of patients), fatigue, and syncope even at rest.
- Inspection of the carotid artery may show a rapidly rising carotid arterial pulse.
- Palpation of peripheral arteries reveals a characteristic double impulse (called *pulsus biferiens*).
- Palpation of the chest reveals a double or triple apical impulse, which may be displaced laterally.
- Percussion may reveal bibasilar crackles if heart failure is present.
- Auscultation reveals a harsh systolic murmur, heard after S_1 at the apex near the left sternal border. The murmur is intensified by standing and with Valsalva's maneuver. An S_4 may also be audible.

Diagnostic test results
- Echocardiography shows left ventricular hypertrophy and a thick, asymmetrical intraventricular septum in patients with obstructive hypertrophic cardiomyopathy, whereas hypertrophy affects various ventricular areas in those with nonobstructive hypertrophic cardiomyopathy. The septum may have a ground-glass appearance. Poor septal contraction, abnormal motion of the anterior mitral leaflet during systole, and narrowing or occlusion of the left ven-

tricular outflow tract may also be seen in obstructive hypertrophic cardiomyopathy. The left ventricular cavity appears small, with vigorous posterior-wall motion but reduced septal excursion.

- Cardiac catheterization reveals elevated left ventricular end-diastolic pressure and, possibly, mitral insufficiency. In a rare form of the disease, the left atrium has a slipper-foot shape and the left ventricle a spade shape.
- Electrocardiography usually shows left ventricular hypertrophy; ST-segment and T-wave abnormalities; Q waves in leads II, III, aV_F, and V_4 to V_6 (because of hypertrophy, not infarction); left anterior hemiblock; left-axis deviation; and ventricular and atrial arrhythmias.
- Chest X-rays may show a mild to moderate increase in heart size, and a thallium scan usually reveals myocardial perfusion defects.

Treatment

The goals of treatment are to relax the ventricle and to relieve outflow tract obstruction. Propranolol (Inderal), a beta-adrenergic receptor blocker, is the drug of choice. It slows the heart rate and increases ventricular filling by relaxing the obstructing muscle, thereby reducing angina, syncope, dyspnea, and arrhythmias. However, propranolol may aggravate symptoms of cardiac decompensation.

Atrial fibrillation, a medical emergency with hypertrophic cardiomyopathy, necessitates cardioversion. It also calls for heparin administration before cardioversion and continuing until fibrillation subsides because of the high risk of systemic embolism. Calcium channel blockers (such as verapamil [Calan]) may improve diastolic dysfunction until fibrillation subsides.

If heart failure occurs, amiodarone (Cordarone) may be used, unless an atrioventricular block exists. This drug seems to be effective in reducing ventricular and supraventricular arrhythmias as well. Vasodilators (such as nitroglycerin [Nitro-Bid]), diuretics, and sympathetic stimulators (such as isoproterenol [Isuprel]) are contraindicated.

If drug therapy fails, surgery is indicated. Ventricular myotomy (resection of the hypertrophied septum) alone or combined with mitral valve replacement may ease outflow tract obstruction and relieve symptoms. However, ventricular myotomy is experimental and may cause complications, such as complete heart block and a ventricular septal defect. Dual-chamber pacing may prevent progression of hypertrophy and obstruction. An implantable defibrillator may be used in patients with malignant ventricular arrhythmias.

DISCHARGE TEACHING

TEACHING THE PATIENT WITH HYPERTROPHIC CARDIOMYOPATHY

● Remind the patient and his family that propranolol may cause depression. Notify the practitioner if symptoms occur.

● Instruct the patient to take his drugs as ordered. Tell him to notify any practitioner caring for him that he shouldn't be given nitroglycerin, a cardiac glycoside, or a diuretic because these drugs can worsen an obstruction.

● Inform the patient that before dental work or surgery, he needs antibiotic prophylaxis to prevent subacute bacterial endocarditis.

Nursing interventions

■ Alternate periods of rest with required activities of daily living and treatments. Provide personal care, as needed, to prevent fatigue.

■ Provide active or passive range-of-motion exercises to prevent muscle atrophy if the patient must maintain bed rest.

■ If propranolol is discontinued, don't stop the drug abruptly; doing so may cause rebound effects, resulting in a myocardial infarction or sudden death. To determine the patient's tolerance for an increased dose of propranolol, take his pulse to check for bradycardia, and have him stand and walk around slowly to check for orthostatic hypotension.

■ Therapeutic restrictions and an uncertain prognosis usually cause profound anxiety and depression; offer support and let the patient express his feelings. Be flexible with visiting hours. If confinement to a facility is prolonged, try to obtain permission for the patient to spend occasional weekends at home.

■ Allow the patient and his family to express their fears and concerns. As needed, help them identify effective coping strategies. (See *Teaching the patient with hypertrophic cardiomyopathy*.)

RED FLAG Warn the patient against strenuous activity, which may precipitate syncope or sudden death. Also, advise him to avoid Valsalva's maneuver or sudden position changes; both may worsen an obstruction. Urge his family to learn cardiopulmonary resuscitation.

PULMONARY HYPERTENSION

Pulmonary hypertension occurs when pulmonary artery pressure (PAP) rises above normal for reasons other than aging or altitude. No definitive set of values is used to diagnose pulmonary hypertension, but the National Institutes of Health requires a mean PAP of 25 mm Hg or more.

Primary or idiopathic pulmonary hypertension is characterized by increased PAP and increased pulmonary vascular resistance, both without an obvious cause. This form is most common in females ages 20 to 40 and is usually fatal within 4 years.

RED FLAG Mortality is highest in pregnant women.

Secondary pulmonary hypertension results from existing cardiac or pulmonary disease or both. The prognosis in secondary pulmonary hypertension depends on the severity of the underlying disorder.

Pathophysiology

In primary pulmonary hypertension, the smooth muscle in the pulmonary artery wall hypertrophies for no reason, narrowing the small pulmonary artery (arterioles) or obliterating it completely. Fibrous lesions also form around vessels, impairing distensibility and increasing vascular resistance. Pressures in the left ventricle, which receives blood from the lungs, remain normal. However, the increased pressures generated in the lungs are transmitted to the right ventricle, which supplies the pulmonary artery. Eventually, the right ventricle fails (cor pulmonale). Although oxygenation isn't severely affected initially, hypoxia and cyanosis eventually occur. Death results from cor pulmonale.

Alveolar hypoventilation can result from diseases caused by alveolar destruction or from disorders that prevent the chest wall from expanding sufficiently to allow air into the alveoli. The resulting decreased ventilation increases pulmonary vascular resistance. Hypoxemia resulting from this ventilation-perfusion mismatch also causes vasoconstriction, further increasing vascular resistance and resulting in pulmonary hypertension.

Coronary artery disease or mitral valvular disease causing increased left ventricular filling pressures may cause secondary pulmonary hypertension. Ventricular septal defect (VSD) and patent ductus arteriosus (PDA) cause secondary hypertension by increasing blood flow through the pulmonary circulation through left-to-right shunting. Pulmonary emboli and chronic destruction of alveolar walls, as in emphysema, cause secondary pulmonary hypertension by obliterating or obstructing the pulmonary vascular bed. Secondary pulmonary hypertension can also occur by vasoconstriction of the vascular bed, such as through hypoxemia, acidosis, or both. Conditions resulting in vascular obstruction can also cause pulmonary hypertension because blood isn't allowed to flow appropriately through the vessels.

Secondary pulmonary hypertension can be reversed if the disorder is resolved. If hypertension persists, hypertrophy occurs in the medial smooth-muscle layer of the arterioles. The larger arteries stiffen, and hypertension progresses. Pulmonary pressure begins to equal systemic blood pressure, causing right ventricular hypertrophy and, eventually, cor pulmonale.

Primary cardiac disease may be congenital or acquired. Congenital defects cause a left-to-right shunting, rerouting blood through the lungs twice and causing pulmonary hypertension. Acquired cardiac diseases, such as rheumatic valvular disease and mitral stenosis, result in left-sided heart failure that diminishes the flow of oxygenated blood from the lungs. This increases pulmonary vascular resistance and right ventricular pressure.

The causes of primary pulmonary hypertension are unknown but are thought to include altered immune mechanisms and hereditary factors.

Secondary pulmonary hypertension results from hypoxemia caused by various conditions, including acquired cardiac disease, such as mitral stenosis and rheumatic valvular disease; alveolar hypoventilation resulting from chronic obstructive pulmonary disorders, diffuse interstitial pneumonia, kyphoscoliosis, malignant metastases, obesity, sarcoidosis, or scleroderma; primary cardiac disease resulting from atrial septal defect, PDA, or VSD; and vascular obstruction resulting from fibrosing mediastinitis, idiopathic veno-occlusive disease, left atrial myxoma, mediastinal neoplasm, pulmonary embolism, and vasculitis.

Complications
- Cor pulmonale
- Cardiac failure
- Cardiac arrest

Assessment findings
- The patient with primary pulmonary hypertension may have no signs or symptoms until lung damage becomes severe. (In fact, the disorder may not be diagnosed until autopsy.)

- Usually, a patient with pulmonary hypertension complains of increasing dyspnea on exertion, weakness, syncope, and fatigue. He may also have difficulty breathing, feel short of breath, and report that breathing causes pain. Such signs may result from left-sided heart failure.
- Inspection may show signs of right-sided heart failure, including ascites and jugular vein distention.
- The patient may appear restless and agitated and have a decreased level of consciousness (LOC). He may be confused and have memory loss.
- You may observe decreased diaphragmatic excursion and respiration, and the point of maximal impulse may be displaced beyond the midclavicular line.
- On palpation, you may also note signs of right-sided heart failure such as peripheral edema. The patient typically has an easily palpable right ventricular lift and a reduced carotid pulse. He may also have a palpable and tender liver and tachycardia.
- Auscultation findings are specific to the underlying disorder but may include a systolic ejection murmur, a widely split S_2 sound, and S_3 and S_4 sounds. You may also hear decreased breath sounds and loud tubular sounds.
- Breath sounds are commonly decreased because of fluid in the lungs, or loud tubular sounds may be heard.
- The patient may have decreased blood pressure.

Diagnostic test results

- Arterial blood gas (ABG) analysis reveals hypoxemia (decreased partial pressure of arterial oxygen).
- Electrocardiography, in right ventricular hypertrophy, shows right axis deviation and tall or peaked P waves in inferior leads.
- Cardiac catheterization discloses increased PAP, with a systolic pressure greater than 30 mm Hg. It may also show an increased pulmonary artery wedge pressure (PAWP) if the underlying cause is left atrial myxoma, mitral stenosis, or left-sided heart failure; otherwise, PAWP is normal.
- Pulmonary angiography reveals filling defects in the pulmonary vasculature such as those that develop with pulmonary emboli.
- Pulmonary function tests show decreased flow rates and increased residual volume in underlying obstructive disease; in underlying restrictive disease, they may show reduced total lung capacity.
- Radionuclide imaging allows assessment of right and left ventricular function.

- Open lung biopsy may determine the type of disorder.
- Echocardiography allows the assessment of ventricular wall motion and possible valvular dysfunction. It can also demonstrate right ventricular enlargement, abnormal septal configuration consistent with right ventricular pressure overload, and a reduction in left ventricular cavity size.
- Perfusion lung scan may produce normal or abnormal results, with multiple patchy and diffuse filling defects that don't suggest pulmonary thromboembolism.

Treatment

Oxygen therapy decreases hypoxemia and resulting pulmonary vascular resistance. For patients with right-sided heart failure, treatment also includes fluid restriction, cardiac glycosides to increase cardiac output, and diuretics to decrease intravascular volume and extravascular fluid accumulation. Vasodilators and calcium channel blockers can reduce myocardial workload and oxygen consumption. Bronchodilators and beta-adrenergic agents may also be prescribed. A patient with primary pulmonary hypertension usually responds to epoprostenol (PGI_2) as a continuous home infusion.

For a patient with secondary pulmonary hypertension, treatment must also aim to correct the underlying cause. If that isn't possible and the disease progresses, the patient may need a heart-lung transplant.

Nursing interventions

- Give oxygen therapy, and observe the patient's response. Report signs of increasing dyspnea so the practitioner can adjust treatment accordingly.
- Monitor ABG levels for acidosis and hypoxemia. Report a change in the patient's LOC immediately.
- When caring for a patient with right-sided heart failure, especially one receiving diuretics, record weight daily, carefully measure intake and output, and explain all medications and diet restrictions. Check for increasing jugular vein distention, which may signal fluid overload.
- Monitor the patient's vital signs, especially his blood pressure and heart rate. If hypotension or tachycardia develops, notify the practitioner. If the patient has a pulmonary artery catheter, monitor his PAP and PAWP as ordered and report changes.
- Make sure the patient alternates periods of rest and activity to reduce the body's oxygen demand and prevent fatigue.
- Arrange for diversional activities. The type of activity—whether active or passive—depends on the patient's physical condition.

- Before discharge, help the patient adjust to the limitations imposed by this disorder. (See *Teaching the patient with pulmonary hypertension.*)
- Listen to the patient's fears and concerns, and remain with him during periods of extreme stress and anxiety.
- Answer questions the patient has as best as you can. Encourage him to identify care measures and activities that make him comfortable and relaxed. Perform these measures, and encourage the patient to do so as well.
- Include the patient in care decisions, and include family members in all phases of his care.

RESTRICTIVE CARDIOMYOPATHY

Restrictive cardiomyopathy, a disorder of the myocardial musculature, is characterized by restricted ventricular filling (the result of left ventricular hypertrophy) and endocardial fibrosis and thickening. If severe, it's irreversible.

Pathophysiology

An extremely rare disorder, the cause of primary restrictive cardiomyopathy is unknown. However, restrictive cardiomyopathy syndrome, a manifestation of amyloidosis, results from infiltration of amyloid into the intracellular spaces in the myocardium, endocardium, and subendocardium.

In both forms of restrictive cardiomyopathy, the myocardium becomes rigid, with poor distention during diastole, inhibiting complete ventricular filling, and fails to contract completely during systole, resulting in low cardiac output.

Restrictive cardiomyopathy is rare. It's most common in children and young adults. There's no racial predilection, but people living in Africa, South America, and India are at increased risk.

Complications
- Heart failure
- Arrhythmias
- Systemic or pulmonary embolization
- Sudden death

Assessment findings
- Fatigue, dyspnea, orthopnea, chest pain, edema, liver engorgement, peripheral cyanosis, pallor, and S_3 or S_4 gallop rhythms due to heart failure
- Systolic murmurs caused by mitral and tricuspid insufficiency

Diagnostic test results
- In advanced stages of this disease, chest X-ray shows massive cardiomegaly, affecting all four chambers of the heart; pericardial effusion; and pulmonary congestion.
- Echocardiography, computed tomography scan, or magnetic resonance imaging rules out constrictive pericarditis as the cause of restricted filling by detecting increased left ventricular muscle mass and differences in end-diastolic pressures between the ventricles.
- Electrocardiography may show low-voltage complexes, hypertrophy, atrioventricular conduction defects, or arrhythmias.
- Arterial pulsation reveals blunt carotid upstroke with small volume.
- Cardiac catheterization shows increased left ventricular end-diastolic pressure and rules out constrictive pericarditis as the cause of restricted filling.

Restrictive cardiomyopathy may be difficult to differentiate from constrictive pericarditis. A biopsy of heart muscle may be used to confirm the diagnosis. Cardiac catheterization can also help differentiate the type of cardiomyopathy through simultaneous left- and right-heart catheterization. In some cases, surgical exploration and biopsies are the only means to distinguish the type of cardiomyopathy or to differentiate it from pericarditis.

Treatment

Although no therapy exists for restricted ventricular filling, a cardiac glycoside, a diuretic, and a restricted sodium diet are beneficial by easing the symptoms of heart failure.

An oral vasodilator—such as isosorbide dinitrate (Isordil), prazosin (Minipress), or hydralazine (Apresoline)—may control intractable heart failure. Anticoagulant therapy may be necessary to prevent thrombophlebitis in the patient on prolonged bed rest. A steroid or chemotherapy may help with underlying disease. A heart transplant may be considered in those with poor myocardial functioning.

Nursing interventions

- In the acute phase, monitor heart rate and rhythm, blood pressure, urine output, and pulmonary artery pressure readings to help guide treatment.
- Give psychological support. Provide appropriate diversionary activities for the patient restricted to prolonged bed rest. Because a poor prognosis may cause profound anxiety and depression, be especially supportive and understanding, and encourage the patient to express his fears. Refer him for psychosocial counseling, as necessary, for assistance in coping with his restricted lifestyle. Be flexible with visiting hours whenever possible. (See *Teaching the patient with restrictive cardiomyopathy*.)

9

Vascular disorders

Vascular disorders can affect the arteries, the veins, or both types of vessels. Arterial disorders include aneurysms, which result from a weakening of the arterial wall; arterial occlusive disease, which commonly results from atherosclerotic narrowing of the artery's lumen; and Raynaud's disease, which may be linked to immunologic dysfunction. Thrombophlebitis, a venous disorder, results from inflammation or occlusion of the affected vessel.

ABDOMINAL AORTIC ANEURYSM

Abdominal aortic aneurysm (AAA), an abnormal dilation in the arterial wall, generally occurs in the aorta between the renal arteries and iliac branches. Rupture, in which the aneurysm breaks open, resulting in profuse bleeding, is a common complication that occurs in larger aneurysm. Dissection occurs when the artery's lining tears and blood leaks into the walls.

AAA is four times more common in men than in women and is most prevalent in whites ages 40 to 70. Less than half of people with a ruptured AAA survive.

Pathophysiology

Aortic aneurysms develop slowly. First, a focal weakness in the muscular layer of the aorta (tunica media), caused by degenerative changes, allows the inner layer (tunica intima) and outer layer (tunica adventitia) to stretch outward. Blood pressure within the aorta progressively weakens the vessel walls and enlarges the aneurysm.

Nearly all AAAs are fusiform, which causes the arterial walls to balloon on all sides. The resulting sac fills with necrotic debris and thrombi.

443

About 95% of abdominal aneurysms result from arteriosclerosis or atherosclerosis; the rest, from cystic medial necrosis, trauma, hypertension, blunt abdominal injury, syphilis, and other infections.

Complications

- Rupture
- Obstruction of blood flow to other organs
- Embolization to a peripheral artery
- Diminished blood supply to vital organs resulting in organ failure (with rupture)

Assessment findings

- Most patients with abdominal aneurysms are asymptomatic until the aneurysm enlarges and compresses surrounding tissue.
- A large aneurysm may produce signs and symptoms that mimic renal calculi, lumbar disk disease, and duodenal compression.
- The patient may complain of gnawing, generalized, steady abdominal pain or low back pain that's unaffected by movement. He may have a sensation of gastric or abdominal fullness caused by pressure on the GI structures.

RED FLAG Sudden onset of severe abdominal pain or lumbar pain that radiates to the flank and groin from pressure on lumbar nerves may signify enlargement and imminent rupture. If the aneurysm ruptures into the peritoneal cavity, severe and persistent abdominal and back pain, mimicking renal or ureteral colic, occurs. If it ruptures into the duodenum, GI bleeding occurs with massive hematemesis and melena.

- The patient may have a syncopal episode when an aneurysm ruptures, causing hypovolemia and a subsequent drop in blood pressure. Once a clot forms and the bleeding stops, he may again be asymptomatic or have abdominal pain because of bleeding into the peritoneum.
- Inspection of the patient with an intact abdominal aneurysm usually reveals no significant findings. However, if the patient isn't obese, you may notice a pulsating mass in the periumbilical area.
- If the aneurysm has ruptured, you may notice signs of hypovolemic shock, such as skin mottling, decreased level of consciousness (LOC), diaphoresis, and oliguria.
- The abdomen may appear distended, and an ecchymosis or hematoma may be present in the abdominal, flank, or groin area.
- Paraplegia may occur if the aneurysm rupture reduces blood flow to the spine.

- Auscultation of the abdomen may reveal a systolic bruit over the aorta caused by turbulent blood flow in the widened arterial segment. Hypotension occurs with aneurysm rupture.
- Palpation of the abdomen may disclose some tenderness over the affected area. A pulsatile mass may be felt; however, avoid deep palpation to locate the mass because this may cause the aneurysm to rupture.
- Palpation of the peripheral pulses may reveal absent pulses distal to a ruptured aneurysm.

Diagnostic test results

Because an abdominal aneurysm seldom produces symptoms, it's typically detected accidentally on an X-ray or during a routine physical examination.

Several tests can confirm suspected abdominal aneurysm:
- Abdominal ultrasonography or echocardiography can help determine the size, shape, and location of the aneurysm.
- Anteroposterior and lateral X-rays of the abdomen can be used to detect aortic calcification, which outlines the mass, at least 75% of the time.
- A computed tomography scan can be used to visualize the aneurysm's effect on nearby organs, particularly the position of the renal arteries in relation to the aneurysm.
- Aortography shows the condition of vessels proximal and distal to the aneurysm and the extent of the aneurysm, but the diameter of the aneurysm may be underestimated because aortography shows only the flow channel and not the surrounding clot.
- Magnetic resonance imagining can be used as an alternative to aortography.

Treatment

Usually, abdominal aneurysm requires resection of the aneurysm and Dacron graft replacement of the aortic section. If the aneurysm is small and produces no symptoms, surgery may be delayed; however, small aneurysms can rupture. A beta-adrenergic receptor blocker may be given to decrease the rate of growth of the aneurysm. Regular physical examination and ultrasound checks help monitor progression of the aneurysm. Large aneurysms or those that produce symptoms risk rupture and require immediate repair. In asymptomatic patients, surgery is advised when the aneurysm is 5 to 6 cm in diameter. In symptomatic patients, repair is indicated regardless of size. In patients with

REPAIRING ABDOMINAL AORTIC ANEURYSMS WITH ENDOVASCULAR GRAFTING

Endovascular grafting is a minimally invasive procedure used to repair abdominal
aortic aneurysms. Such grafting reinforces
the walls of the aorta to prevent rupture
and prevents expansion of the aneurysm.

    The procedure is performed with fluo-
roscopic guidance, with a delivery catheter
with an attached compressed graft inserted through a small incision into the
femoral or iliac artery over a guide wire.
The delivery catheter is advanced into the
aorta, where it's positioned across the
aneurysm. A balloon on the catheter ex-
pands the graft and affixes it to the vessel
wall. The procedure generally takes 2 to 3
hours to perform. Patients are instructed to
walk the first day after surgery and are discharged from the facility in 1 to 3 days.

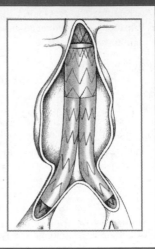

poor perfusion distal to the aneurysm, external grafting may be done.
(See *Repairing abdominal aortic aneurysms with endovascular grafting.*)

    For patients with acute dissection, emergency treatment before
surgery includes resuscitation with fluid and blood replacement, I.V.
propranolol (Inderal) to reduce myocardial contractility, I.V. nitroprusside (Nitropress) to reduce and maintain blood pressure to 100 to
120 mm Hg systolic, and an analgesic to relieve pain. An arterial line
and indwelling urinary catheter are inserted to monitor the patient's
condition.

Nursing interventions

IN A NONACUTE SITUATION

- Allow the patient to express his fears and concerns. Help him identify effective coping strategies as he attempts to deal with his diagnosis.
- Offer the patient and his family psychological support. Answer all
  questions honestly and provide reassurance.

- Before elective surgery, weigh the patient, insert an indwelling urinary catheter and an I.V. line, and assist with insertion of the arterial line and pulmonary artery catheter to monitor hemodynamic balance.
- Give a prophylactic antibiotic as ordered.

IN AN ACUTE SITUATION

- Monitor the patient's vital signs on his admission to the intensive care unit (ICU).
- Insert an I.V. line with at least a 18G needle to facilitate blood replacement.
- Obtain blood samples for kidney function tests (such as blood urea nitrogen, creatinine, and electrolyte levels), a complete blood count with differential, blood typing and crossmatching, and arterial blood gas (ABG) levels.
- Monitor the patient's cardiac rhythm strip. Insert an arterial line to allow for continuous blood pressure monitoring. Assist with insertion of a pulmonary artery line to monitor for hemodynamic balance.
- Give drugs, such as an antihypertensive and a beta-adrenergic receptor blocker to control aneurysm progression and an analgesic to relieve pain.
- Look for signs of rupture, which may be immediately fatal. Watch closely for signs of acute blood loss (such as decreasing blood pressure, increasing pulse and respiratory rates, restlessness, decreased sensorium, and cool, clammy skin).
- If rupture occurs, get the patient to surgery immediately. Medical antishock trousers may be used while transporting him to surgery.

AFTER SURGERY

- With the patient in the ICU, closely monitor vital signs, intake and hourly output, neurologic status (such as LOC, pupil size, and sensation in arms and legs), and ABG levels.
- Assess fluid status, and replace fluids as needed to ensure adequate hydration.
- Watch for signs of bleeding (such as increased pulse and respiratory rates, and hypotension), which may occur retroperitoneally from the graft site.
- Check abdominal dressings for excessive bleeding or drainage. Assess the wound site for evidence of infection. Be alert for temperature elevations and other signs of infection. Use sterile technique to change dressings.

- After nasogastric intubation for intestinal decompression, irrigate the tube frequently to ensure patency. Record the amount and type of drainage.
- Large amounts of blood may be needed during the resuscitative period to replace blood loss. Thus, renal failure due to ischemia is a major postoperative complication, possibly requiring hemodialysis.

  RED FLAG Assess for return of severe back pain, which can indicate that the graft is tearing.

- Mechanical ventilation is required after surgery. Assess the depth, rate, and character of respirations and breath sounds at least every hour. Have the patient cough, or suction the endotracheal tube, as needed, to maintain a clear airway. If the patient can breathe unassisted and has good breath sounds and adequate ABG levels, tidal volume, and vital capacity 24 hours after surgery, he will be extubated and will require oxygen by mask.
- Weigh the patient daily to evaluate fluid balance.
- Provide frequent turning, and help the patient walk as soon as he's able (generally the second day after surgery). (See *Teaching the patient with an abdominal aortic aneurysm.*)

FEMORAL AND POPLITEAL ANEURYSMS

Because femoral and popliteal aneurysms occur in the two major peripheral arteries, they're also known as peripheral arterial aneurysms.

This condition is most common in men older than age 50. Elective surgery before complications arise greatly improves the prognosis.

Causes

Femoral and popliteal aneurysms may be fusiform (spindle-shaped) or saccular (pouchlike). Fusiform types are three times more common. Aneurysms may be singular or multiple segmental lesions, in many instances affecting both legs, and may accompany other arterial aneurysms located in the abdominal aorta or iliac arteries.

Femoral and popliteal aneurysms usually result from progressive atherosclerotic changes in the arterial walls (medial layer). Rarely, they result from congenital weakness in the arterial wall. They may also result from blunt or penetrating trauma, bacterial infection, or peripheral vascular reconstructive surgery (which causes pseudoaneurysms, also called *false aneurysms,* where a blood clot forms a second lumen).

Complications

- Thrombosis
- Emboli
- Gangrene
- Poor tissue perfusion to areas distal to the aneurysm may require amputation

Assessment findings

- The patient may report pain in the popliteal space when a popliteal aneurysm is large enough to compress the medial popliteal nerve.
- Inspection may reveal edema and venous distention if the vein is compressed.
- Femoral and popliteal aneurysms can produce signs and symptoms of severe ischemia in the leg or foot resulting from acute thrombosis within the aneurysmal sac, embolization of mural thrombus fragments and, rarely, rupture.
- A patient with acute aneurysmal thrombosis may report severe pain.
- Inspection may reveal distal petechial hemorrhages from aneurysmal emboli. The affected leg or foot may show loss of color.
- Palpation of the affected leg or foot may indicate coldness and a loss of pulse. Gangrene may develop.
- Bilateral palpation that reveals a pulsating mass above or below the inguinal ligament in femoral aneurysm and behind the knee in popliteal aneurysm usually confirms the diagnosis. When thrombosis has occurred, palpation detects a firm, nonpulsating mass.

Diagnostic test results

- Arteriography or ultrasonography may help resolve doubtful situations. Arteriography may also detect associated aneurysms, especially those in the abdominal aorta and the iliac arteries.
- Ultrasonography may also help determine the size of the femoral or popliteal artery.

Treatment

Femoral and popliteal aneurysms require surgical bypass and reconstruction of the artery, usually with an autogenous saphenous vein graft replacement. Arterial occlusion that causes severe ischemia and gangrene may require leg amputation.

Nursing interventions

BEFORE ARTERIAL SURGERY

- Assess and record the patient's circulatory status, noting the location and quality of peripheral pulses in the affected leg.
- Give a prophylactic antibiotic or anticoagulant.
- Discuss expected postoperative procedures, review the explanation of the surgery, and answer the patient's questions.

AFTER ARTERIAL SURGERY

- Carefully monitor the patient for early signs and symptoms of thrombosis or graft occlusion (such as loss of pulse, decreased skin temperature and sensation, and severe pain) and infection (such as fever).

- Palpate distal pulses at least every hour for the first 24 hours and then as often as ordered. Correlate these findings with the preoperative circulatory assessment. Mark the sites on the patient's skin where pulses are palpable to facilitate repeated checks.
- Help the patient walk soon after surgery to prevent venous stasis and, possibly, thrombus formation. (See *Teaching the patient with femoral and popliteal aneurysm.*)

PERIPHERAL ARTERIAL OCCLUSIVE DISEASE

Peripheral arterial occlusive disease is an obstruction or narrowing of the lumen of the aorta and its major branches, which interrupts blood flow, usually to the legs and feet. Arterial occlusive disease may affect the carotid, vertebral, innominate, subclavian, mesenteric, and celiac arteries. (See *Possible sites of major artery occlusion,* page 452.)

Peripheral arterial occlusive disease is more common in men than in women. The prognosis depends on the location of the occlusion, the development of collateral circulation to counteract reduced blood flow and, in patients with acute disease, the time elapsed between the development of the occlusion and its removal.

Pathophysiology

Peripheral arterial occlusive disease is almost always the result of atherosclerosis in which fatty, fibrous plaques narrow the lumen of blood vessels. This occlusion can occur acutely or progressively over 20 to 40 years, with areas of vessel branching, or bifurcation, being the most common sites. The narrowing of the lumens reduces the blood volume that can flow through them, causing arterial insufficiency to the affected area. Ischemia usually occurs after the vessel lumens have narrowed by at least 50%, reducing blood flow to levels which no longer meet the needs of tissues and nerves.

Arterial occlusive disease is a common complication of atherosclerosis. The occlusive mechanisms may be endogenous, due to emboli formation or thrombosis, or exogenous, due to trauma or fracture. (See *What causes acute arterial occlusion?* page 453.)

Predisposing factors include smoking; aging; conditions such as hypertension, hyperlipidemia, and diabetes mellitus; and family history of vascular disorders, myocardial infarction, or stroke.

AGE AWARE Aging causes sclerotic changes in blood vessels, which leads to decreased elasticity and narrowing of the lumen, further contributing to the development of peripheral arterial occlusive disease.

POSSIBLE SITES OF MAJOR ARTERY OCCLUSION

Listed below are some of the possible sites of major artery occlusions.

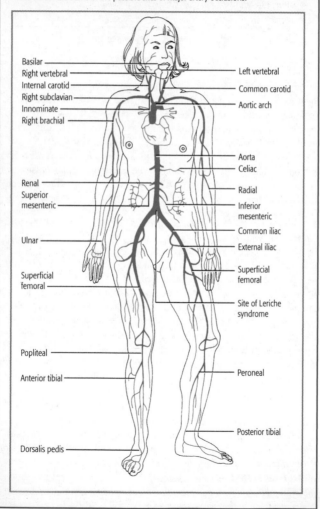

Basilar
Right vertebral
Internal carotid
Right subclavian
Innominate
Right brachial

Left vertebral
Common carotid
Aortic arch

Aorta
Celiac

Renal
Superior mesenteric

Radial
Inferior mesenteric
Common iliac
External iliac

Ulnar

Superficial femoral

Superficial femoral

Site of Leriche syndrome

Popliteal

Anterior tibial

Peroneal

Posterior tibial

Dorsalis pedis

WHAT CAUSES ACUTE ARTERIAL OCCLUSION?

The most common cause of acute arterial occlusion is obstruction of a major artery by a clot. The occlusive mechanism may be endogenous, resulting from emboli formation, thrombosis, or plaques, or exogenous, resulting from trauma or fracture.

Embolism

Often the obstruction results from an embolus originating in the heart. Emboli typically lodge in the arms and legs, where blood vessels narrow or branch. In the arms, emboli usually lodge in the brachial artery but may occlude the subclavian or axillary arteries. Common leg sites include the iliac, femoral, and popliteal arteries. Emboli originating in the heart can cause neurologic damage if they enter the cerebral circulation.

Thrombosis

In a patient with atherosclerosis and marked arterial narrowing, thrombosis may cause acute intrinsic arterial occlusion. This complication typically arises in areas with severely stenotic vessels, especially in a patient who also has heart failure, hypovolemia, polycythemia, or traumatic injury.

Plaques

Atheromatous debris (plaques) from proximal arterial lesions may also intermittently obstruct small vessels (usually in the hands or feet). These plaques may also develop in the brachiocephalic vessels and travel to the cerebral circulation, where they may lead to transient cerebral ischemia or infarction.

Exogenous causes

Acute arterial occlusion may stem from insertion of an indwelling arterial catheter or intra-arterial drug abuse.

Extrinsic arterial occlusion can also result from direct blunt or penetrating trauma to the artery.

In people older than age 70, the prevalence of the disease is estimated to be 10% to 18%.

Complications
- Severe ischemia and necrosis
- Skin ulceration
- Gangrene, which can lead to limb amputation
- Impaired nail and hair growth
- Stroke or transient ischemic attack
- Peripheral or systemic embolism

Assessment findings

Varied assessment findings depend on the vessel involved. (See *Signs and symptoms of peripheral arterial occlusive disease*, pages 454 and 455.)

SIGNS AND SYMPTOMS OF PERIPHERAL ARTERIAL OCCLUSIVE DISEASE

A patient with arterial occlusive disease may have a wide variety of signs and symptoms depending on which portion of the vasculature is affected by the disorder.

SITE OF OCCLUSION	SIGNS AND SYMPTOMS
Internal and external carotid arteries	Transient ischemic attacks (TIAs) due to reduced cerebral circulation produce unilateral sensory or motor dysfunction (transient monocular blindness, hemiparesis), possible aphasia or dysarthria, confusion, decreased mentation, and headache (these recurrent clinical features usually last for 5 to 10 minutes but may persist for up to 24 hours and may herald a stroke; absent or decreased pulsation with an auscultatory bruit over the affected vessels)
Vertebral and basilar arteries	TIAs of brain stem and cerebellum (less common than carotid TIA), producing binocular visual disturbances, vertigo, dysarthria, and falling down without loss of consciousness
Innominate (brachiocephalic) artery	Signs and symptoms of vertebrobasilar occlusion, indications of ischemia (claudication) of right arm, possible bruit over right side of neck
Subclavian artery	Subclavian steal syndrome characterized by backflow of blood from the brain through the vertebral artery on the same side as the occlusion, into the subclavian artery distal to the occlusion, clinical effects of vertebrobasilar occlusion and exercise-induced arm claudication, possible gangrene (usually limited to the digits)
Mesenteric artery	Bowel ischemia, infarct necrosis, and gangrene; sudden, acute abdominal pain; nausea and vomiting; diarrhea; leukocytosis; shock due to massive intraluminal and plasma loss
Aortic bifurcation (saddle block occlusion, a medical emergency associated with cardiac embolization)	Sensory and motor deficits (muscle weakness, numbness, paresthesia, paralysis), signs and symptoms of ischemia (sudden pain; cold, pale legs with decreased or absent peripheral pulses) in both legs

SIGNS AND SYMPTOMS OF PERIPHERAL ARTERIAL OCCLUSIVE DISEASE *(continued)*

SITE OF OCCLUSION	SIGNS AND SYMPTOMS
Iliac artery (Leriche's syndrome)	Intermittent claudication of lower back, buttocks, and thighs, relieved by rest; absent or reduced femoral or distal pulses; shiny, scaly skin, subcutaneous tissue loss, and no body hair on affected limb; nail deformities; increased capillary refill time; blanching of feet on elevation; possible bruit over femoral arteries; impotence in males
Femoral and popliteal arteries (associated with aneurysm formation)	Intermittent claudication of the calves on exertion; ischemic pain in feet; pretrophic pain (heralds necrosis and ulceration); leg pallor and coolness; shiny, scaly skin, subcutaneous tissue loss, and no body hair on affected limb; nail deformities; increased capillary refill time; blanching of feet on elevation; gangrene; no palpable pulses distal to occlusion (auscultation over affected area may reveal a bruit)

Peripheral cute arterial occlusion occurs suddenly, in many cases without warning. However, peripheral occlusion can usually be recognized by the five Ps:

- Pain, the most common symptom, occurs suddenly and is localized to the affected arm or leg.
- Pallor results from vasoconstriction distal to the occlusion.
- Pulselessness occurs distal to the occlusion.
- Paralysis and paresthesia occur in the affected arm or leg from disturbed nerve endings or skeletal muscles.

A sixth P, known as *poikilothermy,* refers to temperature changes that occur distal to the occlusion, making the skin feel cool.

Diagnostic test results

- Arteriography demonstrates the type, location, and degree of obstruction and the establishment of collateral circulation. It's particularly useful for monitoring patients with chronic disease and for evaluating candidates for reconstructive surgery.

- Ultrasonography and plethysmography are noninvasive tests that, in patients with acute disease, show decreased blood flow distal to the occlusion.
- Doppler ultrasonography typically reveals a relatively low-pitched sound and a monophasic waveform.
- Segmental limb pressures and pulse volume measurements help evaluate the location and extent of the occlusion.
- Ophthalmodynamometry helps determine the degree of obstruction in the internal carotid artery by comparing ophthalmic artery pressure with brachial artery pressure on the affected side. More than a 20% difference between pressures suggests arterial insufficiency.
- Electroencephalography and a computed tomography scan may be necessary to rule out brain lesions.

Treatment

In patients with mild chronic disease, treatment usually consists of supportive measures: smoking cessation, hypertension control, walking, and foot and leg care. In patients with carotid artery occlusion, antiplatelet therapy may begin with dipyridamole (Persantine) and aspirin or clopidogrel (Plavix). For those patients with intermittent claudication caused by chronic peripheral arterial occlusive disease, pentoxifylline (Trental) may improve blood flow through the capillaries. This drug is particularly useful for those who aren't good surgical candidates.

Thrombolytics—such as urokinase (Abbokinase), streptokinase (Streptase), and alteplase (Activase)—can dissolve clots and relieve the obstruction caused by a thrombus.

Acute peripheral arterial occlusive disease usually requires surgery, such as:

- embolectomy. A balloon-tipped catheter is used to remove thrombotic material from the artery. Embolectomy is used mainly for mesenteric, femoral, or popliteal artery occlusion.
- thromboendarterectomy. This involves the opening of the artery and removal of the obstructing thrombus and the medial layer of the arterial wall. Plaque deposits remain intact. Thromboendarterectomy is usually performed after angiography and is commonly used with autogenous vein or Dacron bypass surgery (femoropopliteal or aortofemoral).
- atherectomy. Plaque is excised using a drill or slicing mechanism.
- balloon angioplasty. The obstruction is compressed using balloon inflation.

- laser angioplasty. Excision and a hot-tip laser are used to vaporize the destruction.
- stents. A mesh of wires that stretch and mold to the arterial walls are inserted to prevent reocclusion.
- combined therapy. Any of the above treatments may be used concomitantly.
- percutaneous transluminal coronary angioplasty (PTCA). Using fluoroscopy and a special balloon catheter, the stenosis or occluded artery is dilated to a predetermined diameter without overdistending it.
- laser surgery. An excimer or a hot-tip laser obliterates the clot and plaque by vaporizing it.
- patch grafting. This involves removal of the thrombosed arterial segment and replacement with an autogenous vein or Dacron graft.
- bypass graft. Blood flow is diverted through an anastomosed autogenous or woven Dacron graft to bypass the thrombosed arterial segment.

Amputation may be necessary if arterial reconstructive surgery fails or if gangrene, uncontrollable infection, or intractable pain develops.

Other therapy includes heparin to prevent emboli (for embolic occlusion) and bowel resection after restoration of blood flow (for mesenteric artery occlusion).

Nursing interventions

FOR PATIENTS WITH CHRONIC PERIPHERAL ARTERIAL OCCLUSIVE DISEASE

- Prevent trauma to the affected extremity. Use minimal pressure mattresses, heel protectors, a foot cradle, or a footboard to reduce pressure that could lead to skin breakdown. Keep the arm or leg warm, but never use heating pads. If the patient is wearing socks, remove them frequently to check the skin.
- Avoid using restrictive clothing such as antiembolism stockings.
- Give an analgesic to relieve pain.
- Allow the patient to express fears and concerns, and help him identify and use effective coping strategies.

FOR PREOPERATIVE CARE DURING AN ACUTE EPISODE

- Assess the patient's circulatory status by checking for the most distal pulses and by inspecting his skin color and temperature.
- Give an analgesic to relieve pain.

- Give heparin or a thrombolytic by continuous I.V. drip. Use an infusion pump to ensure the proper flow rate.
- Wrap the patient's affected foot in soft cotton batting, and reposition it frequently to prevent pressure on one area.
- Strictly avoid elevating or applying heat to the affected leg.
- Watch for signs of fluid and electrolyte imbalance, and monitor intake and output for signs of renal failure (such as urine output of less than 30 ml/hour).
- If the patient has carotid, innominate, vertebral, or subclavian artery occlusion, monitor him for signs of stroke, such as numbness in an arm or a leg and intermittent blindness.

FOR POSTOPERATIVE CARE
- Monitor the patient's vital signs. Continuously assess his circulatory function by assessing skin color and temperature and by checking for distal pulses. In charting, compare earlier assessments and observations. Watch closely for signs of hemorrhage (such as tachycardia and hypotension), and check dressings for excessive bleeding.
- If the patient has a carotid, innominate, vertebral, or subclavian artery occlusion, assess neurologic status frequently for changes in level of consciousness, pupil size, and muscle strength.
- If the patient has a mesenteric artery occlusion, connect a nasogastric tube to low intermittent suction. Monitor intake and output (low urine output may indicate damage to renal arteries during surgery). Check bowel sounds for the return of peristalsis. Increasing abdominal distention and tenderness may indicate extension of bowel ischemia with resulting gangrene, necessitating further excision, or it may indicate peritonitis.
- If the patient has a saddle block occlusion, check distal pulses for adequate circulation. Watch for signs of renal failure and mesenteric artery occlusion (severe abdominal pain) and for cardiac arrhythmias, which may precipitate embolus formation.
- If PTCA was performed, sheath (catheter) care must be done. The line must be kept open with a heparin infusion; monitor the insertion site for bleeding. Keep the catheterized leg immobile, and keep the patient on strict bed rest. Monitor and record pulses in the catheterized leg. Provide an analgesic for back pain associated with catheter placement.
- If the patient has an iliac artery occlusion, monitor urine output for signs of renal failure from decreased perfusion to the kidneys as a result of surgery. Provide meticulous catheter care.

TEACHING THE PATIENT WITH PERIPHERAL ARTERIAL OCCLUSIVE DISEASE

● When preparing the patient for discharge, instruct him to watch for signs and symptoms of recurrence (such as pain, pallor, numbness, paralysis, or absence of pulse) that can result from graft occlusion or occlusion at another site. Caution against wearing constrictive clothing, crossing legs, bumping affected limbs, and wearing garters.

● Warn the patient to avoid all tobacco products.

● Tell the patient to avoid temperature extremes. If he must go outside in the cold, remind him to dress warmly and take special care to keep his feet warm.

● Instruct the patient to wash his feet daily and inspect them for signs of injury or infection. Remind him to report abnormalities to the practitioner.

● Advise the patient to wear sturdy, properly fitting shoes. Refer him to a podiatrist for foot problems.

● Teach the patient about preventive measures, such as smoking cessation, regular exercise, weight control, reduction of dietary fat intake, and avoidance of pressure and constriction to extremities. These measures may reduce the risk of arterial occlusive disease, especially in patients with a history of cardiovascular disease.

■ If the patient has a femoral or popliteal artery occlusion, assist with early ambulation, and don't allow the patient to sit for an extended period.

■ When caring for a patient who has undergone amputation, check the stump carefully for drainage. If drainage occurs, note and record its color and amount, and the time. Elevate the stump, if indicated, and give an analgesic as needed. Because phantom limb pain is common, explain this phenomenon to the patient. (See *Teaching the patient with peripheral arterial occlusive disease*.)

RAYNAUD'S DISEASE

Raynaud's disease—also known as *vasospastic arterial disease*—is one of several primary arteriospastic disorders. These disorders are characterized by episodic vasospasm in the small peripheral arteries and arterioles precipitated by exposure to cold or stress.

Raynaud's disease occurs bilaterally and usually affects the hands or, less commonly, the feet and, rarely, the earlobes and the tip of the nose. The disease is five times more common in women than in men,

CAUSES OF RAYNAUD'S PHENOMENON

Patients with the primary or idiopathic form of Raynaud's phenomenon have Raynaud's disease. Raynaud's phenomenon, on the other hand, may occur secondary to the following diseases and conditions as well as with the use of certain drugs.

Collagen vascular disease

- Dermatomyositis
- Polymyositis
- Rheumatoid arthritis
- Scleroderma
- Systemic lupus erythematosus

Arterial occlusive disease

- Acute arterial occlusion
- Atherosclerosis of the extremities
- Thoracic outlet syndrome
- Thromboangiitis obliterans

Neurologic disorders

- Carpal tunnel syndrome
- Invertebral disk disease
- Poliomyelitis
- Spinal cord tumors
- Stroke
- Syringomyelia

Blood dyscrasias

- Cold agglutinins
- Cryofibrinogenemia
- Myeloproliferative disorders
- Waldenström's disease

Trauma

- Cold injury
- Electric shock
- Hammering
- Keyboarding
- Piano playing
- Vibration injury

Drugs

- Beta-adrenergic receptor blockers
- Bleomycin
- Cisplatin
- Ergot derivatives such as ergotamine
- Methysergide
- Vinblastine

Other

- Pulmonary hypertension

particularly between late adolescence and age 40. The disorder is benign, requiring no specific treatment and with no serious effects.

Raynaud's phenomenon, however, is a condition commonly associated with several connective tissue disorders, such as scleroderma, systemic lupus erythematosus, and polymyositis. The concurrent disorders have a progressive course, leading to ischemia, gangrene, and amputation. (For other disorders and conditions associated with Raynaud's phenomenon, see *Causes of Raynaud's phenomenon.*)

Pathophysiology

Although the cause is unknown, several conditions account for the reduced blood flow to the digits: intrinsic vascular wall hyperactivity to cold, ineffective basal heat production, increased vasomotor tone from sympathetic stimulation, stress, and an antigen-antibody immune response (the most probable theory because abnormal immunologic test results accompany Raynaud's phenomenon).

Complications
- Ischemia, gangrene, and amputation resulting from severe, persistent vasoconstriction
- Amputation of one or more phalanges with full-thickness tissue necrosis and gangrene (although extremely uncommon)

Assessment findings
- The patient with Raynaud's disease may report skin color changes induced by cold or stress.
- The response to cold and stress is typically triphasic. Initially, the skin of affected areas appears markedly pale from severe vasoconstriction. During this phase, the patient may report numbness and tingling. In the second phase, the skin appears cyanotic, resulting from dilation of cutaneous arterioles and venules.

  Because vasoconstriction is diminished, reactive hyperemia results, so the skin in the third phase appears red and feels warm. During this phase, the patient may report a throbbing, burning, and painful sensation.
- Between attacks, the affected areas usually appear normal, although they may feel cool and perspire excessively. In patients with long-standing disease, you may notice trophic changes, such as sclerodactyly and ulcerations.

Diagnostic test results
- Diagnosis is based primarily on presenting symptoms. Before Raynaud's phenomenon can be diagnosed, secondary diseases, such as chronic arterial occlusive disease and connective tissue disease, must be ruled out.
- Arteriography and digital photoplethysmography may also help diagnose the presence of Raynaud's disease or phenomenon.

Treatment
Initially, treatment consists of avoidance of cold, mechanical, or chemical injury; cessation of smoking; and reassurance that symptoms are benign. Because adverse reactions to drugs, especially vasodilators, may be more bothersome than the disease itself, drug therapy is reserved for unusually severe signs and symptoms. Such therapy may include phenoxybenzamine (Dibenzyline), nifedipine (Procardia), or reserpine and prazosin (Minipress). Biofeedback therapy may be useful if signs and symptoms are caused by stress.

TEACHING THE PATIENT WITH RAYNAUD'S DISEASE

● Warn against exposure to the cold. Tell the patient to wear mittens or gloves in cold weather or when handling cold items or defrosting the freezer.

● Advise the patient to avoid stress and to stop smoking. Refer her to a smoking-cessation program if needed.

● Instruct the patient to inspect her skin frequently and to seek immediate care for signs of skin breakdown or infection.

● Teach the patient about prescribed drugs, their proper use, and their adverse effects. Tell her to report adverse reactions to her practitioner.

Sympathectomy may be helpful when conservative treatment fails to prevent ischemic ulcers (occurring in less than 25% of patients).

Nursing interventions

■ If signs and symptoms are caused by stress, help the patient identify stress-producing areas of her life and effective coping strategies. If appropriate, refer her to a biofeedback program to help control signs and symptoms related to stress.

■ Provide psychological support and reassurance to allay the patient's fear of amputation and disfigurement.

■ Evaluate the patient's occupation and its effect on symptom occurrence. If needed, refer the patient to occupational rehabilitation to prevent progression to untreatable complications. (See *Teaching the patient with Raynaud's disease.*)

THORACIC AORTIC ANEURYSM

Thoracic aortic aneurysm is a potentially life-threatening disorder characterized by abnormal widening of the ascending, transverse, or descending part of the aorta. The aneurysm may be saccular, an out-pouching of the arterial wall, with a narrow neck, involving only a portion of the vessel circumference; or fusiform, a spindle-shaped enlargement, encompassing the entire aortic circumference.

Dissection of the aneurysm is the circumferential or transverse tear of the aortic wall intima, usually within the medial layer. It occurs in about 60% of patients, is usually an emergency, and has a poor prognosis. (See *Classifying aortic dissection.*)

CLASSIFYING AORTIC DISSECTION

These drawings illustrate the DeBakey classification of aortic dissections (shaded areas) according to location. Dissections can also be classified by their location in relation to the aortic valve. Thus, types I and II are proximal; type III, distal.

Type I

In type I, the most common and lethal type of dissection, intimal tearing occurs in the ascending aorta, and the dissection extends into the descending aorta.

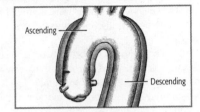

Type II

In type II, which appears most commonly with Marfan syndrome, dissection is limited to the ascending aorta.

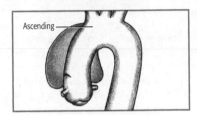

Type III

Type III dissection includes two formations. In the first, type IIIa, the intimal tear is located in the descending aorta with distal propagation of the dissection that's confined to the thorax. The second, type IIIb, has the same origin site, but may extend beyond the diaphragm.

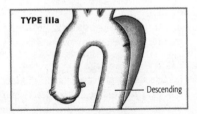

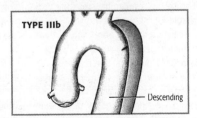

The ascending thoracic aorta is the most common site for the aneurysm, which occurs predominantly in men younger than age 60 who have coexisting hypertension. Descending thoracic aortic aneurysms are most common in younger patients who have had chest trauma.

Pathophysiology

Commonly, ascending thoracic aortic aneurysm results from atherosclerosis, which weakens the aortic wall and gradually distends the lumen in this area. It's also closely associated with cigarette smoking and hypertension.

Descending thoracic aortic aneurysm usually occurs after blunt chest trauma that shears the aorta transversely (acceleration-deceleration injury), such as in a motor vehicle accident, or after a penetrating chest injury, such as a knife wound. It may also be caused by hypertension.

Mycotic aneurysm develops from staphylococcal, streptococcal, or salmonella infections, usually at an atherosclerotic plaque.

Cystic medial necrosis caused by degeneration of the collagen and elastic fibers in the media of the aorta causes aneurysms during pregnancy and in patients with hypertension and Marfan syndrome. However, it can also be the cause without any underlying condition.

Other causes include congenital disorders, such as coarctation of the aorta, syphilis infection, and rheumatic vasculitis.

Complications

- Rupture of untreated thoracic dissecting aneurysm into the pericardium, with resulting cardiac tamponade

Assessment findings

- Thoracic aortic aneurysms fail to produce signs and symptoms until they expand and begin to dissect. Pain and other symptoms result from compression of the surrounding structures or from dissection of the aneurysm. (See *Clinical characteristics of thoracic dissection*.)
- The patient may complain of hoarseness, dyspnea, throat pain, dysphagia, and a dry cough when a transverse aneurysm compresses the surrounding structures.
- Dissection of the aneurysm causes sudden pain and possibly syncope.
- In dissecting ascending aneurysm, the patient may complain of pain with a boring, tearing, or ripping sensation in the thorax or the right anterior chest. It may extend to the neck, shoulders, lower

CLINICAL CHARACTERISTICS OF THORACIC DISSECTION

ASCENDING AORTA	DESCENDING AORTA	TRANSVERSE AORTA
CHARACTERISTIC OF PAIN		
Severe, boring, ripping, extending to neck, shoulders, lower back, and abdomen (rarely to jaw and arms); more severe on right side	Sudden onset; sharp, tearing, usually between the shoulder blades; may radiate to the chest; most diagnostic feature	Sudden onset; sharp, boring, tearing; radiates to shoulders
OTHER SYMPTOMS AND EFFECTS		
If dissection involves carotid arteries, abrupt onset of neurologic deficit (usually intermittent); bradycardia, aortic insufficiency, and hemopericardium detected by pericardial friction rub; unequal intensity of right and left carotid pulses and radial pulses; difference in blood pressure, especially systolic, between right and left arms	Aortic insufficiency without murmur, hemopericardium, or pleural friction rub; carotid and radial pulses and blood pressure in both arms typically equal	Hoarseness, dyspnea, pain, dysphagia, and dry cough from compression of surrounding structures
DIAGNOSTIC FEATURES		
CHEST X-RAY		
Best diagnostic tool; shows widening of mediastinum, enlargement of ascending aorta	Widening of mediastinum; descending aorta larger than ascending section	Widening of mediastinum; descending aorta larger than ascending section; widened transverse arch
AORTOGRAPHY		
False lumen; narrowing of lumen of aorta in ascending section	False lumen; narrowing of lumen of aorta in descending section	False lumen; narrowing of lumen of aorta in transverse arch

(continued)

CLINICAL CHARACTERISTICS OF
THORACIC DISSECTION *(continued)*

ASCENDING AORTA	DESCENDING AORTA	TRANSVERSE AORTA
TREATMENT		
Surgical repair needed; this is a medical emergency that requires immediate aggressive treatment to reduce blood pressure (usually with nitroprusside or trimethaphan)	Surgical repair required but less urgent than for the ascending dissection; to control hypertension, nitroprusside and propranolol may be used if bradycardia and heart failure are absent	Immediate surgical repair (mortality as high as 50%), control of hypertension

back, and abdomen but seldom radiates to the jaw and arms. The pain is most intense at its onset and is commonly misdiagnosed as a transmural myocardial infarction (MI).

- In dissecting descending aneurysm, the pain is sharp, tearing, and located between the shoulder blades, and in many cases radiates to the chest.
- In dissecting transverse aneurysm, the pain is sharp, boring, and tearing and radiates to the shoulders.
- In a patient with a thoracic aortic aneurysm, you may find pallor, diaphoresis, dyspnea, cyanosis, leg weakness or transient paralysis, and an abrupt onset of intermittent neurologic deficits.
- Palpation of peripheral pulses in dissecting ascending aneurysm may disclose abrupt loss of radial and femoral pulses and right and left carotid pulses.
- In dissecting descending aneurysm, carotid and radial pulses may be present and equal bilaterally.
- Percussion of the chest may reveal an increasing area of flatness over the heart, suggesting cardiac tamponade and hemopericardium.
- Auscultation of the heart in dissecting ascending aneurysm may disclose a murmur of aortic insufficiency, a diastolic murmur, and (if hemopericardium is present) a pericardial friction rub.

- Blood pressure may be normal or significantly elevated, with a large difference in systolic blood pressure between the right and left arms.
- In dissecting descending aneurysm, systolic blood pressure is equal bilaterally, and you hear no murmur of aortic insufficiency or pericardial friction rub. You may detect bilateral crackles and rhonchi if pulmonary edema is present.

Diagnostic test results

In an asymptomatic patient, the diagnosis commonly occurs accidentally, through posteroanterior and oblique chest X-rays showing widening of the aorta and mediastinum.

Several tests can help confirm the aneurysm:

- Aortography, the most definitive test, shows the lumen of the aneurysm, its size, and its location.
- Magnetic resonance imaging and computed tomography scanning help confirm and locate the presence of aortic dissection.
- Electrocardiography (ECG) helps rule out the presence of MI as the cause of the symptoms, and echocardiography may help identify dissecting aneurysm of the aortic root.
- Transesophageal echocardiography can be used to measure the aneurysm in both the ascending and the descending aorta.
- Hemoglobin levels may be normal or decreased, resulting from blood loss from a leaking aneurysm.

Treatment

For long-term treatment, beta-adrenergic receptor blockers and other agents can control hypertension and cardiac output. In an emergency, antihypertensives such as nitroprusside, negative inotropic agents such as propanolol, oxygen for respiratory distress, opioids for pain, I.V. fluids, and whole blood transfusions, if needed, may be used.

In dissecting ascending aortic aneurysm—an extreme emergency—surgical resection of the aneurysm can restore normal blood flow through a Dacron or Teflon graft replacement. With aortic valve insufficiency, surgery consists of replacing the aortic valve.

Postoperative measures include careful monitoring and continuous assessment in the intensive care unit, antibiotics, insertion of endotracheal (ET) and chest tubes, ECG monitoring and, in many instances, pulmonary artery catheterization and monitoring.

Nursing interventions

- In a nonemergency situation when a patient is diagnosed with a thoracic aneurysm, allow him to express his fears and concerns. Help him identify and use effective coping strategies.
- Offer the patient and his family psychological support. Answer all questions honestly and provide reassurance.
- In an acute situation, monitor blood pressure, pulmonary artery wedge pressure (PAWP), and central venous pressure (CVP). Assess pain, breathing, and carotid, radial, and femoral pulses.
- Give analgesics to relieve pain.
- Explain diagnostic tests. If surgery is scheduled, explain the procedure and expected postoperative care (I.V. lines, ET and drainage tubes, cardiac monitoring, and ventilation).
- Make sure laboratory tests include a complete blood count with differential, electrolyte measurements, typing and crossmatching for whole blood, arterial blood gas analysis, and urinalysis.
- Insert an indwelling urinary catheter to monitor hourly outputs. Give dextrose 5% in water or lactated Ringer's solution, and antibiotic. Carefully monitor nitroprusside I.V.; use a separate I.V. line for infusion. Adjust the dose by slowly increasing the infusion rate. Meanwhile, check blood pressure every 5 minutes until it stabilizes. With suspected bleeding from an aneurysm, give whole blood transfusions as ordered.

AFTER REPAIR OF THORACIC ANEURYSM

- Carefully assess the patient's level of consciousness. Monitor vital signs, pulmonary artery pressure, CVP, PAWP, pulse rate, urine output, and pain.
- Check respiratory function. Carefully observe and record type and amount of chest tube drainage, and assess heart and breath sounds frequently.
- Monitor I.V. therapy and intake and output to determine the adequacy of renal function.
- Give an analgesic, especially before the patient performs breathing exercises or is moved.
- After stabilization of vital signs, encourage and assist the patient in turning, coughing, and deep breathing. If necessary, provide intermittent positive-pressure breathing to promote lung expansion. Help the patient walk as soon as he's able. (See *Teaching the patient with thoracic aortic aneurysm.*)

DISCHARGE TEACHING

TEACHING THE PATIENT WITH THORACIC AORTIC ANEURYSM

● Ensure compliance with antihypertensive therapy by explaining the need for such drugs and the expected adverse effects.
● Direct the patient to call the practitioner immediately if he experiences sharp pain in the chest or back of the neck.
● Teach the patient how to monitor his blood pressure.
● Refer him to community agencies for continued support and assistance as needed.

■ Watch for signs of infection, especially fever, and excessive drainage on the dressing. Monitor for signs that resemble those of the initial dissecting aneurysm, suggesting a tear at the graft site.
■ Assist with range-of-motion exercises of legs to prevent thromboemboli from venostasis during prolonged bed rest.

THROMBOPHLEBITIS

Thrombophlebitis is an acute condition characterized by inflammation and thrombus formation. It may occur in deep or superficial veins. Deep vein thrombosis (DVT) affects small veins, such as the lesser saphenous vein, or large veins, such as the vena cava and the iliac, femoral, and popliteal veins. It's more serious than superficial vein thrombophlebitis because it affects the veins deep in the leg musculature that carry most of the venous outflow from the leg. (See *Major venous pathways of the leg,* page 470.) Thrombophlebitis is typically progressive, leading to pulmonary embolism, a potentially life-threatening complication. Superficial thrombophlebitis is usually self-limiting and seldom leads to pulmonary embolism. Thrombophlebitis typically begins with localized inflammation alone (phlebitis), but such inflammation rapidly provokes thrombus formations. Rarely, venous thrombosis develops without associated inflammation of the vein (phlebothrombosis).

Causes

A thrombus occurs when an alteration in the epithelial lining causes platelet aggregation and consequent fibrin entrapment of red and white blood cells and additional platelets. Thrombus formation is more rapid in areas where blood flow is slower, resulting from greater

MAJOR VENOUS PATHWAYS OF THE LEG

Thrombophlebitis can occur in any leg vein. It most commonly occurs at valve sites.

Inferior vena cava
External iliac
Common femoral
Deep femoral
Superficial femoral
Popliteal
Communicating (perforator)
Anterior tibial

Common iliac
Internal iliac
Greater saphenous
Lesser saphenous
Posterior tibial

contact between platelet and thrombin accumulation. The rapidly expanding thrombus initiates a chemical inflammatory process in the vessel epithelium, which leads to fibrosis. The enlarging clot may occlude the vessel lumen partially or totally, or it may detach and embolize to lodge elsewhere in systemic circulation.

Deep vein thrombophlebitis may be idiopathic, but it usually results from endothelial damage, accelerated blood clotting and reduced blood flow, such as in predisposing factors of prolonged bed rest, trauma, surgery, childbirth, and use of hormonal contraceptives such as estrogens. It's also more likely to occur in the presence of certain diseases, treatments, injuries, or other factors, such as:

- hypercoagulable states—cigarette smoking; circulating lupus anti-coagulant; deficiencies of antithrombin III, protein C, or protein S; disseminated intravascular coagulation; estrogen use; dysfibrino-genemia; myeloproliferative diseases; and systemic infection
- intimal damage—infection, infusion of irritating I.V. solutions, trauma, or venipuncture
- neoplasms—of the lung, ovary, pancreas, stomach, testicles, or urinary tract
- surgery—abdominal, genitourinary, orthopedic, or thoracic
- fracture—of the spine, pelvis, femur, or tibia
- venous stasis—acute myocardial infarction, heart failure, dehydration, immobility, incompetent vein valves, postoperative convalescence, or stroke
- venulitis—Behçet's disease, homocystinuria, or thromboangiitis obliterans
- other—pregnancy or previous deep vein thrombosis.

Complications
- Pulmonary embolism
- Chronic venous insufficiency (see *Dealing with chronic venous insufficiency,* page 472)

Assessment findings
- In both deep vein and superficial vein thrombophlebitis, clinical features vary with the site of inflammation and length of the affected vein. Up to 50% of patients with deep vein thrombophlebitis may be asymptomatic, but others may complain of some tenderness, aching, or severe pain in the affected leg or arm, fever, chills, and malaise. Complete your physical examination carefully because much of the patient's subsequent care depends on your findings.
- Inspection may reveal redness, swelling, and cyanosis of the affected leg or arm.
- Some patients with deep vein thrombophlebitis of a leg vein may have a positive Homans' sign (pain on dorsiflexion of the foot), but this is considered an unreliable sign.
- A positive cuff sign (elicited by inflating a blood pressure cuff until pain occurs) may be present in deep vein thrombophlebitis of either the arm or leg.
- When palpated, the affected leg or arm may feel warm.
- Patients with superficial vein thrombophlebitis may also be asymptomatic, or they may complain of pain localized to the thrombus site.

DEALING WITH CHRONIC VENOUS INSUFFICIENCY

Chronic venous insufficiency results from the valvular destruction of deep vein thrombophlebitis, usually in the iliac and femoral veins and occasionally in the saphenous veins. It's commonly accompanied by incompetence of the communicating veins of the ankle, causing increased venous pressure and fluid migration into the interstitial tissue.

Signs and symptoms

Chronic venous insufficiency causes chronic swelling of the affected leg from edema, leading to tissue fibrosis and induration, skin discoloration from extravasation of blood in subcutaneous tissue, and stasis ulcers around the ankle.

Treatment

Appropriate treatment for small stasis ulcers is bed rest, elevation of the legs, warm soaks, and antimicrobial therapy for infection.

Treatment to counteract increased venous pressure, the result of reflux from the deep venous system to superficial veins, may include compression dressings or a zinc gelatin boot (Unna boot). This therapy begins after massive swelling subsides.

Large stasis ulcers unresponsive to conservative treatment may require excision and skin grafting. Care includes daily inspection to assess healing and measures similar to those for varicose veins.

- Inspection may disclose redness and swelling at the site and surrounding area.
- When palpated, the area feels warm, and a tender, hard cord extends over the affected vein's length.
- Extensive vein involvement may cause lymphadenitis.
- Physical examination aids the differential diagnosis, especially in superficial thrombophlebitis. The initial findings are redness and warmth over the affected area, palpable veins, and pain during palpation or compression.

Diagnostic test results

Diagnosis must rule out arterial occlusive disease, lymphangitis, cellulitis, and myositis. Diagnosis of superficial vein thrombophlebitis is based on physical findings, whereas diagnosis of deep vein thrombophlebitis is based on the following characteristic test findings:

- Doppler ultrasonography identifies reduced blood flow to a specific area and obstruction to venous flow, particularly in iliofemoral deep vein thrombophlebitis.

- Plethysmography shows decreased circulation distal to the affected area; it's more sensitive than ultrasonography in detecting deep vein thrombophlebitis.
- Phlebography usually confirms the diagnosis and shows filling defects and diverted blood flow.
- D-dimer results indicate an abnormally high level of fibrin degradation products, reflective of significant clot formation and breakdown in the body; however, it doesn't reveal location or cause.

Treatment

In deep vein thrombophlebitis, treatment includes bed rest, with elevation of the affected arm or leg; application of warm, moist compresses to the affected area; and analgesics. After the acute episode subsides, the patient may begin to ambulate while wearing antiembolism stockings (applied before he gets out of bed).

Treatment may include anticoagulants (initially, heparin; later, warfarin) to prolong clotting time. However, the full anticoagulant dose must be discontinued during surgery to avoid the risk of hemorrhage. After some types of surgery, especially major abdominal or pelvic operations, prophylactic doses of anticoagulants may reduce the risk of deep vein thrombophlebitis.

For lysis of acute, extensive deep vein thrombophlebitis, treatment should include streptokinase or urokinase, if the risk of bleeding doesn't outweigh the potential benefits of thrombolytic treatment.

Rarely, deep vein thrombophlebitis may cause complete venous occlusion, which necessitates venous interruption through simple ligation to vein plication, or clipping. Embolectomy may be done if clots are being shed to the pulmonary and systemic vasculature and other treatment is unsuccessful. Caval interruption with transvenous placement of an umbrella filter can trap emboli, preventing them from traveling to the pulmonary vasculature.

Therapy for severe superficial vein thrombophlebitis may include an anti-inflammatory drug such as indomethacin along with antiembolism stockings, warm compresses, and elevating the patient's leg.

Nursing interventions

- Enforce bed rest as ordered, and elevate the patient's affected arm or leg. If you plan to use pillows for elevating the leg, place them so they support its entire length to avoid compressing the popliteal space.
- Apply warm compresses or a covered aquamatic K pad to increase circulation to the affected area and to relieve pain and inflammation. Give analgesics to relieve pain as ordered.

DISCHARGE TEACHING

TEACHING THE PATIENT WITH THROMBOPHLEBITIS

● Before discharge, emphasize the importance of follow-up blood studies to monitor anticoagulant therapy.

● If the patient is being discharged on heparin therapy, teach him or his family how to give subcutaneous injections. If he requires further assistance, arrange for a home health care nurse.

● Tell the patient to avoid prolonged sitting or standing to help prevent a recurrence.

● Teach the patient how to properly apply and use antiembolism stockings. Tell him to report complications such as cold, blue toes.

● To prevent bleeding, encourage the patient to use an electric razor and to avoid drugs that contain aspirin.

■ Mark, measure, and record the circumference of the affected arm or leg daily, and compare this measurement with that of the other arm or leg. To ensure accuracy and consistency of serial measurements, mark the skin over the area, and measure at the same spot daily.

■ Give I.V. heparin with an infusion monitor or pump to control the flow rate if necessary.

■ Measure partial thromboplastin time regularly for the patient on heparin therapy. Measure prothrombin time for the patient on warfarin (therapeutic anticoagulation values for both are 1½ to 2 times control values).

■ Watch for signs and symptoms of bleeding, such as tarry stools, coffee-ground vomitus, and ecchymoses. Watch for oozing of blood at I.V. sites, and assess gums for excessive bleeding.

■ Be alert for signs of pulmonary emboli (such as crackles, dyspnea, hemoptysis, sudden changes in mental status, restlessness, and hypotension).

■ To prevent thrombophlebitis in high-risk patients, perform range-of-motion exercises while the patient is on bed rest, use intermittent pneumatic calf massage during lengthy surgical or diagnostic procedures, apply antiembolism stockings postoperatively, and encourage early ambulation. (See *Teaching the patient with thrombophlebitis.*)

Cardiovascular complications

CARDIAC TAMPONADE

Cardiac tamponade involves a rapid increase in intrapericardial pressure, which impairs diastolic filling of the heart and reduces cardiac output. The increase in pressure usually results from blood or fluid accumulation in the pericardial sac. If fluid accumulates rapidly, as little as 250 ml can create an emergency situation.

Prognosis depends on the rate of fluid accumulation. If it accumulates rapidly, cardiac tamponade requires emergency life-saving measures to prevent death. Slow accumulation and an increase in pressure, as in pericardial effusion associated with cancer, may not produce immediate signs and symptoms because the fibrous wall of the pericardial sac can gradually stretch to accommodate as much as 1 to 2 L of fluid.

Pathophysiology

In cardiac tamponade, the progressive accumulation of fluid in the pericardial sac causes compression of the heart chambers. This compression obstructs blood flow into the ventricles and reduces the amount of blood that can be pumped out of the heart with each contraction. (See *Understanding cardiac tamponade,* page 476.)

Each time the ventricles contract, more fluid accumulates in the pericardial sac. This further limits the amount of blood that can fill the ventricular chambers—especially the left ventricle—during the next cardiac cycle.

RED FLAG Cardiac tamponade may cause a cardiac condition called pulseless electrical activity (PEA). In PEA, isolated electrical activity occurs sporadically without evidence of myocardial contraction. Unless

UNDERSTANDING CARDIAC TAMPONADE

The pericardial sac, which surrounds and protects the heart, is composed of several layers. The *fibrous pericardium* is the tough outermost membrane; the inner membrane, called the *serous membrane,* consists of the visceral and parietal layers. The visceral layer clings to the heart and is also known as the *epicardial layer of the heart.* The *parietal layer* lies between the visceral layer and the fibrous pericardium. The pericardial space—between the visceral and parietal layers—contains 10 to 30 ml of pericardial fluid. This fluid lubricates the layers and minimizes friction when the heart contracts.

NORMAL HEART AND PERICARDIUM

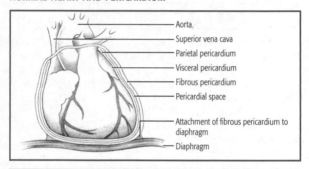

- Aorta
- Superior vena cava
- Parietal pericardium
- Visceral pericardium
- Fibrous pericardium
- Pericardial space
- Attachment of fibrous pericardium to diaphragm
- Diaphragm

In cardiac tamponade, blood or fluid fills the pericardial space, compressing the heart chambers, increasing intracardiac pressure, and obstructing venous return. As blood flow into the ventricles falls, so does cardiac output. Without prompt treatment, low cardiac output can be fatal.

CARDIAC TAMPONADE

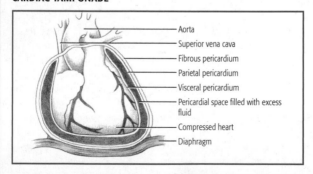

- Aorta
- Superior vena cava
- Fibrous pericardium
- Parietal pericardium
- Visceral pericardium
- Pericardial space filled with excess fluid
- Compressed heart
- Diaphragm

the underlying cardiac tamponade is identified and treated quickly, PEA results in death.

The amount of fluid necessary to cause cardiac tamponade varies greatly; it may be as little as 50 ml when the fluid accumulates rapidly or more than 2 L when the fluid accumulates slowly and the pericardium stretches to adapt.

Cardiac tamponade may be idiopathic (Dressler's syndrome) or may result from:

- effusion (in patients with cancer, bacterial infection, tuberculosis or, rarely, acute rheumatic fever)
- hemorrhage from trauma (such as a gunshot or stab wound to the chest and perforation by catheter during cardiac or central venous catheterization, or after cardiac surgery)
- hemorrhage from nontraumatic causes (such as rupture of the heart or great vessels, or anticoagulant therapy in a patient with pericarditis)
- viral, postirradiation, or idiopathic pericarditis
- acute myocardial infarction
- chronic renal failure during dialysis
- pneumothorax causing pressure against the heart
- drug reaction (such as with procainamide, hydralazine, minoxidil, isoniazid, penicillin, methysergide, and daunorubicin)
- a connective tissue disorder (such as rheumatoid arthritis, systemic lupus erythematosus, rheumatic fever, vasculitis, or scleroderma).

Complications
- Reduced cardiac output (fatal without prompt treatment)

Assessment findings
- The patient's history may show a disorder that can cause cardiac tamponade.
- He may report acute pain and dyspnea, sitting upright and leaning forward to facilitate breathing and lessen the pain. He may be orthopneic, diaphoretic, anxious, and restless, and appear pale or cyanotic.
- You may note jugular vein distention produced by increased venous pressure, although this may not be present if the patient is hypovolemic.
- Palpation of the peripheral pulses may disclose rapid, weak pulses. Palpation of the upper quadrant may reveal hepatomegaly.
- Percussion may disclose a widening area of flatness across the anterior chest wall, indicating a large effusion. Hepatomegaly may also be noted.

- Auscultation of the blood pressure may demonstrate a decreased arterial blood pressure, paradoxical pulse (an abnormal inspiratory drop in systemic blood pressure greater than 15 mm Hg), and narrow pulse pressure.
- Heart sounds may be muffled. A quiet heart with faint sounds usually accompanies only severe tamponade and occurs within minutes of the tamponade, as happens with cardiac rupture or trauma. The lungs are clear.

Diagnostic test results

The following test results are characteristic of cardiac tamponade:

- Chest X-rays show slightly widened mediastinum and enlargement of the cardiac silhouette.
- Electrocardiography (ECG) is useful to rule out other cardiac disorders. The QRS complex may be reduced, and electrical alternans of the P wave, QRS complex, and T wave may be present. Generalized ST-segment elevation is noted in all leads.
- Pulmonary artery pressure monitoring detects increased right atrial pressure, right ventricular diastolic pressure, and central venous pressure (CVP).
- Echocardiography records pericardial effusion with signs of right ventricular and atrial compression.

Treatment

The goal of treatment is to relieve intrapericardial pressure and cardiac compression by removing accumulated blood or fluid. Pericardiocentesis (needle aspiration of the pericardial cavity) or surgical creation of an opening dramatically improves systemic arterial pressure and cardiac output with aspiration of as little as 25 ml of fluid. A drain may be inserted into the pericardial sac to drain the effusion. (See *Aspirating pericardial fluid*.) This may be left in until the effusion process stops or the corrective action (pericardial window) is performed.

If tamponade or effusions or adhesions from chronic pericarditis recur, a portion or all of the pericardium may need to be removed to allow adequate ventricular filling and contraction. A pericardial window may be performed, which involves removing a portion of the pericardium to permit excess pericardial fluid to drain into the pleural space. In more severe cases, removal of the toughened encasing pericardium (pericardectomy) may be necessary.

In the hypotensive patient, trial volume loading with I.V. normal saline solution with albumin and, perhaps, an inotropic drug such as dopamine is necessary to maintain cardiac output.

ASPIRATING PERICARDIAL FLUID

In pericardiocentesis, a needle and syringe assembly is inserted through the chest wall into the pericardial sac, as illustrated here. Electrocardiographic monitoring with a lead-wire attached to the needle and electrodes placed on the limbs (right arm [RA], right leg [RL], left arm [LA], and left leg [LL]) helps to ensure proper needle placement and to avoid damage to the heart.

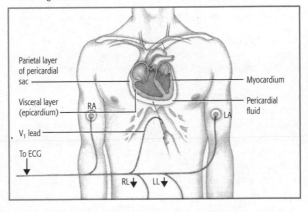

Depending on the cause of tamponade, additional treatment may include:

- for traumatic injury, blood transfusion or a thoracotomy to drain reaccumulating fluid or to repair bleeding sites
- for heparin-induced tamponade, the heparin antagonist protamine
- for warfarin-induced tamponade, vitamin K.

Nursing interventions

- Monitor the patient with cardiac tamponade in the intensive care unit. Check for signs of increasing tamponade, increasing dyspnea, and arrhythmias.

FOR A PATIENT WHO HAS UNDERGONE PERICARDIOCENTESIS

- Reassure the patient to reduce his anxiety.
- Gather a pericardiocentesis tray, an ECG machine, and an emergency cart with a defibrillator at the bedside. Make sure the equipment is turned on and ready to be used. Position the patient at a

45- to 60-degree angle. Connect the precordial ECG lead to the hub of the aspiration needle with an alligator clamp and connecting wire, and assist with fluid aspiration. When the needle touches the myocardium, you see ST-segment elevation or premature ventricular contractions.

■ Monitor blood pressure and CVP during and after pericardiocentesis. Infuse I.V. solutions, as ordered, to maintain blood pressure. Watch for a decrease in CVP and a concomitant increase in blood pressure, which indicate relief of cardiac compression.

■ Administer oxygen therapy as needed.

RED FLAG Watch for complications of pericardiocentesis, such as ventricular fibrillation, vasovagal arrest, and coronary artery or cardiac chamber puncture. Closely monitor cardiac rhythm strip changes, blood pressure, pulse rate, level of consciousness, and urine output.

FOR A PATIENT WHO HAS UNDERGONE THORACOTOMY

■ Give an antibiotic, protamine, or vitamin K.

■ Postoperatively monitor critical parameters, such as vital signs and arterial blood gas levels, and assess heart and breath sounds. Give an analgesic as ordered. Maintain the chest drainage system, and be alert for complications, such as hemorrhage and arrhythmias. (See *Teaching the patient with cardiac tamponade*.)

CARDIOGENIC SHOCK

Cardiogenic shock is a condition of diminished cardiac output that severely impairs tissue perfusion. It's sometimes called pump failure. Cardiogenic shock can occur as a serious complication in nearly 15% of all patients who are hospitalized with acute myocardial infarction (MI). It typically affects patients whose area of infarction involves 40%

or more of left ventricular muscle mass; in such patients, mortality may exceed 85%.

Pathophysiology

In cardiogenic shock, the left ventricle can't maintain adequate cardiac output. Compensatory mechanisms increase heart rate, strengthen myocardial contractions, promote sodium and water retention, and cause selective vasoconstriction. However, these mechanisms increase myocardial workload and oxygen consumption, which reduces the heart's ability to pump blood, especially if the patient has myocardial ischemia. Consequently, blood backs up, resulting in pulmonary edema. Eventually, cardiac output falls and multisystem organ failure develops as the compensatory mechanisms fail to maintain perfusion.

Cardiogenic shock can result from any condition that causes significant left ventricular dysfunction with reduced cardiac output, such as an MI (most common), myocardial ischemia, papillary muscle dysfunction, and end-stage cardiomyopathy.

Other causes include myocarditis and depression of myocardial contractility after cardiac arrest and prolonged cardiac surgery. Mechanical abnormalities of the ventricle, such as acute mitral or aortic insufficiency or an acutely acquired ventricular septal defect or ventricular aneurysm, may also result in cardiogenic shock.

Complications

- Acute respiratory distress syndrome
- Acute tubular necrosis
- Disseminated intravascular coagulation
- Cerebral hypoxia
- Death

Assessment findings

- Typically, the patient's history includes a disorder that severely decreases left ventricular function, such as an MI or cardiomyopathy.
- Patients with underlying cardiac disease may complain of angina because of decreased myocardial perfusion and oxygenation.
- Urine output is usually less than 20 ml/hour.
- Inspection usually reveals pale skin, decreased sensorium, and rapid, shallow respirations.
- Palpation of peripheral pulses may reveal a rapid, thready pulse. The skin feels cold and clammy.
- Auscultation of blood pressure usually discloses a mean arterial pressure of less than 60 mm Hg in adults and a narrowing pulse pressure.

CLASSIFYING SHOCK

TYPE	DESCRIPTION
Cardiogenic	Results from a direct or indirect pump failure with decreasing cardiac output. Total body fluid isn't decreased. Causes include valvular stenosis or insufficiency, myocardial infarction, cardiomyopathy, arrhythmias, cardiac arrest, cardiac tamponade, pericarditis, pulmonary hypertension, and pulmonary emboli.
Distributive	Results from inadequate vascular tone that leads to massive vasodilation. Vascular volume remains normal and heart pumps adequately, but size of vascular space increases. Result is maldistribution of blood within the circulatory system. It includes the following subtypes: ● *Anaphylactic shock:* characterized by massive vasodilation and increased capillary permeability secondary to a hypersensitivity reaction to an antigen. ● *Neurogenic shock:* characterized by massive vasodilation from loss or suppression of sympathetic tone. Causes include head trauma, spinal cord injuries, anesthesia, and stress. ● *Septic shock:* a form of severe sepsis characterized by hypotension and altered tissue perfusion. Vascular tone is lost and cardiac output may be decreased.
Hypovolemic	Results from a decrease in central vascular volume. Total body fluids may or may not be decreased. Causes include hemorrhage, dehydration, and fluid shifts (caused by trauma, burns, or anaphylaxis).

- In a patient with chronic hypotension, the mean pressure may fall below 50 mm Hg before he exhibits signs of shock.
- The heart is auscultated to detect gallop rhythm, faint heart sounds and, possibly (if shock results from rupture of the ventricular septum or papillary muscles), a holosystolic murmur.
- Although many of these clinical features also occur in heart failure and other shock syndromes, they are usually more profound in cardiogenic shock. (See *Classifying shock*.)
- Patients with pericardial tamponade may have distant heart sounds.

Diagnostic test results

- Pulmonary artery pressure (PAP) monitoring reveals increased PAP and pulmonary artery wedge pressure (PAWP), reflecting an increase in left ventricular end-diastolic pressure (preload) and heightened resistance to left ventricular emptying (afterload) caused by ineffective pumping and increased peripheral vascular resistance. Thermodilution catheterization reveals a reduced cardiac index (less than 1.8 L/minute/ml).

■ Invasive arterial pressure monitoring shows hypotension caused by impaired ventricular ejection.

■ Arterial blood gas analysis may show metabolic and respiratory acidosis and hypoxia.

■ Electrocardiography demonstrates possible evidence of an acute MI, ischemia, or a ventricular aneurysm.

■ Serum enzyme measurements display elevated levels of creatine kinase (CK), aspartate aminotransferase, and alanine aminotransferase, which point to an MI or ischemia and suggest heart failure or shock. CK isoenzyme levels may confirm an acute MI.

■ Cardiac catheterization and echocardiography reveal other conditions that can lead to pump dysfunction and failure, such as cardiac tamponade, papillary muscle infarct or rupture, ventricular septal rupture, pulmonary emboli, venous pooling (associated with venodilators and continuous intermittent positive pressure breathing), and hypovolemia.

Treatment

Treatment aims to enhance cardiovascular status by increasing cardiac output, improving myocardial perfusion, and decreasing cardiac workload with combinations of cardiovascular drugs and mechanical-assist techniques.

I.V. drug therapy may include dopamine (Inocor), a vasopressor to increase cardiac output, blood pressure, and renal blood flow; milrinone (Primacor) or dobutamine (Dobutrex), an inotropic agent to increase myocardial contractility; and norepinephrine (Levophed), when a more potent vasoconstrictor is necessary. Nitroprusside, a vasodilator, may be used with a vasopressor to further improve cardiac output by decreasing peripheral vascular resistance (afterload) and reducing left ventricular end-diastolic pressure (preload). The patient's blood pressure must be adequate to support nitroprusside therapy and must be monitored closely. Furosemide (Lasix) is used to decrease pulmonary congestion.

Treatment may also include the intra-aortic balloon pump (IABP), a mechanical-assist device that attempts to improve coronary artery perfusion and decrease cardiac workload. The inflatable balloon pump is inserted through the femoral artery into the descending thoracic aorta. The balloon inflates during diastole to increase coronary artery perfusion pressure and deflates before systole (before the aortic valve opens) to reduce resistance to ejection (afterload) and, therefore, lessen cardiac workload. Improved ventricular ejection, which significantly improves cardiac output, and a subsequent vasodilation in the peripheral vessels lead to lower preload volume.

When drug therapy and IABP insertion fail, a ventricular assist device may be used.

Nursing interventions

- In the intensive care unit, start I.V. infusions with normal saline solution or lactated Ringer's solution, using a large-bore (14G to 18G) catheter, which allows easier administration of later blood transfusions.

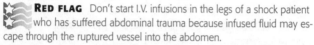 **RED FLAG** Don't start I.V. infusions in the legs of a shock patient who has suffered abdominal trauma because infused fluid may escape through the ruptured vessel into the abdomen.

- Monitor and record blood pressure, pulse and respiratory rates, and peripheral pulses every 1 to 5 minutes until the patient's condition is stabilized. Record hemodynamic pressure readings every 15 minutes. Monitor cardiac rhythm continuously. Systolic blood pressure less than 80 mm Hg usually results in inadequate coronary artery blood flow, cardiac ischemia, arrhythmias, and further complications of low cardiac output. When blood pressure drops below 80 mm Hg, increase the oxygen flow rate, and notify the practitioner immediately.
- A progressive drop in blood pressure accompanied by a thready pulse generally signals inadequate cardiac output from reduced intravascular volume. Notify the practitioner, and increase the infusion rate.
- Using a pulmonary artery catheter, closely monitor PAP, PAWP, and cardiac output. A high PAWP indicates heart failure, increased systemic vascular resistance, decreased cardiac output, and decreased cardiac index and should be reported immediately.
- Insert an indwelling urinary catheter if necessary to measure hourly urine output. If the output is less than 30 ml/hour in an adult, increase the fluid infusion rate, but watch for signs of fluid overload such as an increase in PAWP. Notify the practitioner if the patient's urine output doesn't improve.
- Give an osmotic diuretic, such as mannitol, to increase renal blood flow and urine output. Determine how much fluid to give by checking blood pressure, urine output, central venous pressure (CVP), or PAWP. To increase accuracy, measure CVP at the level of the right atrium, using the same reference point on the chest each time.

DISCHARGE TEACHING

TEACHING THE PATIENT WITH CARDIOGENIC SHOCK

● Teach the patient the early warning signs of myocardial infarction and how to access emergency care.
● Educate the patient about signs and symptoms of heart failure and cardiac arrhythmias.
● Review home care instructions, medications, and special equipment needs such as oxygen.

■ Draw an arterial blood sample to measure blood gas levels. Administer oxygen by face mask or airway to ensure adequate oxygenation of tissues. Adjust the oxygen flow rate to a higher or lower level as blood gas measurements indicate. Many patients need 100% oxygen, and some require 5 to 15 cm H_2O of positive end-expiratory or continuous positive airway pressure ventilation.

■ Monitor complete blood count and electrolyte levels.

■ During therapy, assess skin color and temperature, and note any changes. Cold, clammy skin may be a sign of continuing peripheral vascular constriction, indicating progressive shock.

RED FLAG When a patient is on the IABP, move him as little as possible. Never flex the patient's leg at the hip because this may displace or fracture the catheter. Never place the patient in a sitting position (including for chest X-rays) while the balloon is inflated; the balloon may tear through the aorta and cause immediate death. Assess pedal pulses and skin temperature and color to make sure circulation to the leg is adequate. Check the dressing on the insertion site frequently for bleeding, and change it according to facility protocol. Also check the site for hematoma or signs of infection, and culture any drainage.

■ If the patient becomes hemodynamically stable, gradually reduce the frequency of balloon inflation to wean him from the IABP. During weaning, carefully watch for monitor changes, chest pain, and other signs and symptoms of recurring cardiac ischemia and shock.

■ To ease emotional stress, plan your care to allow frequent rest periods, and provide for as much privacy as possible. Allow family members to visit and comfort the patient as much as possible.

■ Allow the family to express their anger, anxiety, and fear. (See *Teaching the patient with cardiogenic shock.*)

HYPOVOLEMIC SHOCK

Hypovolemic shock is a potentially life-threatening situation in which reduced intravascular blood volume causes circulatory dysfunction and inadequate tissue perfusion. Tissue anoxia prompts a shift in cellular metabolism from aerobic to anaerobic pathways. This produces an accumulation of lactic acid, resulting in metabolic acidosis.

Without sufficient blood or fluid replacement, hypovolemic shock may lead to irreversible cerebral and renal damage, cardiac arrest and, ultimately, death. (See *How hypovolemic shock progresses*.) Hypovolemic shock necessitates early recognition of signs and symptoms and prompt, aggressive treatment to improve the prognosis.

Pathophysiology

In hypovolemic shock, venous return to the heart is reduced when fluid is lost from the intravascular space through external losses or the shift of fluid from the vessels to the intersitial or intracellular spaces. This reduction in preload decreases ventricular filling, leading to a drop in stroke volume. Then, cardiac output falls, causing reduced perfusion of the tissues and organs.

Hypovolemic shock usually results from acute blood loss—about one-fifth of total volume. Massive blood loss may result from GI bleeding, internal hemorrhage (such as hemothorax or hemoperitoneum), external hemorrhage (caused by accidental or surgical trauma), or any condition (such as severe burns) that reduces circulating intravascular plasma volume or other body fluids.

Other causes of hypovolemic shock include intestinal obstruction, peritonitis, acute pancreatitis, ascites and dehydration from excessive perspiration, severe diarrhea or protracted vomiting, diabetes insipidus, diuresis, and inadequate fluid intake.

Complications

- Acute respiratory distress syndrome
- Acute tubular necrosis and renal failure
- Disseminated intravascular coagulation (DIC)
- Multiple-organ-dysfunction syndrome

Assessment findings

- The patient's history includes disorders or conditions that reduce blood volume, such as GI hemorrhage, trauma, and severe diarrhea and vomiting.
- A patient with cardiac disease may complain of angina because of decreased myocardial perfusion and oxygenation.

HOW HYPOVOLEMIC SHOCK PROGRESSES

Vascular fluid volume loss causes the extreme tissue hypoperfusion that characterizes hypovolemic shock. *Internal fluid loss* results from internal hemorrhage (such as GI bleeding) and third-space fluid shifting (such as in diabetic ketoacidosis). *External fluid loss* results from severe bleeding or from severe diarrhea, diuresis, or vomiting.

Inadequate vascular volume leads to decreased venous return and cardiac output. The resulting drop in arterial blood pressure activates the body's compensatory mechanisms in an attempt to increase vascular volume. If compensation is unsuccessful, decompensation and death may rapidly ensue.

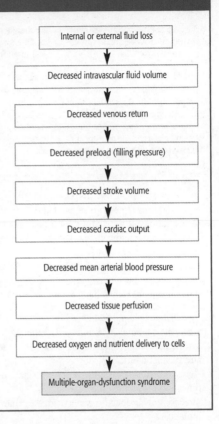

Internal or external fluid loss

↓

Decreased intravascular fluid volume

↓

Decreased venous return

↓

Decreased preload (filling pressure)

↓

Decreased stroke volume

↓

Decreased cardiac output

↓

Decreased mean arterial blood pressure

↓

Decreased tissue perfusion

↓

Decreased oxygen and nutrient delivery to cells

↓

Multiple-organ-dysfunction syndrome

- Inspection may reveal pale skin, decreased sensorium, and rapid, shallow respirations.
- Urine output is usually less than 20 ml/hour.
- Palpation of peripheral pulses may disclose a rapid, thready pulse; the skin feels cold and clammy.
- Auscultation of blood pressure usually detects a mean arterial pressure of less than 60 mm Hg in adults and a narrowing pulse pressure.

CHECKING FOR EARLY HYPOVOLEMIC SHOCK

Orthostatic vital signs and tilt test results can help assess for the possibility of impending hypovolemic shock.

Orthostatic vital signs

Measure the patient's blood pressure and pulse rate while lying in a supine position, sitting, and standing. Wait at least 1 minute between each position change. A systolic blood pressure decrease of 10 mm Hg or more between positions or a pulse rate increase of 10 beats/minute or more is a sign of volume depletion and impending hypovolemic shock.

Tilt test

With the patient lying in a supine position, raise his legs above heart level. If his blood pressure increases significantly, the test is positive, indicating volume depletion and impending hypovolemic shock.

- In patients with chronic hypotension, the mean pressure may fall below 50 mm Hg before signs of shock appear.
- Orthostatic vital signs and the tilt test may help determine the presence of hypovolemic shock. (See *Checking for early hypovolemic shock*.)
- Central venous pressure (CVP), right atrial pressure, pulmonary artery pressure, pulmonary artery wedge pressure (PAWP), and cardiac output are reduced.

Diagnostic test results

Characteristic laboratory findings include:
- low hematocrit and decreased hemoglobin level and red blood cell and platelet counts
- elevated serum potassium, sodium, lactate dehydrogenase, creatinine, and blood urea nitrogen levels
- increased urine specific gravity (greater than 1.020) and urine osmolality
- decreased urine creatinine levels
- decreased pH and partial pressure of arterial oxygen and increased partial pressure of carbon dioxide.
    Tests to identify internal bleeding sites include:
- X-rays
- aspiration of gastric contents through a nasogastric tube
- tests for occult blood
- coagulation studies may detect coagulopathy from DIC.

Treatment

Emergency treatment measures include prompt and adequate blood and fluid replacement to restore intravascular volume and to raise blood pressure and maintain it above 60 mm Hg. Infusion of normal saline solution or lactated Ringer's solution and then possibly plasma proteins (albumin) or other plasma expanders may produce adequate volume expansion until packed cells can be matched. A rapid solution infusion system can provide these crystalloids or colloids at high flow rates.

For severe cases, an intra-aortic balloon pump, ventricular assist device, or pneumatic antishock garment may be helpful.

Treatment may also include oxygen administration, bleeding control by direct application of pressure and related measures, dopamine or another inotropic agent, and possibly surgery to correct the underlying problem. To be effective, dopamine or other inotropics must be used with vigorous fluid resuscitation.

Nursing interventions

- Check for a patent airway and adequate circulation. If blood pressure and heart rate are absent, start cardiopulmonary resuscitation.
- Record the patient's blood pressure, pulse and respiratory rates, and peripheral pulses every 15 minutes until the patient's condition is stabilized. Monitor cardiac rhythm continuously.
- When systolic blood pressure drops below 80 mm Hg, increase the oxygen flow rate, and notify the practitioner immediately because systolic blood pressure less than 80 mm Hg usually results in inadequate coronary artery blood flow, cardiac ischemia, arrhythmias, and further complications of low cardiac output.
- Start an I.V. infusion with normal saline solution or lactated Ringer's solution, using a large-bore (14G to 18G) catheter, which allows easier administration of later blood transfusions.

RED FLAG Don't start an I.V. infusion in the legs of a shock patient who has suffered abdominal trauma because infused fluid may escape through the ruptured vessel into the abdomen.

- Notify the practitioner and increase the infusion rate if the patient has a progressive drop in blood pressure accompanied by a thready pulse. This generally signals inadequate cardiac output from reduced intravascular volume.
- Insert an indwelling urinary catheter if necessary to measure hourly urine output. If output is less than 30 ml/hour in adults, increase the fluid infusion rate, but watch for signs of fluid overload such as

an increase in PAWP. Notify the practitioner if urine output doesn't improve.

- An osmotic diuretic, such as mannitol, may be ordered to increase renal blood flow and urine output. Determine how much fluid to give by checking blood pressure, urine output, CVP, or PAWP. (To increase accuracy, CVP should be measured at the level of the right atrium, using the same reference point on the chest each time.)
- Draw an arterial blood sample to measure blood gas levels. Administer oxygen by face mask or endotracheal tube to ensure adequate tissue oxygenation. Adjust the oxygen flow rate to a higher or lower level, as blood gas measurements indicate.
- Draw venous blood for a complete blood count, electrolyte measurements, typing and crossmatching, and coagulation studies.
- During therapy, assess skin color and temperature, and note any changes. Cold, clammy skin may be a sign of continuing peripheral vascular constriction, indicating progressive shock.
- Watch for signs of impending coagulopathy (petechiae, bruising, bleeding or oozing from gums or venipuncture sites).
- Provide emotional support to the patient and his family. (See *Teaching the patient with hypovolemic shock*.)
- Members of some groups (such as Jehovah's Witnesses) are opposed to blood transfusion and may refuse this type of treatment because of religious reasons. In an emergency, a court order may be obtained to allow such treatment if it's in the patient's best interest.

VENTRICULAR ANEURYSM

Ventricular aneurysm is a potentially life-threatening condition that involves an outpouching—almost always of the left ventricle—that produces ventricular wall dysfunction in 10% to 20% of patients after a myocardial infarction (MI). It may develop within days to weeks after an MI or may be delayed for years. Resection improves the prognosis in patients with ventricular failure or ventricular arrhythmias.

Pathophysiology

MI causes ventricular aneurysm. When an MI destroys a large muscular section of the left ventricle, necrosis reduces the ventricular wall to a thin sheath of fibrous tissue. Under intracardiac pressure, this thin layer stretches and forms a separate noncontractile sac (aneurysm). Abnormal muscle-wall movement accompanies ventricular aneurysm. (See *Understanding ventricular aneurysm,* page 492.)

During systolic ejection, the abnormal muscle-wall movements associated with the aneurysm cause the remaining normally functioning myocardial fibers to increase the force of contraction to maintain stroke volume and cardiac output. At the same time, a portion of the stroke volume is lost to passive distention of the noncontractile sac.

Complications

- Ventricular arrhythmias
- Cerebral embolization
- Heart failure
- Death

Assessment findings

- The patient may have a history of a previous MI. However, sometimes an MI is silent, so the patient may be unaware of having had one. He may complain of palpitations and angina.
- If the patient has developed heart failure as a result of the aneurysm, he may report dyspnea, fatigue, and edema.
- Inspection of the chest may reveal a visible or palpable systolic precordial bulge.
- Jugular vein distention may be apparent if heart failure is present.
- Palpation of peripheral pulses may reveal an irregular rhythm caused by arrhythmias (such as premature ventricular contractions). An alternating pulse may be felt.
- Palpation of the chest usually detects a double, diffuse, or displaced apical impulse.
- Auscultation of the heart may detect an irregular rhythm and a gallop rhythm.
- Crackles and rhonchi may be present in the lung if heart failure is present.

UNDERSTANDING VENTRICULAR ANEURYSM

When myocardial infarction destroys a large, muscular section of the left ventricle, necrosis reduces the ventricular wall to a thin layer of fibrous tissue. The thin wall stretches under intracardiac pressure and forms a ventricular aneurysm. Ventricular aneurysms usually occur on the anterior or apical surface of the heart.

Ventricular aneurysms balloon outward with each systole (dyskinesia). Blood is diverted to the distended muscle wall of the aneurysm, which doesn't contract (akinesia). Mural thrombus is present about half of the time—thromboembolism rarely is. Calcification of the thrombus is common.

To maintain stroke volume and cardiac output, the remaining normally functioning myocardial fibers increase contractile force. If they can't, overall ventricular function is impaired and complications, such as heart failure and ventricular arrhythmias, may develop.

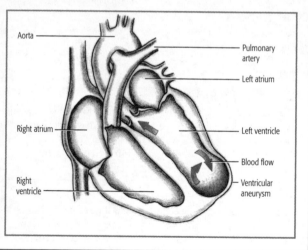

- Aorta
- Pulmonary artery
- Left atrium
- Right atrium
- Left ventricle
- Blood flow
- Right ventricle
- Ventricular aneurysm

Diagnostic test results

The following tests may determine the presence of a ventricular aneurysm:

- Echocardiography demonstrates abnormal motion in the left ventricular wall.

- Left ventriculography reveals left ventricular enlargement, with an area of akinesia or dyskinesia (during cineangiocardiography) and diminished cardiac function.
- Electrocardiography may show persistent ST-segment and T-wave elevations at rest. ST-segment elevation over the aneurysm creates an elevated rounded appearance.
- Chest X-rays may disclose an abnormal bulge distorting the heart's contour if the aneurysm is large; X-rays may be normal if the aneurysm is small.
- Noninvasive nuclear cardiology scan may indicate the site of infarction and suggest the area of aneurysm.

Treatment

Depending on the size of the aneurysm and the presence of complications, treatment may require only routine medical examination to follow the patient's condition, or aggressive measures for intractable ventricular arrhythmias, heart failure, and emboli.

Emergency treatment of ventricular arrhythmia includes an I.V. antiarrhythmic, cardioversion, and defibrillation. Preventive treatment continues with an oral antiarrhythmic, such as procainamide (Procan), quinidine, or disopyramide (Norpace).

Emergency treatment for heart failure with pulmonary edema includes oxygen, I.V. digoxin, I.V. furosemide, potassium replacement, I.V. morphine sulfate and, when necessary, I.V. nitroprusside and endotracheal (ET) intubation. Maintenance therapy may include an oral nitrate and an angiotensin-converting enzyme inhibitor, such as captopril (Capoten) or enalapril (Vasotec).

Systemic embolization requires anticoagulation therapy or embolectomy. Refractory ventricular tachycardia, heart failure, recurrent arterial embolization, and persistent angina with coronary artery occlusion may require surgery. The most effective surgery is aneurysmectomy with myocardial revascularization.

Nursing interventions

- In a patient with heart failure, closely monitor vital signs, heart sounds, intake and output, fluid and electrolyte balance, and blood urea nitrogen and serum creatinine levels.
- Be alert for sudden sensory changes that indicate cerebral embolization and for signs that suggest renal failure or MI.
- Arrhythmias require elective cardioversion. If the patient is conscious, give diazepam I.V. as ordered before cardioversion.

TEACHING THE PATIENT WITH VENTRICULAR ANEURYSM

● Teach the patient how to check for pulse irregularity and rate changes. Encourage him to follow his prescribed drug regimen—even during the night—and to watch for adverse reactions.

● Because arrhythmias can cause sudden death, refer the family to a community-based cardiopulmonary resuscitation training program.

■ If the patient is receiving an antiarrhythmic, check appropriate laboratory results. For instance, if the patient takes procainamide, check for antinuclear antibodies because the drug may induce signs and symptoms that mimic lupus erythematosus.

■ Provide psychological support for the patient and his family to reduce anxiety. (See *Teaching the patient with ventricular aneurysm.*)

■ If the patient is scheduled to undergo resection, explain expected postoperative care in the intensive care unit (such as an ET tube, a ventilator, hemodynamic monitoring, and chest tubes).

■ After surgery, monitor vital signs, intake and output, heart sounds, and pulmonary artery catheter. Watch for signs of infection, such as fever and drainage.

Selected references
Index

Selected references

─────────────────○─────────────────

Angerstein, R.L., et al. "Preventing Sudden Cardiac Death in Post
    Myocardial Infarction Patients with Left Ventricular Dysfunction,"
    Journal of Cardiovascular Nursing 20(6):397-404, November-
    December 2005.

Berra, K., et al. "Cardiovascular Disease Prevention and Disease
    Management: A Critical Role for Nursing," *Journal of
    Cardiopulmonary Rehabilitation* 26(4):197-206, July-August 2006.

Cardiovascular Care Made Incredibly Easy. Philadelphia: Lippincott
    Williams & Wilkins, 2004.

Diepenbrock, N.H. *Quick Reference to Critical Care,* 2nd ed. Philadelphia:
    Lippincott Williams & Wilkins, 2004.

Diseases: A Nursing Process Approach to Excellent Care, 4th ed. Philadel-
    phia: Lippincott Williams & Wilkins, 2006.

Dumont, C.J. "Predictors of Vascular Complications Post Diagnostic
    Cardiac Catheterization and Percutaneous Coronary Interventions,"
    Dimensions in Critical Care Nursing 25(3):137-42, May-June 2006.

Frodsham, R. "Cardiac Resynchronisation Therapy for Patients with Heart
    Failure," *Nursing Standard* 19(45):46-50, July 2005.

Goldstine, L.B., et al. "Primary Prevention of Ischemic Stroke: A
    Guideline from the American Heart Association/American Stroke
    Association Stroke Council: cosponsored by the Atherosclerotic
    Peripheral Vascular Disease Interdisciplinary Working Group;
    Cardiovascular Nursing Council; Clinical Cardiology Council;
    Nutrition, Physical Activity, and Metabolism Council; and the
    Quality of Care and Outcomes Research Interdisciplinary Working
    Group," *Circulation* 113(24):e873-923, June 2006.

Haraden, J., and Jaenicke, C. "Correlation of Preoperative Ankle-Brachial
    Index and Pulse Volume Recording with Impaired Saphenous Vein
    Incisional Wound Healing Post Coronary Artery Bypass Surgery,"
    Journal of Vascular Nursing 24(2):35-45, June 2006.

Hayman, L.L., and Reineke, P.R. "Promoting Cardiovascular Health in Children and Adolescents," *Journal of Cardiovascular Nursing* 21(4):269-75, July-August, 2006.

Headley, J.M. "Arterial Pressure-based Technologies: A New Trend in Cardiac Output Monitoring," *Critical Care Nursing Clinics of North America* 18(2):179-87, June 2006.

Heger, J.W., et al. *Cardiology,* 5th ed. Philadelphia: Lippincott Williams & Wilkins, 2004.

Karch. A.M. *2007 Lippincott's Nursing Drug Guide.* Philadelphia: Lippincott Williams & Wilkins, 2007.

Moser, D.K., et al., "Reducing Delay in Seeking Treatment by Patients with Acute Coronary Syndrome and Stroke: A Scientific Statement from the American Heart Association Council on Cardiovascular Nursing and Stroke Council," *Circulation* 114(2):168-82, July 2006.

Prentice, D., and Sona, C. "Esophageal Doppler Monitoring for Hemodynamic Assessment," *Critical Care Nursing Clinics of North America* 18(2):189-93, June 2006.

Professional Guide to Diagnostic Tests. Philadelphia: Lippincott Williams & Wilkins, 2005.

Professional Guide to Pathophysiology, 2nd ed. Philadelphia: Lippincott Williams & Wilkins, 2007.

Schoenhagen, P., and Nissen SE. "Identification of the Metabolic Syndrome and Imaging of Subclinical Coronary Artery Disease: Early Markers of Cardiovascular Risk," *Journal of Cardiovascular Nursing* 21(4):291-97, July-August, 2006.

Sharis, P.J., and Cannon, C.P. *Evidence-Based Cardiology,* 2nd ed. Philadelphia: Lippincott Williams & Wilkins, 2006.

Todd, B.A., and Higgins, K. "Recognizing Aortic and Mitral Valve Disease," *Nursing* 35(6):58-63, June 2005.

Xu, Y., and Whitmer, K. "C-reactive Protein and Cardiovascular Disease in People with Diabetes: High-sensitivity CRP Testing Can Help Assess Risk for Future Cardiovascular Disease Events in This Population," *AJN* 106(8):66-72, August 2006.

Index

i refers to an illustration; t refers to a table.

---

i refers to an illustration; t refers to a table.

---

i refers to an illustration; t refers to a table.

i refers to an illustration; t refers to a table.

---

i refers to an illustration; t refers to a table.

i refers to an illustration; t refers to a table.
